REFERENCE EDITION

ENDOCRINE BOARD REVIEW 2023

Frances J. Hayes, MB BCh BAO
Program Chair
Associate Clinical Chief of Endocrinology
Massachusetts General Hospital
Associate Professor of Medicine
Harvard Medical School

John D. Carmichael, MD
Co-Director, USC Pituitary Center
Associate Professor of Clinical Medicine
Division of Endocrinology, Diabetes, and Metabolism
Keck School of Medicine of University of Southern California

Natalie E. Cusano, MD, MS
Professor of Medicine
Zucker School of Medicine at Hofstra/Northwell
Director of the Bone Metabolism Program
Division of Endocrinology at Lenox Hill Hospital

Tobias Else, MD
Associate Professor
Division of Metabolism, Endocrinology, and Diabetes
University of Michigan

Jacqueline Jonklaas, MD, PhD, MPH
Professor
Division of Endocrinology
Georgetown University Medical Center

Sangeeta R. Kashyap, MD
Assistant Chief of Clinical Affairs
Division of Endocrinology, Diabetes, and Metabolism
Weill Cornell Medicine New York Presbyterian

Margaret Flynn Lippincott, MD
Assistant Professor of Medicine
Harvard Medical School
Physician Investigator
Reproductive Endocrine Unit
Massachusetts General Hospital

Marie E. McDonnell, MD
Section Chief, Diabetes Section
Division of Endocrinology Diabetes and Hypertension
Brigham and Women's Hospital
Associate Professor of Medicine
Harvard Medical School

Stephanie Page, MD, PhD
Professor/Head, Division of Metabolism, Endocrinology, and Nutrition
Co-Director, UW Medicine Diabetes Institute
Robert B. McMillen Professor of Lipid Research
University of Washington School of Medicine

Anne L. Peters, MD
Professor of Clinical Medicine
Keck School of Medicine of University of Southern California

Abbie L. Young, MS, CGC, ELS(D)
Medical Editor

Endocrine Society
2055 L Street NW, Suite 600, Washington, DC 20036
1-888-ENDOCRINE • www.endocrine.org

ENDOCRINE SOCIETY

The Endocrine Society is the world's largest, oldest, and most active organization working to advance the clinical practice of endocrinology and hormone research. Founded in 1916, the Society now has more than 18,000 global members across a range of disciplines. The Society has earned an international reputation for excellence in the quality of its peer-reviewed journals, educational resources, meetings, and programs that improve public health through the practice and science of endocrinology.

For between-edition updates, visit us at:
https://www.endocrine.org/education-and-training/book-updates

Other publications:
endocrine.org/publications

ISBN: 978-1-936704-17-0
Library of Congress Control Number: 2022951735

On the Cover: © Shutterstock. Medical stethoscope on computer keyboard with clipboard

OVERVIEW

Endocrine Board Review (EBR) 15th Edition (2023) is a board examination preparation book designed for endocrine fellows who have completed or are nearing completion of their fellowship and are preparing to sit for the board certification exam, and for practicing endocrinologists in search of a comprehensive self-assessment of endocrinology, either to prepare for recertification or to update their practice. EBR consists of approximately 220 case-based, American Board of Internal Medicine (ABIM) style, multiple-choice questions. Each section follows the ABIM Endocrinology, Diabetes, and Metabolism Certification Examination blueprint, covering the breadth and depth of the certification and recertification examinations. Each case is discussed in detail with detailed answer explanations and references provided.

The EBR 15th Edition (2023) reference book is intended primarily for consultation and self-assessment of knowledge relating to endocrinology. As a reference book, educational credits are not available upon completion of the multiple-choice questions included. For information on educational products that include educational credit, please visit endocrine.org/store.

LEARNING OBJECTIVES

Upon completion of this educational activity, learners will be able to demonstrate enhanced medical knowledge and clinical skills across all major areas of endocrinology; apply knowledge and skills in diagnosing, managing, and treating a wide spectrum of endocrine disorders; and successfully complete the board examination for certification or recertification in the subspecialty of endocrinology, diabetes, and metabolism.

TARGET AUDIENCE

This activity should be of substantial interest to endocrinologists, internists, and endocrine fellows preparing for the board examination or recertification; or endocrinologists and other health care practitioners seeking a review in endocrinology.

STATEMENT OF INDEPENDENCE

The Endocrine Society has a policy of ensuring that the content and quality of this educational activity are balanced, independent, objective, and scientifically rigorous. The scientific content of this activity was developed under the supervision of the Endocrine Society's EBR faculty. There are no commercial supporters of this activity and no commercial entities have had an influence over the planning of this activity.

DISCLOSURE POLICY

The faculty, committee members, and staff who are in position to control the content of this activity are required to disclose to the Endocrine Society and to learners any relevant financial relationship(s) of the individual or spouse/partner that have occurred within the last 12 months with any commercial interest(s) whose products or services are related to the content. Financial relationships are defined by remuneration in any amount from the commercial interest(s) in the form of grants; research support; consulting fees; salary; ownership interest (eg, stocks, stock options, or ownership interest excluding diversified mutual funds); honoraria or other payments for participation in speakers' bureaus, advisory boards, or boards of directors; or other financial benefits. The intent of this disclosure is not to prevent planners with relevant financial relationships from planning or delivery of content, but rather to provide learners with information that allows them to make their own judgments of whether these financial relationships may have influenced the educational activity with regard to exposition or conclusion.

The Endocrine Society has reviewed all disclosures and resolved or managed all identified conflicts of interest, as applicable.

The faculty reported the following relevant financial relationship(s) during the content development process for this activity:

John D. Carmichael, MD, has served as an advisory board member for Novo Nordisk, Recordati, and Camurus.

Natalie E. Cusano, MD, MS, has served as a research investigator for Shire/Takeda, a speaker for Alexion Pharmaceuticals, and a consultant for Ascendis Pharma.

Tobias Else, MD, has served as a co-investigator for Corcept Pharmaceuticals and Merck; an advisory board member for Merck and Lantheus; and a committee member for VHL Alliance.

Sangeeta R. Kashyap, MD, has served as a consultant and coinvestigator to GI Dynamics; she has received research funding from Fractyl, Inc; and she is Chief Medical Officer of Gila Therapeutics.

Stephanie Page, MD, PhD, is an editor at UpToDate.

Anne L. Peters, MD, has served as an advisory board member for Abbott Diabetes Care, Medscape, Novo Nordisk, Vertex, and Zealand and as a consultant for Blue Circle Health. She has received research support from Dexcom, Insulet, and Abbott Diabetes Care. She has stock options in Omada Health and Teladoc.

Marie E. McDonnell, MD, has served as a trial event adjudicator for a trial conducted by Eisai and receives research funding from Lilly, Inc, that is paid to her institution.

The following faculty reported no relevant financial relationships: Frances J. Hayes, MB BCh BAO; Jacqueline Jonklaas, MD, PhD, MPH; and Margaret Flynn Lippincott, MD

The medical editor for this activity reported no relevant financial relationships: Abbie L. Young, MS, CGC, ELS(D)

Endocrine Society staff associated with the development of content for this activity reported no relevant financial relationships.

DISCLAIMERS

The information presented in this activity represents the opinion of the faculty and is not necessarily the official position of the Endocrine Society.

Use of professional judgment:

The educational content in this activity relates to basic principles of diagnosis and therapy and does not substitute for individual patient assessment based on the health care provider's examination of the patient and consideration of laboratory data and other factors unique to the patient. Standards in medicine change as new data become available.

Drugs and dosages:

When prescribing medications, the physician is advised to check the product information sheet accompanying each drug to verify conditions of use and to identify any changes in drug dosage schedule or contraindications.

POLICY ON UNLABELED/OFF-LABEL USE

The Endocrine Society has determined that disclosure of unlabeled/off-label or investigational use of commercial product(s) is informative for audiences and therefore requires this information to be disclosed to the learners at the beginning of the presentation. Uses of specific therapeutic agents, devices, and other products discussed in this educational activity may not be the same as those indicated in product labeling approved by the Food and Drug Administration (FDA). The Endocrine Society requires that any discussions of such "off-label" use be based on scientific research that conforms to generally accepted standards of experimental design, data collection, and data analysis. Before recommending or prescribing any therapeutic agent or device, learners should review the complete prescribing information, including indications, contraindications, warnings, precautions, and adverse events.

ACKNOWLEDGMENT OF COMMERCIAL SUPPORT

The activity is not supported by educational grant(s) or other funds from any commercial supporters.

Publication Date: August 2023

Contents

For between-edition updates, visit us at: https://www.endocrine.org/education-and-training/book-updates.

LABORATORY REFERENCE RANGES

Reference ranges vary among laboratories. Conventional units are listed first with SI units in parentheses.

Lipid Values

High-density lipoprotein (HDL) cholesterol

- Optimal ---------- >60 mg/dL (SI: >1.55 mmol/L)
- Normal ---------- 40-60 mg/dL (SI: 1.04-1.55 mmol/L)
- Low ---------- <40 mg/dL (SI: <1.04 mmol/L)

Low-density lipoprotein (LDL) cholesterol

- Optimal ----------
  <100 mg/dL (SI: <2.59 mmol/L) (for primary prevention);
  <70 mg/dL (SI: <1.81 mmol/L) (for secondary prevention)
- Low ---------- 100-129 mg/dL (SI: 2.59-3.34 mmol/L)
- Borderline-high ---------- 130-159 mg/dL (SI: 3.37-4.12 mmol/L)
- High ---------- 160-189 mg/dL (SI: 4.14-4.90 mmol/L)
- Very high ---------- ≥190 mg/dL (SI: ≥4.92 mmol/L)

Non-HDL cholesterol

- Optimal ---------- <130 mg/dL (SI: <3.37 mmol/L)
- Borderline-high ---------- 130-159 mg/dL (SI: 3.37-4.12 mmol/L)
- High ---------- ≥240 mg/dL (SI: ≥6.22 mmol/L)

Total cholesterol

- Optimal ---------- <200 mg/dL (SI: <5.18 mmol/L)
- Borderline-high ---------- 200-239 mg/dL (SI: 5.18-6.19 mmol/L)
- High ---------- ≥240 mg/dL (SI: ≥6.22 mmol/L)

Triglycerides

- Optimal ---------- <150 mg/dL (SI: <1.70 mmol/L)
- Borderline-high ---------- 150-199 mg/dL (SI: 1.70-2.25 mmol/L)
- High ---------- 200-499 mg/dL (SI: 2.26-5.64 mmol/L)
- Very high ---------- ≥500 mg/dL (SI: ≥5.65 mmol/L)

Lipoprotein (a) ---------- ≤30 mg/dL (SI: ≤1.07 μmol/L)

Apolipoprotein B ---------- 50-110 mg/dL (SI: 0.5-1.1 g/L)

Hematologic Values

Erythrocyte sedimentation rate ---------- 0-20 mm/h

Haptoglobin ---------- 30-200 mg/dL (SI: 300-2000 mg/L)

Hematocrit ---------- 41%-51% (SI: 0.41-0.51) (male); 35%-45% (SI: 0.35-0.45) (female)

Hemoglobin A_{1c} ---------- 4.0%-5.6% (20-38 mmol/mol)

Hemoglobin ---------- 13.8-17.2 g/dL (SI: 138-172 g/L) (male); 12.1-15.1 g/dL (SI: 121-151 g/L) (female)

International normalized ratio ---------- 0.8-1.2

Mean corpuscular volume (MCV ---------- 80-100 μm^3 (SI: 80-100 fL)

Platelet count ---------- 150-450 x 10^3/μL (SI: 150-450 x 10^9/L)

Protein (total) ---------- 6.3-7.9 g/dL (SI: 63-79 g/L)

Reticulocyte count - 0.5%-1.5% of red blood cells (SI: 0.005-0.015)

White blood cell count ---------- 4500-11,000/μL (SI: 4.5-11.0 x 10^9/L)

Thyroid Values

Thyroglobulin ---------- 3-42 ng/mL (SI: 3-42 μg/L) (after surgery and radioactive iodine treatment: <1.0 ng/mL [SI: <1.0 μg/L])

Thyroglobulin antibodies ---------- ≤4.0 IU/mL (SI: ≤4.0 kIU/L)

Thyrotropin (TSH) ---------- 0.5-5.0 mIU/L

Thyrotropin-receptor antibodies (TRAb) ---------- ≤1.75 IU/L

Thyroid-stimulating immunoglobulin ---------- ≤120% of basal activity

Thyroperoxidase (TPO) antibodies ---------- <2.0 IU/mL (SI: <2.0 kIU/L)

Thyroxine (T_4) (free) ---------- 0.8-1.8 ng/dL (SI: 10.30-23.17 pmol/L)

Thyroxine (T_4) (total) ---------- 5.5-12.5 μg/dL (SI: 94.02-213.68 nmol/L)

Free thyroxine (T_4) index ---------- 4-12

Triiodothyronine (T_3) (free) ---------- 2.3-4.2 pg/mL (SI: 3.53-6.45 pmol/L)

Triiodothyronine (T_3) (total) ---------- 70-200 ng/dL (SI: 1.08-3.08 nmol/L)

Triiodothyronine (T_3), reverse ---------- 10-24 ng/dL (SI: 0.15-0.37 nmol/L)

Triiodothyronine uptake, resin ---------- 25%-38%

Radioactive iodine uptake ---------- 3%-16% (6 hours); 15%-30% (24 hours)

Endocrine Values

Serum

Aldosterone ---------- 4-21 ng/dL (SI: 111.0-582.5 pmol/L)

Alkaline phosphatase ---------- 50-120 U/L (SI: 0.84-2.00 μkat/L)

Alkaline phosphatase (bone-specific) ----------
≤20 μg/L (adult male); ≤14 μg/L (premenopausal female);
≤22 μg/L (postmenopausal female)

Androstenedione ----------
65-210 ng/dL (SI: 2.27-7.33 nmol/L) (adult male);
30-200 ng/dL (SI:1.05-6.98 nmol/L) (adult female)

Antimullerian hormone ----------
0.7-19.0 ng/mL (SI: 5.0-135.7 pmol/L) (male, >12 years);
0.9-9.5 ng/mL (SI: 6.4-67.9 pmol/L) (female, 13-45 years);
<1.0 ng/mL (SI: <7.1 pmol/L) (female, >45 years)

Calcitonin ---------- <16 pg/mL (SI: <4.67 pmol/L) (basal, male);
<8 pg/mL (SI: <2.34 pmol/L) (basal, female);
≤130 pg/mL (SI: ≤37.96 pmol/L) (peak calcium infusion, male);
≤90 pg/mL (SI: ≤26.28 pmol/L) (peak calcium infusion, female)

Carcinoembryonic antigen ---------- <2.5 ng/mL (SI: <2.5 μg/L)

Chromogranin A ---------- <93 ng/mL (SI: <93 μg/L)

Corticosterone 53-1560 ng/dL (SI: 1.53-45.08 nmol/L) (>18 years)

Corticotropin (ACTH) ---------- 10-60 pg/mL (SI: 2.2-13.2 pmol/L)

Cortisol (8 AM) ------------- 5-25 μg/dL (SI: 137.9-689.7 nmol/L)

Cortisol (4 PM)----------------2-14 μg/dL (SI: 55.2-386.2 nmol/L)

C-peptide ------------------- 0.5-2.0 ng/mL (SI: 0.17-0.66 nmol/L)

C-reactive protein -----------0.8-3.1 mg/L (SI: 7.62-29.52 nmol/L)

Cross-linked N-telopeptide of type 1 collagen -------------------

5.4-24.2 nmol BCE/mmol creat (male);

6.2-19.0 nmol BCE/mmol creat (female)

Dehydroepiandrosterone sulfate (DHEA-S)

Patient Age	Female	Male
18-29 years	44-332 μg/dL (SI: 1.19-9.00 μmol/L)	89-457 μg/dL (SI: 2.41-12.38 μmol/L)
30-39 years	31-228 μg/dL (SI: 0.84-6.78 μmol/L)	65-334 μg/dL (SI: 1.76-9.05 μmol/L)
40-49 years	18-244 μg/dL (SI: 0.49-6.61 μmol/L)	48-244 μg/dL (SI: 1.30-6.61 μmol/L)
50-59 years	15-200 μg/dL (SI: 0.41-5.42 μmol/L)	35-179 μg/dL (SI: 0.95-4.85 μmol/L)
≥60 years	15-157 μg/dL (SI: 0.41-4.25 μmol/L)	25-131 μg/dL (SI: 0.68-3.55 μmol/L)

Deoxycorticosterone ----<10 ng/dL (SI: <0.30 nmol/L) (>18 years)

1,25-Dihydroxyvitamin D_3---16-65 pg/mL (SI: 41.6-169.0 pmol/L)

Estradiol ------------10-40 pg/mL (SI: 36.7-146.8 pmol/L) (male);

10-180 pg/mL (SI: 36.7-660.8 pmol/L) (follicular, female);

100-300 pg/mL (SI: 367.1-1101.3 pmol/L) (midcycle, female);

40-200 pg/mL (SI: 146.8-734.2 pmol/L) (luteal, female);

<20 pg/mL (SI: <73.4 pmol/L) (postmenopausal, female)

Estrone -------------10-60 pg/mL (SI: 37.0-221.9 pmol/L) (male);

17-200 pg/mL (SI: 62.9-739.6 pmol/L) (premenopausal female);

7-40 pg/mL (SI: 25.9-147.9 pmol/L) (postmenopausal female)

α-Fetoprotein ------------------------------ <6 ng/mL (SI: <6 μg/L)

Follicle-stimulating hormone (FSH) ------------------------------

1.0-13.0 mIU/mL (SI: 1.0-13.0 IU/L) (male);

<3.0 mIU/mL (SI: <3.0 IU/L) (prepuberty, female);

2.0-12.0 mIU/mL (SI: 2.0-12.0 IU/L) (follicular, female);

4.0-36.0 mIU/mL (SI: 4.0-36.0 IU/L) (midcycle, female);

1.0-9.0 mIU/mL (SI: 1.0-9.0 IU/L) (luteal, female);

>30.0 mIU/mL (SI: >30.0 IU/L) (postmenopausal, female)

Free fatty acids ------------- 10.6-18.0 mg/dL (SI: 0.4-0.7 nmol/L)

Gastrin------------------------------- <100 pg/mL (SI: <100 ng/L)

Growth hormone (GH)-- 0.01-0.97 ng/mL (SI: 0.01-0.97 μg/L) (male);

0.01-3.61 ng/mL (SI: 0.01-3.61 μg/L) (female)

Homocysteine ----------------------- ≤1.76 mg/L (SI: ≤13 μmol/L)

β-Human chorionic gonadotropin (β-hCG) -----------------------

<3.0 mIU/mL (SI: <3.0 IU/L) (nonpregnant female);

>25 mIU/mL (SI: >25 IU/L) indicates a positive pregnancy test

β-Hydroxybutyrate ---------------<3.0 mg/dL (SI: <288.2 μmol/L)

17-Hydroxypregnenolone --- 29-189 ng/dL (SI: 0.87-5.69 nmol/L)

17α-Hydroxyprogesterone --------------------------------------

<220 ng/dL (SI: <6.67 nmol/L) (adult male);

<80 ng/dL (SI: <2.42 nmol/L) (follicular, female);

<285 ng/dL (SI: <8.64 nmol/L) (luteal, female);

<51 ng/dL (SI: <1.55 nmol/L) (postmenopausal, female)

25-Hydroxyvitamin D ---

<20 ng/mL (SI: <49.9 nmol/L) (deficiency);

21-29 ng/mL (SI: 52.4-72.4 nmol/L) (insufficiency);

30-80 ng/mL (SI: 74.9-199.7 nmol/L) (optimal levels);

>80 ng/mL (SI: >199.7 nmol/L) (toxicity possible)

Inhibin B ------------------------15-300 pg/mL (SI: 15-300 ng/L)

Insulinlike growth factor 1 (IGF-1)

Patient Age	Female	Male
18 years	162-541 ng/mL (SI: 21.2-70.9 nmol/L)	170-640 ng/mL (SI: 22.3-83.8 nmol/L)
19 years	138-442 ng/mL (SI: 18.1-57.9 nmol/L)	147-527 ng/mL (SI: 19.3-69.0 nmol/L)
20 years	122-384 ng/mL (SI: 16.0-50.3 nmol/L)	132-457 ng/mL (SI: 17.3-59.9 nmol/L)
21-25 years	116-341 ng/mL (SI: 15.2-44.7 nmol/L)	116-341 ng/mL (SI: 15.2-44.7 nmol/L)
26-30 years	117-321 ng/mL (SI: 15.3-42.1 nmol/L)	117-321 ng/mL (SI: 15.3-42.1 nmol/L)
31-35 years	113-297 ng/mL (SI: 14.8-38.9 nmol/L)	113-297 ng/mL (SI: 14.8-38.9 nmol/L)
36-40 years	106-277 ng/mL (SI: 13.9-36.3 nmol/L)	106-277 ng/mL (SI: 13.9-36.3 nmol/L)
41-45 years	98-261 ng/mL (SI: 12.8-34.2 nmol/L)	98-261 ng/mL (SI: 12.8-34.2 nmol/L)
46-50 years	91-246 ng/mL (SI: 11.9-32.2 nmol/L)	91-246 ng/mL (SI: 11.9-32.2 nmol/L)
51-55 years	84-233 ng/mL (SI: 11.0-30.5 nmol/L)	84-233 ng/mL (SI: 11.0-30.5 nmol/L)
56-60 years	78-220 ng/mL (SI: 10.2-28.8 nmol/L)	78-220 ng/mL (SI: 10.2-28.8 nmol/L)
61-65 years	72-207 ng/mL (SI: 9.4-27.1 nmol/L)	72-207 ng/mL (SI: 9.4-27.1 nmol/L)
66-70 years	67-195 ng/mL (SI: 8.8-25.5 nmol/L)	67-195 ng/mL (SI: 8.8-25.5 nmol/L)
71-75 years	62-184 ng/mL (SI: 8.1-24.1 nmol/L)	62-184 ng/mL (SI: 8.1-24.1 nmol/L)

Patient Age	Female	Male
76-80 years	57-172 ng/mL (SI: 7.5-22.5 nmol/L)	57-172 ng/mL (SI: 7.5-22.5 nmol/L)
>80 years	53-162 ng/mL (SI: 6.9-21.2 nmol/L)	53-162 ng/mL (SI: 6.9-21.2 nmol/L)

Insulinlike growth factor binding protein 3 ----------- 2.5-4.8 mg/L

Insulin---------------------- 1.4-14.0 μIU/mL (SI: 9.7-97.2 pmol/L)

Islet-cell antibody assay---- 0 Juvenile Diabetes Foundation units

Luteinizing hormone (LH)---

1.0-9.0 mIU/mL (SI: 1.0-9.0 IU/L) (male);

<1.0 mIU/mL (SI: <1.0 IU/L) (prepuberty, female);

1.0-18.0 mIU/mL (SI: 1.0-18.0 IU/L) (follicular, female);

20.0-80.0 mIU/mL (SI: 20.0-80.0 IU/L) (midcycle, female);

0.5-18.0 mIU/mL (SI: 0.5-18.0 IU/L) (luteal, female);

>30.0 mIU/mL (SI: >30.0 IU/L) (postmenopausal, female)

Metanephrines (plasma fractionated)

Metanephrine--------------------<99 pg/mL (SI: <0.50 nmol/L)

Normetanephrine------------- <165 pg/mL (SI: <0.90 nmol/L)

75-g oral glucose tolerance test blood glucose values -----------

60-100 mg/dL (SI: 3.3-5.6 mmol/L) (fasting);

<200 mg/dL (SI: <11.1 mmol/L) (1 hour);

<140 mg/dL (SI: <7.8 mmol/L) (2 hour);

between 140-200 mg/dL (SI: 7.8-11.1 mmol/L) is considered impaired glucose tolerance or prediabetes; greater than 200 mg/dL (SI: >11.1 mmol/L) is a sign of diabetes mellitus

50-g oral glucose tolerance test for gestational diabetes --------

<140 mg/dL (SI: <7.8 mmol/L) (1 hour)

100-g oral glucose tolerance test for gestational diabetes -------

<95 mg/dL (SI: <5.3 mmol/L) (fasting);

<180 mg/dL (SI: <10.0 mmol/L) (1 hour);

<155 mg/dL (SI: <8.6 mmol/L) (2 hour);

<140 mg/dL (SI: <7.8 mmol/L) (3 hour)

Osteocalcin ---------------------9.0-42.0 ng/mL (SI: 9.0-42.0 μg/L)

Parathyroid hormone, intact (PTH) - 10-65 pg/mL (SI: 10-65 ng/L)

Parathyroid hormone–related protein (PTHrP) -------- <2.0 pmol/L

Progesterone -----------------≤1.2 ng/mL (SI: ≤3.8 nmol/L) (male);

≤1.0 ng/mL (SI: ≤3.2 nmol/L) (follicular, female);

2.0-20.0 ng/mL (SI: 6.4-63.6 nmol/L) (luteal, female);

≤1.1 ng/mL (SI: ≤3.5 nmol/L) (postmenopausal, female);

>10.0 ng/mL (SI: >31.8 nmol/L) (evidence of ovulatory adequacy)

Proinsulin ----------------- 26.5-176.4 pg/mL (SI: 3.0-20.0 pmol/L)

Prolactin ----------------4-23 ng/mL (SI: 0.17-1.00 nmol/L) (male);

4-30 ng/mL (SI: 0.17-1.30 nmol/L) (nonlactating female);

10-200 ng/mL (SI: 0.43-8.70 nmol/L) (lactating female)

Prostate-specific antigen (PSA) ----------------------------------

<2.0 ng/mL (SI: <2.0 μg/L) (≤40 years);

<2.8 ng/mL (SI: <2.8 μg/L) (≤50 years);

<3.8 ng/mL (SI: <3.8 μg/L) (≤60 years);

<5.3 ng/mL (SI: <5.3 μg/L) (≤70 years);

<7.0 ng/mL (SI: <7.0 μg/L) (≤79 years);

<7.2 ng/mL (SI: <7.2 μg/L) (≥80 years)

Renin activity, plasma, sodium replete, ambulatory --------------

0.6-4.3 ng/mL per h

Renin, direct concentration ------- 4-44 pg/mL (SI: 0.1-1.0 pmol/L)

Sex hormone–binding globulin (SHBG) ---------------------------

1.1-6.7 μg/mL (SI: 10-60 nmol/L) (male);

2.2-14.6 μg/mL (SI: 20-130 nmol/L) (female)

α-Subunit of pituitary glycoprotein hormones --------------------

<1.2 ng/mL (SI: <1.2 μg/L)

Testosterone (bioavailable)---------------------------------------

0.8-4.0 ng/dL (SI: 0.03-0.14 nmol/L)

(20-50 years, female on oral estrogen);

0.8-10.0 ng/dL (SI: 0.03-0.35 nmol/L)

(20-50 years, female not on oral estrogen);

83.0-257.0 ng/dL (SI: 2.88-8.92 nmol/L) (male 20-29 years);

72.0-235.0 ng/dL (SI: 2.50-8.15 nmol/L) (male 30-39 years);

61.0-213.0 ng/dL (SI: 2.12-7.39 nmol/L) (male 40-49 years);

50.0-190.0 ng/dL (SI: 1.74-6.59 nmol/L) (male 50-59 years);

40.0-168.0 ng/dL (SI: 1.39-5.83 nmol/L) (male 60-69 years)

Testosterone (free)-- 9.0-30.0 ng/dL (SI: 0.31-1.04 nmol/L) (male);

0.3-1.9 ng/dL (SI: 0.01-0.07 nmol/L) (female)

Testosterone (total) - 300-900 ng/dL (SI: 10.4-31.2 nmol/L) (male);

8-60 ng/dL (SI: 0.3-2.1 nmol/L) (female)

Vitamin B_{12} ---------------- 180-914 pg/mL (SI: 133-674 pmol/L)

Chemistry Values

Alanine aminotransferase ------- 10-40 U/L (SI: 0.17-0.67 μkat/L)

Albumin--------------------------------3.5-5.0 g/dL (SI: 35-50 g/L)

Amylase ------------------------ 26-102 U/L (SI: 0.43-1.70 μkat/L)

Anion gap ------------------------- 3-11 mEq/L (SI: 3-11 mmol/L)

Aspartate aminotransferase ---- 20-48 U/L (SI: 0.33-0.80 μkat/L)

Bicarbonate -------------------- 21-28 mEq/L (SI: 21-28 mmol/L)

Bilirubin (total)---------------- 0.3-1.2 mg/dL (SI: 5.1-20.5 μmol/L)

Blood gases

Po_2, arterial blood ---------80-100 mm Hg (SI: 10.6-13.3 kPa)

Pco_2, arterial blood ------------35-45 mm Hg (SI: 4.7-6.0 kPa)

Blood pH--- 7.35-7.45

Calcium -----------------------8.2-10.2 mg/dL (SI: 2.1-2.6 mmol/L)

Calcium (ionized) ----------- 4.60-5.08 mg/dL (SI: 1.2-1.3 mmol/L)

Carbon dioxide ------------------ 22-28 mEq/L (SI: 22-28 mmol/L)

CD_4 cell count--------------------500-1400/μL (SI: 0.5-1.4 x 10^9/L)

Chloride----------------------- 96-106 mEq/L (SI: 96-106 mmol/L)

Creatine kinase ----------------- 50-200 U/L (SI: 0.84-3.34 μkat/L)

Creatinine-----------0.7-1.3 mg/dL (SI: 61.9-114.9 μmol/L) (male); 0.6-1.1 mg/dL (SI: 53.0-97.2 μmol/L) (female)

Ferritin -------------------- 15-200 ng/mL (SI: 33.7-449.4 pmol/L)

Folate ---------------------------------- ≥4.0 ng/mL (SI: ≥4.0 μg/L)

Glucose ------------------------ 70-99 mg/dL (SI: 3.9-5.5 mmol/L)

γ-Glutamyltransferase ----------- 2-30 U/L (SI: 0.03-0.50 μkat/L)

Iron --
50-150 μg/dL (SI: 9.0-26.8 μmol/L) (male);
35-145 μg/dL (SI: 6.3-26.0 μmol/L) (female)

Lactate dehydrogenase --------- 100-200 U/L (SI: 1.7-3.3 μkat/L)

Lactic acid --------------------5.4-20.7 mg/dL (SI: 0.6-2.3 mmol/L)

Lipase -------------------------- 10-73 U/L (SI: 0.17-1.22 μkat/L)

Magnesium -------------------- 1.5-2.3 mg/dL (SI: 0.6-0.9 mmol/L)

Osmolality ------------275-295 mOsm/kg (SI: 275-295 mmol/kg)

Phosphate -------------------- 2.3-4.7 mg/dL (SI: 0.7-1.5 mmol/L)

Potassium -------------------- 3.5-5.0 mEq/L (SI: 3.5-5.0 mmol/L)

Prothrombin time -------------------------------------8.3-10.8 s

Serum urea nitrogen-------------8-23 mg/dL (SI: 2.9-8.2 mmol/L)

Sodium ------------------- 136-142 mEq/L (SI: 136-142 mmol/L)

Transferrin saturation --------------------------------- 14%-50%

Troponin I ------------------------------ <0.6 ng/mL (SI: <0.6 μg/L)

Tryptase ---------------------------- <11.5 ng/mL (SI: <11.5 μg/L)

Uric acid ----------------- 3.5-7.0 mg/dL (SI: 208.2-416.4 μmol/L)

Urine

Albumin-----------30-300 μg/mg creat (SI: 3.4-33.9 μg/mol creat)

Albumin-to-creatinine ratio ----------------------- <30 mg/g creat

Aldosterone------------------- 3-20 μg/24 h (SI: 8.3-55.4 nmol/d) (should be <12 μg/24 h [SI: <33.2 nmol/d] with oral sodium loading—confirmed with 24-hour urinary sodium >200 mEq)

Calcium ------------------- 100-300 mg/24 h (SI: 2.5-7.5 mmol/d)

Catecholamine fractionation

Normotensive normal ranges:

Dopamine ------------------<400 μg/24 h (SI: <2610 nmol/d)

Epinephrine --------------------<21 μg/24 h (SI: <115 nmol/d)

Norepinephrine ----------------<80 μg/24 h (SI: <473 nmol/d)

Citrate ---------------- 320-1240 mg/24 h (SI: 16.7-64.5 mmol/d)

Cortisol ------------------------ 4-50 μg/24 h (SI: 11-138 nmol/d)

Cortisol following dexamethasone suppression test (low-dose: 2 day, 2 mg daily)-- <10 μg/24 h (SI: <27.6 nmol/d)

Creatinine------------------- 1.0-2.0 g/24 h (SI: 8.8-17.7 mmol/d)

Glomerular filtration rate (estimated) ---->60 mL/min per 1.73 m^2

5-Hydroxyindole acetic acid---2-9 mg/24 h (SI: 10.5-47.1 μmol/d)

Iodine (random)--->100 μg/L

17-Ketosteroids - 6.0-21.0 mg/24 h (SI: 20.8-72.9 μmol/d) (male); 4.0-17.0 mg/24 h (SI: 13.9-59.0 μmol/d) (female)

Metanephrine fractionation

Normotensive normal ranges:

Metanephrine-------- <261 μg/24 h (SI: <1323 nmol/d) (male); <180 μg/24 h (SI: <913 nmol/d) (female)

Normetanephrine-------------------- age and sex dependent

Total metanephrine------------------ age and sex dependent

Osmolality --------- 150-1150 mOsm/kg (SI: 150-1150 mmol/kg)

Oxalate ------------------------- <40 mg/24 h (SI: <456 mmol/d)

Phosphate ----------------- 0.9-1.3 g/24 h (SI: 29.1-42.0 mmol/d)

Potassium -------------------17-77 mEq/24 h (SI: 17-77 mmol/d)

Sodium ------------------40-217 mEq/24 h (SI: 40-217 mmol/d)

Uric acid ------------------------<800 mg/24 h (SI: <4.7 mmol/d)

Saliva

Cortisol (salivary), midnight --------- <0.13 μg/dL (SI: <3.6 nmol/L)

Semen

Semen analysis------------->20 million sperm/mL; >50% motility

COMMON ABBREVIATIONS USED IN ENDOCRINE BOARD REVIEW

ACTH = corticotropin
ACE inhibitor = angiotensin-converting enzyme inhibitor
ALT = alanine aminotransferase
AST = aspartate aminotransferase
BMI = body mass index
CNS = central nervous system
CT = computed tomography
DHEA = dehydroepiandrosterone
DHEA-S = dehydroepiandrosterone sulfate
DNA = deoxyribonucleic acid
DPP-4 inhibitor = dipeptidyl-peptidase 4 inhibitor
DXA = dual-energy x-ray absorptiometry
FDA = Food and Drug Administration
FGF-23 = fibroblast growth factor 23
FNA = fine-needle aspiration
FSH = follicle-stimulating hormone
GH = growth hormone
GHRH = growth hormone–releasing hormone
GLP-1 receptor agonist = glucagonlike peptide 1 receptor agonist
GnRH = gonadotropin-releasing hormone
hCG = human chorionic gonadotropin
HDL = high-density lipoprotein
HIV = human immunodeficiency virus
HMG-CoA reductase inhibitor = 3-hydroxy-3-methylglutaryl coenzyme A reductase inhibitor
IGF-1 = insulinlike growth factor 1
LDL = low-density lipoprotein
LH = luteinizing hormone
MCV = mean corpuscular volume
MIBG = *meta*-iodobenzylguanidine
MRI = magnetic resonance imaging
NPH insulin = neutral protamine Hagedorn insulin
PCSK9 inhibitor = proprotein convertase subtilisin/kexin 9 inhibitor
PET = positron emission tomography
PSA = prostate-specific antigen
PTH = parathyroid hormone
PTHrP = parathyroid hormone–related protein
SGLT-2 inhibitor = sodium-glucose cotransporter 2 inhibitor
SHBG = sex hormone–binding globulin
T_3 = triiodothyronine
T_4 = thyroxine
TPO antibodies = thyroperoxidase antibodies
TRH = thyrotropin-releasing hormone
TRAb = TSH-receptor antibodies
TSH = thyrotropin
VLDL = very low-density lipoprotein

ENDOCRINE BOARD REVIEW

QUESTIONS

Adrenal Board Review

Tobias Else, MD

1 A 69-year-old woman presents to the emergency department with abdominal pain, lethargy, fatigue, and nausea. Symptoms started 3 days ago and have been worsening. She had a hip replacement 10 days ago without complications.

She has hypertension, which is controlled with lisinopril, 20 mg daily. She has no history of diabetes mellitus or osteoporosis. She does not smoke cigarettes.

On physical examination, her blood pressure is 92/52 mm Hg and pulse rate is 86 beats/min. She appears ill. There is no hyperpigmentation. Her abdomen is diffusely tender, and there is a healing scar on her right hip.

Abdominal CT (with contrast) shows bilateral adrenal masses (60 Hounsfield units) (*see image, arrows*), and an endocrine consultation is sought.

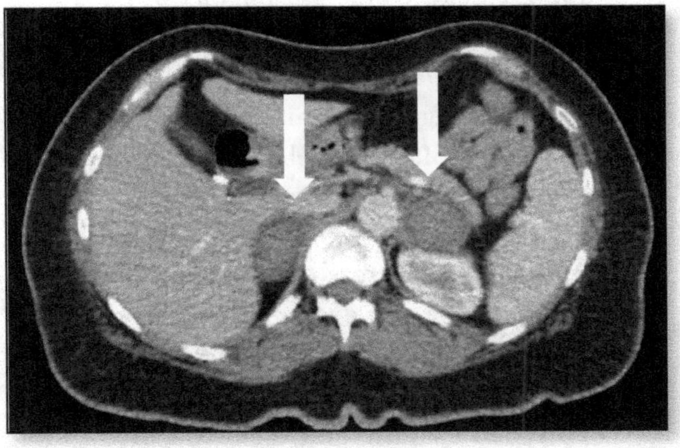

Laboratory test results:

- Sodium = 128 mEq/L (136-142 mEq/L) (SI: 128 mmol/L [136-142 mmol/L])
- Potassium = 5.4 mEq/L (3.5-5.0 mEq/L) (SI: 5.4 mmol/L [3.5-5.0 mmol/L])
- Serum cortisol (8 AM) = 1.8 µg/dL (5-25 µg/dL) (SI: 49.7 nmol/L [137.9-689.7 nmol/L])
- Serum DHEA-S = 48 µg/dL (35-179 µg/dL) (SI: 2.22 µmol/L [0.95-4.85 µmol/L])

The patient is started on hydrocortisone, 50 mg every 8 hours.

Which of the following is the best next step in this patient's management?

A. Adrenal mass biopsy
B. Chest/abdomen/pelvis CT
C. DOTATATE-PET
D. FDG-PET
E. No further imaging or biochemical workup needed

2 A 58-year-old woman is referred for an incidentally discovered adrenal nodule. She had a recent emergency department visit for abdominal pain, which improved without therapy. She is otherwise healthy and does not have hypertension, osteoporosis, or diabetes mellitus. Her only medication is combined hormone replacement therapy, which she has taken since age 49 years.

CT for suspected nephrolithiasis is performed, and it shows a 1.4-cm right adrenal mass with a density of 5 Hounsfield units (*see image, arrow*).

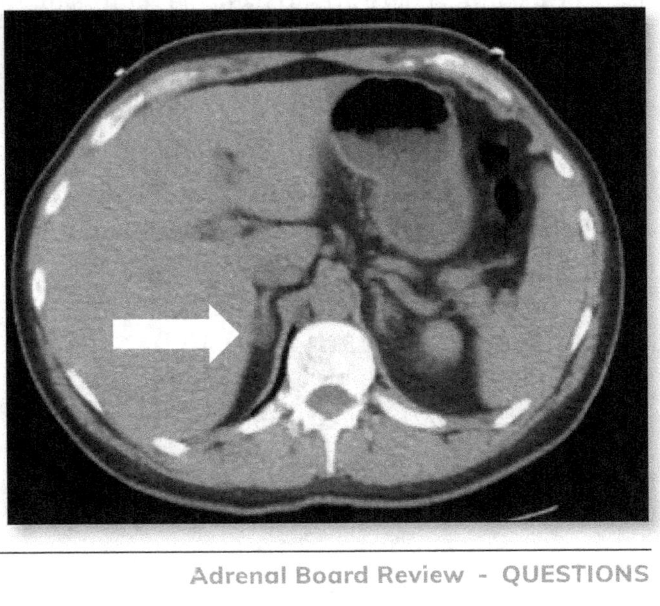

On physical examination, she appears healthy. Her blood pressure is 110/77 mm Hg, and pulse rate is 78 beats/min. Her height is 66.5 in (169 cm), and weight is 132.3 lb (60 kg) (BMI = 21.0 kg/m^2). There is no hyperpigmentation, striae, or bruises.

Laboratory test results:

Cortisol (following a 1-mg dexamethasone-suppression test) = 1.2 µg/dL (SI: 33.1 nmol/L)
Sodium = 137 mEq/L (136-142 mEq/L) (SI: 137 mmol/L [136-142 mmol/L])
Potassium = 4.2 mEq/L (3.5-5.0 mEq/L) (SI: 4.2 mmol/L [3.5-5.0 mmol/L])

Which of the following describes the best follow-up care?

A. Measure aldosterone and renin
B. Measure plasma free metanephrines
C. Perform FDG-PET
D. Recommend no further evaluation now, follow-up with primary care physician
E. Recommend no further evaluation now, return to clinic in 1 year for repeated CT

3 A 56-year-old man with episodic hypertension presents for endocrine evaluation. He describes intermittent episodes of turning pale, headache, and pounding heartbeat. These episodes are accompanied by nausea and last 1 to 4 hours. During one of these episodes, his blood pressure was 220/120 mm Hg with a pulse rate of 111 beats/min.

On physical examination, he appears healthy. His blood pressure is 148/90 mm Hg, and pulse rate is 92 beats/min. There are no palpable tumors on abdominal examination.

Laboratory test results:

Plasma normetanephrine = 328 pg/mL (<165 pg/mL) (SI: 1.79 nmol/L [<0.90 nmol/L])
Plasma metanephrine = 400 pg/mL (<99 pg/mL) (SI: 2.03 nmol/L [<0.50 nmol/L])
Sodium = 140 mEq/L (136-142 mEq/L) (SI: 140 mmol/L [136-142 mmol/L])
Potassium = 3.5 mEq/L (3.5-5.0 mEq/L) (SI: 3.5 mmol/L [3.5-5.0 mmol/L])
Serum aldosterone = 8.1 ng/dL (4-21 ng/dL) (SI: 224.7 pmol/L [111.0-582.5 pmol/L])
Plasma renin activity = 4.4 ng/mL per h (0.6-4.3 ng/mL per h)

Which of the following imaging studies is the best next step in this patient's care?

A. CT of the abdomen
B. DOTATATE-PET
C. FDG-PET
D. MIBG scan
E. Whole-body MRI

4 A 62-year-old woman has suspected adrenal insufficiency. She is currently hospitalized with tiredness, fatigue, nausea, and vomiting. She has an underlying diagnosis of metastatic melanoma and started immunotherapy with nivolumab and ipilimumab 4 months ago. She developed symptoms following her last infusion 3 days ago. The metastatic disease has responded well to therapy; 4 lung nodules have almost completely disappeared and a right adrenal metastasis has decreased from 4.3 cm to 1.4 cm.

Laboratory test results (at hospital admission):

Sodium = 128 mEq/L (136-142 mEq/L) (SI: 128 mmol/L [136-142 mmol/L])
Potassium = 4.4 mEq/L (3.5-5.0 mEq/L) (SI: 4.4 mmol/L [3.5-5.0 mmol/L])
Cortisol = 1.8 µg/dL (30-minute cortisol = 16.2 µg/dL [SI: 49.7 nmol/L]); 60-minute cortisol = 17.9 µg/dL [SI: 493.8 nmol/L])

The patient receives stress-dose steroids (hydrocortisone, 50 mg every 8 hours). On hospital day 3, she is resting comfortably and is feeling much better. Nausea and vomiting have subsided.

On physical examination, she appears healthy. Her blood pressure is 124/81 mm Hg, and pulse rate is 88 beats. She is afebrile, has no hyperpigmentation, and has intact vision.

Which of the following is the best next step in this patient's management?

A. Continue hydrocortisone orally, 20 mg in the morning and 10 mg in the early afternoon, and measure aldosterone and renin in 2 days
B. Measure 21-hydroxylase antibodies
C. Order exogenous steroid panel
D. Perform pituitary MRI
E. Stop hydrocortisone replacement and measure 8-AM cortisol the next day

5 A 64-year-old woman is referred for the incidental finding of a right adrenal nodule. On noncontrast CT, the homogeneous nodule measures 3.9 cm, with a density of 2 Hounsfield units. She has a history of borderline hypertension and postmenopausal osteoporosis, for which she is treated with alendronate, 70 mg weekly. She has gained 15.4 lb (7 kg) over the last 5 years. She has no concerns and feels well. An endocrine laboratory evaluation is done (*see laboratory results*).

After 2 years, she returns to clinic. She continues to take alendronate but has also started lisinopril for hypertension. She struggles with weight loss. She has started metformin.

On physical examination, she has gained an additional 13.2 lb (6 kg). Her height is 63.8 in (162 cm), and weight is 202.8 lb (92 kg) (BMI = 35.0 kg/m^2). Her blood pressure is 132/80 mm Hg, and pulse rate is 80 beats/min) She has no facial plethora, dermal atrophy, bruising, or supraclavicular fat pads.

Laboratory test results:

Analyte	2 years ago	Now
Hemoglobin A_{1c}	6.1% (43 mmol/mol)	6.9% (52 mmol/mol)
ACTH (8 AM)	9 pg/mL (SI: 1.98 pmol/L)	8 pg/mL (SI: 1.76 pmol/L)
DHEA-S	58 µg/dL (SI: 1.57 µmol/L)	<15 µg/dL (SI: <0.41)
Cortisol after 1 mg dexamethasone	4.1 µg/dL (SI: 113.1 nmol/L)	4.1 µg/dL (SI: 113.1 nmol/L)
Urinary free cortisol	22 µg/24 h (SI: 60.7 nmol/d)	28 µg/24 h (SI: 77.3 nmol/d)

Which of the following is the best next step in this patient's care?

A. Delay medical or surgical therapy until urinary free cortisol is clearly elevated
B. Measure cortisol after a high-dose (8-mg) dexamethasone-suppression test
C. Perform FDG-PET to evaluate for malignant transformation
D. Refer for laparoscopic right adrenalectomy
E. Start osilodrostat, 2 mg twice daily

6 A 49-year-old woman is diagnosed with an adrenal tumor. She has noticed weight gain, active striae, and easy bruising.

On physical examination, she has stigmata of active Cushing syndrome.

Initial laboratory test results:

Cortisol (8 AM) = 24 µg/dL (5-25 µg/dL) (SI: 662.1 nmol/L [137.9-689.7 nmol/L])
ACTH = 8 pg/mL (10-60 pg/mL) (SI: 1.8 pmol/L [2.2-13.2 pmol/L])
Urinary cortisol = 112 µg/24 h (4-50 µg/24 h) (SI: 309.1 nmol/d [11-138 nmol/d])
Cortisol (1-mg dexamethasone-suppression test) = 14 µg/dL (SI: 386.2 nmol/L)
ACTH (1-mg dexamethasone-suppression test) = 6 pg/mL (SI: 1.3 pmol/L)
DHEA-S = <15 µg/dL (18-244 µg/dL) (SI: 0.41 µmol/L [0.49-6.61 µmol/L])

CT shows a right adrenal lipid-rich adenoma, and she undergoes surgery with removal of a 4.7-cm adenoma. Four weeks postoperatively, she is taking hydrocortisone, 15 mg in the morning and 5 mg in the early afternoon. She feels worse than before surgery. She has loss of appetite, nausea, and headaches and has lost 4.4 lb (2 kg).

On physical examination, her blood pressure is 134/78 mm Hg and pulse rate is 82 beats/min. Her height is 63.4 in (161 cm), and weight is 242.5 lb (110 kg) (BMI = 42.4 kg/m^2). She has a slightly cushingoid habitus (less than before surgery), no bruises, healing scar on abdomen from laparoscopic surgery, and pale striae.

Laboratory workup (before hydrocortisone morning dose):

Cortisol (8 AM) = 3.1 μg/dL (5-25 μg/dL) (SI: 85.5 nmol/L [137.9-689.7 nmol/L])
ACTH = 79 pg/mL (5-25 pg/mL) (SI: 17.4 pmol/L [2.2-13.2 pmol/L])
Sodium = 138 mEq/L (136-142 mEq/L) (SI: 138 mmol/L [136-142 mmol/L])
Potassium = 3.9 mEq/L (3.5-5.0 mEq/L) (SI: 3.9 mmol/L [3.5-5.0 mmol/L])

Which of the following is the most likely cause of this patient's symptoms?

A. Adrenal androgen deficiency
B. Adrenal insufficiency
C. Cortisol withdrawal syndrome
D. Incomplete removal of the adrenal tumor
E. Missed diagnosis of ACTH-dependent hypercortisolism

7 A 62-year-old woman has had multiple episodes of hyperkalemia (potassium ranging from 4.7 to 5.4 mEq/L [4.7-5.4 mmol/L]). She takes ibuprofen, 800 mg 3 times daily, for back pain. Other medications are metformin, 1000 mg twice daily, and glipizide, 5 mg twice daily, for diabetes mellitus. She has been resistant to any additional therapy for diabetes, and her hemoglobin A_{1c} values have remained between 7.5% and 8.5% (58-69 mmol/mol) over the last 10 years. Blood pressure is treated with metoprolol, 25 mg twice daily.

She presents to the emergency department with back pain, and endocrinology is consulted regarding hyperkalemia.

On physical examination, her blood pressure is 104/72 mm Hg and pulse rate is 94 beats/min. Her height is 65.4 in (166 cm), and weight is 178.6 lb (81 kg) (BMI = 29.4 kg/m^2). She is uncomfortable with back pain but has no abdominal tenderness.

Laboratory test results (5 PM, after 6 hours in the emergency department):

Cortisol = 12.8 μg/dL (2-14 μg/dL) (SI: 353.1 nmol/L [55.2-386.2 nmol/L])
ACTH = 8 pg/mL (5-25 pg/mL) (SI: 1.8 pmol/L [2.2-13.2 pmol/L])
Aldosterone = 2.1 ng/dL (4-21 ng/dL) (SI: 58.3 pmol/L [111.0-582.5 pmol/L])
Plasma renin activity = 2.2 ng/mL per h (0.6-4.3 ng/L per h)
Sodium = 138 mEq/L (136-142 mEq/L) (SI: 138 mmol/L [136-142 mmol/L])
Potassium = 5.4 mEq/L (3.5-5.0 mEq/L) (SI: 5.4 mmol/L [3.5-5.0 mmol/L])
Bicarbonate = 17 mEq/L (21-28 mEq/L) (SI: 17 mmol/L [21-28 mmol/L])
Creatinine = 1.8 mg/dL (0.6-1.1 mg/dL) (SI: 159.1 μmol/L [53.0-97.2 μmol/L])
Glucose = 243 mg/dL (70-99 mg/dL) (SI: 13.5 mmol/L [3.9-5.5 mmol/L])
DHEA-S = 162 μg/dL (15-157 μg/dL) (SI: 4.39 μmol/L [0.41-4.25 μmol/L])
Urine pH = 5.3

Which of the following is the best next step in this patient's care?

A. Administer hydrocortisone, 50 mg intravenously every 8 hours
B. Hold ibuprofen and advise against further use
C. Start hydrocortisone, 20 mg in the morning and 10 mg in the early afternoon, and fludrocortisone, 0.1 mg daily
D. Start fludrocortisone, 0.1 mg daily
E. Stop metformin and advise against further use

8 A 41-year-old man with chronic back pain is incidentally diagnosed with bilateral adrenal enlargement and is referred for further evaluation. He has a history of hypertension and despite therapy with amlodipine, 10 mg daily, and doxazosin, 8 mg daily, his home blood pressure measurements range from 145-182/88-99 mm Hg. He has had no changes in weight or appearance. He has no history of diabetes mellitus.

On physical examination, his blood pressure is 161/91 mm Hg and pulse rate is 77 beats/min. His height is 74.8 in (190 cm), and weight is 178.6 lb (81 kg) (BMI = 22.4 kg/m^2). He appears healthy and has no bruises, striae, or muscle wasting. There is normal fat distribution and muscle strength.

Laboratory test results:

Cortisol (8 AM) (following 1-mg dexamethasone-suppression test) = 4.5 μg/dL (SI: 124.2 nmol/L)
Urinary cortisol = 94 μg/24 h (4-50 μg/24 h) (SI: 259 nmol/d [11-138 nmol/d])
ACTH = 38 pg/mL (5-25 pg/mL) (SI: 8.4 pmol/L [2.2-13.2 pmol/L])
Aldosterone = <2.1 ng/dL (4-21 ng/dL) (SI: <58 pmol/L [111.0-582.5 pmol/L])
Plasma renin activity = <0.6 ng/mL per h (0.6-4.3 ng/L per h)
Sodium = 138 mEq/L (136-142 mEq/L) (SI: 138 mmol/L [136-142 mmol/L])
Potassium = 3.5 mEq/L (3.5-5.0 mEq/L) (SI: 3.5 mmol/L [3.5-5.0 mmol/L])
DHEA-S = 450 μg/dL (48-244 μg/dL) (SI: 12.2 μmol/L [1.30-6.61 μmol/L])

Which of the following is this patient's most likely diagnosis?

A. ACTH resistance
B. Cushing disease due to pituitary tumor
C. Ectopic ACTH syndrome
D. Glucocorticoid resistance
E. 11β-Hydroxylase deficiency

9 A 29-year-old man who was seen in endocrinology clinic 2 years ago presents to the emergency department. The patient is intoxicated, and he has been having abdominal pain and vomiting. The patient says he has adrenal insufficiency and has a wallet card confirming this. The emergency department physician asks for help reviewing the patient's abdominal CT (*see image*). Bilateral 16-cm heterogeneous adrenal masses are visible. Review of the clinic note from 2 years ago indicates that a firm lump in the right testis had been appreciated at that time.

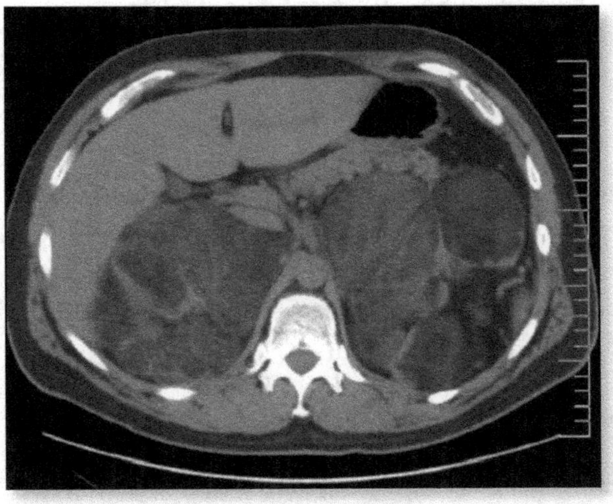

After recommending intravenous hydrocortisone, which of the following diagnoses should the emergency department physician be told that this man most likely has?

A. Autoimmune polyglandular syndrome type 2
B. Bilateral adrenal hemorrhage
C. Bilateral metastases to the adrenal gland from testicular carcinoma
D. Congenital adrenal hyperplasia
E. Histoplasmosis

10 A 61-year-old woman with a 50 pack-year history of cigarette smoking presents with recent-onset hypertension and peripheral edema. She appears to be cachectic and chronically ill. Her blood pressure is 182/104 mm Hg, and pulse rate is 94 beats/min. She has 4+ pretibial edema and severe muscle weakness.

Laboratory test results:

Sodium = 134 mEq/L (136-142 mEq/L) (SI: 134 mmol/L [136-142 mmol/L])
Potassium = 2.0 mEq/L (3.5-5.0 mEq/L) (SI: 2.0 mmol/L [3.5-5.0 mmol/L])
Chloride = 90 mEq/L (96-106 mEq/L) (SI: 90 mEq/L [96-106 mmol/L])
Bicarbonate = 42 mEq/L (21-28 mEq/L) (SI: 42 mmol/L [21-28 mmol/L])
Serum urea nitrogen = 22 mg/dL (8-23 mg/dL) (SI: 7.9 mmol/L [2.9-8.2 mmol/L])
Creatinine = 0.7 mg/dL (0.6-1.1 mg/dL) (SI: 61.9 μmol/L [53.0-97.2 μmol/L])

Aldosterone = <1.0 ng/dL (4-21 ng/dL)
(SI: 27.7 pmol/L [111.0-582.5 pmol/L])
Plasma renin activity = <0.1 ng/mL per h
(0.6-4.3 ng/mL per h)

Spironolactone, potassium chloride, and valsartan are initiated. CT of the chest and abdomen shows bilateral adrenal enlargement, with a 2-cm left adrenal nodule (10 Hounsfield units), and a large left inferior lobe lung mass.

Which of the following is the most likely cause of hypertension and hypokalemia in this patient?

A. Adrenocortical carcinoma with pulmonary metastases
B. Bilateral adrenal hyperplasia, secreting aldosterone
C. Ectopic ACTH-secreting small cell carcinoma of the lung
D. 11-Hydroxylase deficiency
E. Liddle syndrome

11 A 21-year-old man has an appointment for preoperative management of a recently discovered right pheochromocytoma. His father had a bilateral adrenalectomy for pheochromocytomas at age 44 years and died 10 years later of influenza and an adrenal crisis. The patient has recent-onset hypertension and reports having morning headaches. He has been treated with phenoxybenzamine for 3 weeks and he just started therapy with a β-adrenergic blocker.

On physical examination, his blood pressure is 132/78 mm Hg, pulse rate is 78 beats/min, and BMI is 24.7 kg/m^2. He has long, slender arms and pectus carinatum. The following finding is observed (*see image*).

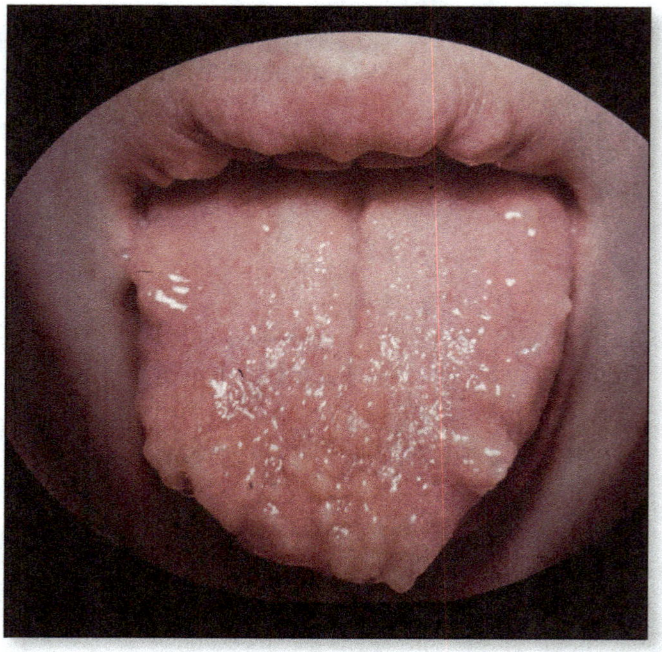

Which of the following syndromes is most likely responsible for the pheochromocytoma in this patient?

A. Carney complex
B. Multiple endocrine neoplasia type 1
C. Multiple endocrine neoplasia type 2B
D. Neurofibromatosis type 1
E. von Hippel–Lindau syndrome

12 A 35-year-old woman with a history of Cushing disease presents for annual follow-up. She developed depression and hypertension 5 years ago, and after diagnosis she underwent transsphenoidal surgery. Her condition improved postoperatively, and she took hydrocortisone for 12 weeks, at which time her adrenal function recovered.

On physical examination today, she has no moon facies, plethora, dorsocervical fat pad, weakness, or bruises. Electrolytes are normal. She has developed borderline hypertension (145/88 mm Hg) and has gained 8.8 lb (4 kg). Her height is 66.1 in (168 cm), and weight is 185.2 lb (84 kg) (BMI = 29.8 kg/m^2).

Which of the following diagnostic procedures should be recommended for further evaluation regarding recurrence in this patient?

A. 1-mg overnight dexamethasone-suppression test
B. 8-mg overnight dexamethasone-suppression test
C. 24-hour urinary free cortisol measurement
D. Inferior petrosal sinus sampling with ovine corticotropin-releasing hormone stimulation
E. Late-night salivary cortisol measurement

13 An 18-year-old college freshman is referred for evaluation of possible adrenal insufficiency. He has a 2-year history of gradually increasing anorexia, fatigue, weakness, and weight loss. He is struggling to get to classes on time and to keep up with his studies. His family history is negative for adrenal disease, but a maternal uncle died suddenly after developing progressive weakness in his 20s.

On physical examination, he is thin, has hyperpigmentation in sun-exposed areas but no vitiligo, and has orthostatic hypotension. He has diffuse muscle weakness, unsteady gait, and brisk deep tendon reflexes.

Initial laboratory test results (from evaluation at the college student health center):

Plasma ACTH = 144 pg/mL (10-60 pg/mL) (SI: 31.7 pmol/L [2.2-13.2 pmol/L])
Serum cortisol = 3.7 μg/dL (SI: 102.1 nmol/L), no increase with cosyntropin
Serum aldosterone = <2 ng/dL (4-21 ng/dL) (SI: <55.5 pmol/L [111.0-582.5 pmol/L])
Plasma renin activity = 24 ng/mL per h (0.6-4.3 ng/mL per h)

Which of the following diagnostic tests will reveal the etiology of his adrenal insufficiency?

A. Adrenal CT
B. Plasma lupus anticoagulant assessment
C. Plasma very long-chain fatty acid measurement
D. Serum 21-hydroxylase antibody assessment
E. Urine synthetic glucocorticoid testing

14 A 45-year-old woman presents with resistant hypertension that has been more difficult to control in the past few years. She has also gained 22 lb (10 kg) over the last 2 years and now has diet-controlled diabetes mellitus. Her medications include amlodipine, hydrochlorothiazide, and lisinopril.

On physical examination, she has subtle facial plethora and dermal atrophy. Proximal muscle strength is normal. She has no dorsocervical fat pad or striae.

Laboratory test results:

Sodium = 138 mEq/L (136-142 mEq/L) (SI: 138 mmol/L [136-142 mmol/L])
Potassium = 3.3 mEq/L (3.5-5.0 mEq/L) (SI: 3.3 mmol/L [3.5-5.0 mmol/L])
Chloride = 103 mEq/L (96-106 mEq/L) (SI: 103 mEq/L [96-106 mmol/L])
Bicarbonate = 23 mEq/L (21-28 mEq/L) (SI: 23 mmol/L [21-28 mmol/L])
Fasting glucose = 157 mg/dL (70-99 mg/dL) (SI: 8.7 mmol/L [3.9-5.5 mmol/L])
Serum aldosterone = 11 ng/dL (4-21 ng/dL) (SI: 305.1 pmol/L [111.0-582.5 pmol/L])
Plasma renin activity = <0.6 ng/mL per h (0.6-4.3 ng/mL per h)
Serum urea nitrogen = 32 mg/dL (8-23 mg/dL) (SI: 11.4 mmol/L [2.9-8.2 mmol/L])
Creatinine = 0.6 mg/dL (0.6-1.1 mg/dL) (SI: 53.0 μmol/L [53.0-97.2 μmol/L])

Repeated laboratory test results after potassium supplementation:

Sodium = 139 mEq/L (SI: 139 mmol/L)
Potassium = 3.7 mEq/L (SI: 3.7 mmol/L)
Serum aldosterone = 14 ng/dL (SI: 388.4 pmol/L)
Plasma renin activity = <0.6 ng/mL per h

CT with contrast of the abdomen demonstrates a 3.8-cm left adrenal mass (8 Hounsfield units) and an atrophic right adrenal gland (*see image, arrows*).

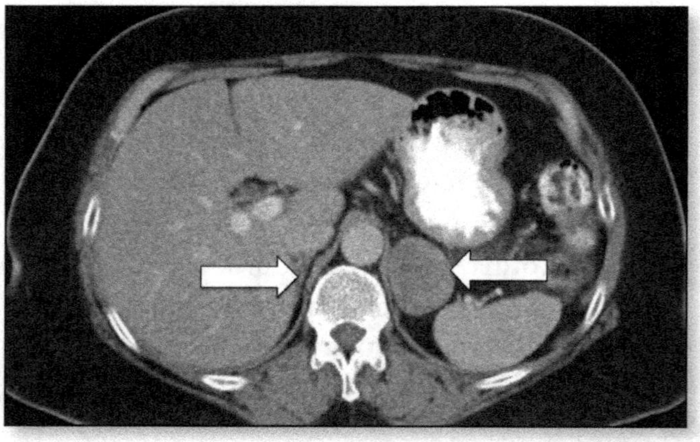

The patient is then referred for further evaluation and recommendations.

Which of the following is the best next step?

A. Measure plasma metanephrines and perform a 1-mg overnight dexamethasone-suppression test
B. Perform left adrenalectomy
C. Perform a saline infusion test measuring aldosterone after administration of 2 L normal saline
D. Prescribe spironolactone, 50 mg daily
E. Schedule adrenal venous sampling to measure aldosterone and cortisol

15 A 43-year-old man is referred for evaluation of resistant hypertension and hypokalemia. His blood pressure while taking amlodipine, carvedilol, lisinopril, metformin, and potassium chloride was 148/96 mm Hg in his primary care physician's office 4 weeks ago. His primary care physician ordered measurement of aldosterone and plasma renin activity, then started spironolactone, 25 mg daily. The patient started spironolactone but did not have his blood drawn until 3 weeks later.

At his appointment today, his blood pressure is 133/86 mm Hg, and he feels well with no adverse effects from his medications.

Laboratory test results:

Sodium = 142 mEq/L (136-142 mEq/L) (SI: 142 mmol/L [136-142 mmol/L])
Potassium = 3.4 mEq/L (3.5-5.0 mEq/L) (SI: 3.4 mmol/L [3.5-5.0 mmol/L])
Serum aldosterone = 35 ng/dL (4-21 ng/dL) (SI: 970.9 pmol/L [111.0-582.5 pmol/L])
Plasma renin activity = <0.6 ng/mL per h (0.6-4.3 ng/mL per h)

Which of the following is the best next step in this patient's evaluation?

A. Perform adrenal CT
B. Perform adrenal MRI
C. Stop carvedilol and lisinopril for 2 weeks and measure aldosterone and renin activity again
D. Stop spironolactone for 6 weeks and measure aldosterone and renin activity again
E. Substitute eplerenone for spironolactone

16 A 51-year-old man is status post right open adrenalectomy for a 6-cm adrenocortical carcinoma that was causing Cushing syndrome. The pathology specimen showed high-grade tumor with vascular invasion, but no inferior vena cava thrombosis or lymph nodes were positive for tumor. Postoperatively, he was treated with hydrocortisone, 20 mg upon waking and 10 mg in the afternoon, and he recovered well with some resolution of cushingoid features. After 4 weeks, adjuvant mitotane was added and titrated up to 6 g daily. At a clinic visit 10 weeks later, his serum mitotane value is now at therapeutic goal, but he reports nausea, anorexia, and fatigue. His blood pressure is 125/82 mm Hg without an orthostatic drop.

Laboratory test results:

Serum mitotane = 16.4 mg/L (therapeutic goal >14 mg/L)
Serum potassium = 4.2 mEq/L (3.5-5.0 mEq/L) (SI: 4.2 mmol/L [3.5-5.0 mmol/L])
Plasma ACTH = <2 pg/mL (10-60 pg/mL) (SI: <0.4 pmol/L [2.2-13.2 pmol/L])
Serum total testosterone = 480 ng/dL (300-900 ng/dL) (SI: 16.7 nmol/L [10.4-31.2 nmol/L])
SHBG = 11.5 μg/mL (1.1-6.7 μg/mL) (SI: 102 nmol/L [10-60 nmol/L])

Which of the following is the best next step in this patient's management?

A. Add fludrocortisone, 0.1 mg daily
B. Add testosterone enanthate, 100 mg weekly
C. Change hydrocortisone dosage to 30 mg in the morning and 20 mg in the afternoon and evening
D. Change hydrocortisone to methylprednisolone, 4 mg daily
E. Reduce mitotane dosage to 0.5 g 4 times daily

17 A 33-year-old woman underwent surgery for Cushing disease 2 years ago. She had normalization of urinary free cortisol but did not experience adrenal insufficiency and stopped hydrocortisone 6 weeks postoperatively. Over the last 6 months, she has noted weight gain, easy bruising, and poor sleep.

Laboratory test results:

Midmorning serum cortisol = 28 µg/dL (5-25 µg/dL) (SI: 773 nmol/L [138-690 nmol/L])
Plasma ACTH = 50 pg/mL (10-60 pg/mL) (SI: 11.0 pmol/L [2.2-13.2 pmol/L])
Serum potassium = 3.8 mEq/L (3.5-5.0 mEq/L) (SI: 3.8 mmol/L [3.5-5.0 mmol/L])
Serum glucose = 180 mg/dL (70-99 mg/dL) (SI: 10.0 mmol/L [3.9-5.5 mmol/L])
Urinary free cortisol = 90 µg/24 h (4-50 µg/24 h) (SI: 249 nmol/d [11-138 nmol/d])

After discussing options, the decision is made to treat her with metyrapone, 500 mg 4 times daily, for inoperable Cushing disease. She returns in 2 weeks with slight weight loss and feels modestly better, but her serum cortisol level is unchanged. Her metyrapone dosage is increased to 750 mg 4 times daily. She returns 2 weeks later with severe fatigue, anorexia, myalgias, and poor sleep.

Laboratory test results while taking metyrapone (performed on hospital autoanalyzer):

Serum cortisol 2 hours after morning metyrapone dose = 25 µg/dL (SI: 690 nmol/L)
Serum potassium = 3.5 mEq/L (SI: 3.5 mmol/L)
Serum glucose = 46 mg/dL (SI: 2.6 mmol/L)

Which of the following tests would help guide adjustment of the metyrapone dosage?

A. Cosyntropin-stimulation test
B. Late-night salivary cortisol measurement
C. Plasma renin activity measurement
D. Serum cortisol and 11-deoxycortisol measurements by tandem mass spectrometry
E. Serum DHEA-S measurement

18 A 28-year-old man is diagnosed with autoimmune adrenal insufficiency and hypothyroidism. He presented with a 25-lb (11.4 kg) weight loss and adrenal crisis during a gastrointestinal illness. He was discharged from the hospital taking hydrocortisone, 20 mg upon waking in the morning and 10 mg in the early afternoon, as well as levothyroxine, 125 mcg daily. He regained most of his lost weight over the next 6 months and remained well without additional crises. For convenience, his glucocorticoid was changed to methylprednisolone, 6 mg upon waking. He has continued to slowly regain his lost weight, but he is now experiencing a generalized feeling of fatigue throughout the day, which does not improve shortly after taking the methylprednisolone. He has even tried dividing his daily dose (3 mg upon waking and 3 mg in the early afternoon), but this has not relieved the fatigue following either dose.

On physical examination, his blood pressure is 104/66 mm Hg and pulse rate is 88 beats/min. He has no purple striae, facial rounding, dermal atrophy, vitiligo, or bruises.

Laboratory test results:

Sodium = 138 mEq/L (136-142 mEq/L) (SI: 138 mmol/L [136-142 mmol/L])
Potassium = 4.9 mEq/L (3.5-5.0 mEq/L) (SI: 4.9 mmol/L [3.5-5.0 mmol/L])
Plasma ACTH = 400 pg/mL (10-60 pg/mL) (SI: 88.0 pmol/L [2.2-13.2 pmol/L])
Plasma renin activity = 13.4 ng/mL per h (0.6-4.3 ng/mL per h)
Serum TSH = 2.2 mIU/L (0.5-5.0 mIU/L)

Which of the following changes is the best management recommendation?

A. Add fludrocortisone acetate, 0.1 mg daily
B. Administer methylprednisolone, 4 mg upon waking and 2 mg at bedtime
C. Reassure him that no changes are necessary
D. Switch methylprednisolone to dexamethasone, 1 mg upon waking
E. Switch methylprednisolone to hydrocortisone, 20 mg upon waking

19 A 53-year-old man is referred for evaluation of primary aldosteronism. He developed resistant hypertension in his late 40s and was found to be hypokalemic 6 months ago on routine blood testing.

Screening laboratory test results:
Sodium = 147 mEq/L (136-142 mEq/L) (SI: 147 mmol/L [136-142 mmol/L])
Potassium = 3.2 mEq/L (3.5-5.0 mEq/L) (SI: 3.2 mmol/L [3.5-5.0 mmol/L])
Serum aldosterone = 33 ng/dL (4-21 ng/dL) (SI: 915 pmol/L [111-583 pmol/L])
Plasma renin activity = <0.6 ng/mL per h (0.6-4.3 ng/mL per h)

On the third day of a high-salt diet:
Urinary sodium = 280 mEq/24 h (SI: 280 mmol/d)
Urinary aldosterone = 40 μg/24 h (SI: 111 nmol/d)

CT with fine cuts of the adrenals shows minor irregularities in both glands but no conclusive tumors. Adrenal venous sampling is delayed for 4 months, and his serum potassium and blood pressure are controlled with spironolactone, 25 mg daily. He is told to stop the spironolactone 2 weeks before adrenal venous sampling.

He undergoes adrenal venous sampling with continuous infusion of cosyntropin at 50 mcg per h. As he is leaving the interventional radiology suite, however, he informs the staff that he forgot to stop the spironolactone, and he took his last dose the previous day. A week later, the laboratory results are received (*see table*).

Measurement	Right Adrenal Vein	Left Adrenal Vein	Inferior Vena Cava
Aldosterone	300 ng/dL (SI: 8322 pmol/L)	8000 ng/dL (SI: 221,920 pmol/L)	44 ng/dL (SI: 1221 pmol/L)
Cortisol	300 μg/dL (SI: 8276 nmol/L)	800 μg/dL (SI: 22,070 nmol/L)	22 μg/dL (SI: 607 nmol/L)
Aldosterone-to-Cortisol Ratio	1.0	10.0	2.0

Which of the following is the most accurate interpretation of the adrenal venous sampling study?

A. Unable to interpret the study and must repeat 2 weeks after stopping spironolactone
B. Left adrenal gland is the source (left adenoma)
C. Both adrenal glands are sources (bilateral, idiopathic hyperaldosteronism)
D. Right adrenal gland is the source (right adenoma)
E. Unsuccessful study, failure to access right adrenal vein

20 A 26-year-old man is referred by his primary care physician for management of classic 21-hydroxylase deficiency. The patient was diagnosed at birth and received treatment with hydrocortisone and fludrocortisone throughout childhood. He stopped all medications at age 22 years. However, he had an adrenal crisis 6 months ago and nearly died. At hospital discharge, he agreed to take prednisone, 7.5 mg daily, and fludrocortisone acetate, 0.1 mg daily. He has been adherent to this regimen and states that he feels better now than when he was untreated.

On physical examination, he appears healthy and has no cushingoid features. He is a short, muscular young man with a blood pressure of 116/81 mm Hg and pulse rate of 66 beats/min.

Laboratory test results:

Serum sodium = 135 mEq/L (136-142 mEq/L) (SI: 135 mmol/L [136-142 mmol/L])
Serum potassium = 4.2 mEq/L (3.5-5.0 mEq/L) (SI: 4.2 mmol/L [3.5-5.0 mmol/L])
Plasma renin activity = 2.4 ng/mL per h (0.6-4.3 ng/mL per h)
Serum androstenedione = 880 ng/dL (65-210 ng/dL) (SI: 30.7 nmol/L [2.3-7.3 nmol/L])
Serum total testosterone = 420 ng/dL (300-900 ng/dL) (SI: 14.6 nmol/L [10.4-31.2 nmol/L])

Which of the following is the most important test to order next?

A. Adrenal MRI
B. Serum aldosterone measurement
C. Serum 17-hydroxyprogesterone measurement
D. Semen analysis
E. Testicular ultrasonography

21 A 44-year-old man has recently been diagnosed with adrenocortical carcinoma. He reports no history of malignancy, but states that his brother had colon cancer at age 38 years and that his mother died of uterine cancer at age 51 years. His mother had 5 siblings: a brother with colon cancer in his late 50s, a sister with stomach cancer in her 40s, and 3 brothers who are alive and well in their 60s without any cancer diagnoses. The patient's maternal grandfather had prostate cancer in his 60s and his maternal grandmother had colon cancer at age 47 years. There are no family members with adrenal tumors.

The patient's family is wondering whether they could have a familial cancer syndrome.

Which hereditary syndrome is most likely in this patient's family?

A. Carney complex
B. Familial adenomatous polyposis
C. Li-Fraumeni syndrome
D. Lynch syndrome (hereditary nonpolyposis colon cancer)
E. Multiple endocrine neoplasia type 1

22 A 24-year-old man is referred for evaluation of hypertension and hypokalemia. He recently moved from the Middle East, where he was treated with potassium supplements and calcium-channel blockers with only fair response.

On physical examination, he is short (59 in [149.9 cm]) and muscular with a full beard. His blood pressure is 152/106 mm Hg, and heart examination reveals a 2/6 holosystolic, nonradiating murmur, and an S_4. He has no edema or flank bruits, and his skin is well-tanned.

Laboratory test results:

Sodium = 144 mEq/L (136-142 mEq/L) (SI: 144 mmol/L [136-142 mmol/L])
Potassium = 3.2 mEq/L (3.5-5.0 mEq/L) (SI: 3.2 mmol/L [3.5-5.0 mmol/L])
Plasma ACTH = 210 pg/mL (10-60 pg/mL) (SI: 46.2 pmol/L [2.2-13.2 pmol/L])
Serum testosterone = 480 ng/dL (300-900 ng/dL) (SI: 16.7 nmol/L [10.4-31.2 nmol/L])
Serum 17-hydroxyprogesterone = 1960 ng/dL (<220 ng/dL) (SI: 59.4 nmol/L [<6.67 nmol/L])
Serum aldosterone = <4 ng/dL (4-21 ng/dL) (SI: <111.0 pmol/L [111.0-582.5 pmol/L])
Plasma renin activity = <0.6 ng/mL per h (0.6-4.3 ng/mL per h)
Serum cortisol = <1 μg/dL (5-25 μg/dL) (SI: <27.6 nmol/L [137.9-689.7 nmol/L])

Which of the following additional laboratory tests is most likely to reveal this patient's diagnosis?

A. Determination of the urinary cortisol-to-cortisone ratio
B. Genotyping the *CYP21A2* gene
C. Serum 11-deoxycortisol measurement
D. Serum 17-hydroxypregnenolone measurement
E. Serum 18-hydroxycortisol measurement

Bone Board Review

Natalie E. Cusano, MD, MS

1 A 70-year-old man presents to his primary care provider with back pain and is diagnosed with an acute atraumatic T7 vertebral fracture. Subsequent bone density testing results are significant for T-scores of −3.0 at the lumbar spine, −2.4 at the femoral neck, and −2.2 at the total hip. He has no history of malignancy or radiation therapy. Results of metabolic evaluation for secondary causes of bone loss are within the normal range, including a complete blood cell count, comprehensive metabolic panel, PTH, TSH, 25-hydroxyvitamin D, and 24-hour urinary calcium excretion. His morning testosterone value is 270 ng/dL (300-900 ng/dL) (SI: 9.4 nmol/L [10.4-31.2 nmol/L]).

Which of the following medications has an FDA/clinical guidelines indication for management of bone disease in this patient?

A. Ibandronate
B. Intranasal calcitonin
C. Romosozumab
D. Teriparatide
E. Testosterone

2 A 71-year-old woman with a history of osteoporosis and a thoracic vertebral fracture is starting romosozumab therapy.

Which of the following represents the approximate expected changes to her lumbar spine bone density and vertebral fracture risk at 12 months based on the pivotal clinical trial leading to drug approval?

Answer	Lumbar spine bone density	Vertebral fracture risk reduction
A.	+5%	50%
B.	+5%	70%
C.	+12%	50%
D.	+12%	70%
E.	+15%	90%

3 A 47-year-old woman with a history of hypothyroidism and hypertension presents to establish care after her previous endocrinologist retired. She is taking levothyroxine, 75 mcg daily, and hydrochlorothiazide, 25 mg daily. She has a history of a right tibial fracture requiring rod placement a few months ago after falling on ice. She has a longstanding history of poor dentition; diffuse joint, bone, and muscle pain; and decreased exercise tolerance dating back to childhood. Review of systems is otherwise negative.

On physical examination, her height is 60 in (152.4 cm) and weight is 110 lb (49.9 kg) (BMI = 21.5 kg/m^2). Examination findings are normal.

Laboratory test results:

Hemoglobin = 12.5 g/dL (12.1-15.1 g/dL) (SI: 125 g/L [121-151 g/L])
Calcium = 8.9 mg/dL (8.2-10.2 mg/dL) (SI: 2.2 mmol/L [2.1-2.6 mmol/L])
Albumin = 4.3 g/dL (3.5-5.0 g/dL) (SI: 43 g/L [35-50 g/L])
Alkaline phosphatase = 13 U/L (50-120 U/L) (SI: 0.22 μkat/L [0.84-2.00 μkat/L])
Phosphate = 2.6 mg/dL (2.3-4.7 mg/dL) (SI: 0.8 mmol/L [0.7-1.5 mmol/L])
Creatinine = 0.7 mg/dL (0.6-1.1 mg/dL) (SI: 61.9 μmol/L [53.0-97.2 μmol/L])

TSH = 5.2 mIU/L (0.5-5.0 mIU/L)
25-Hydroxyvitamin D = 40 ng/mL (30-80 ng/mL [optimal]) (SI: 99.8 nmol/L [62.4-199.7 nmol/L])

Which of the following is the most likely cause of this patient's low alkaline phosphatase?

A. Celiac disease
B. Hypophosphatasia
C. Hypothyroidism
D. Recent fracture
E. X-linked hypophosphatemia

4 A colleague recently heard that the "black box" warning was removed from the label of teriparatide. He asks what that means.

Which of the following is the best explanation to provide this colleague?

A. Patients do not need antiresorptive therapy following a course of teriparatide
B. Patients who have completed 24 months of teriparatide can continue or restart therapy
C. Patients with a history of radiation therapy to the skeleton can be prescribed teriparatide
D. Patients with open epiphyses can be prescribed teriparatide
E. Patients with Paget disease can be prescribed teriparatide

5 A 65-year-old man with bipolar disorder presents for follow-up of hypothyroidism. He has remained on a stable dosage of levothyroxine, 88 mcg daily, for many years. He has been treated with lithium since age 20, and quetiapine was added to his regimen at age 45. He takes vitamin D, 5000 IU daily for vitamin D deficiency. He brings laboratory reports from his primary care provider demonstrating serum calcium values of 10.4 mg/dL and 10.5 mg/dL (2.60 and 2.63 mmol/L) in the past 2 years. He has no history of hypercalcemia.

Current laboratory test results:

Serum calcium = 10.2 mg/dL (8.2-10.2 mg/dL) (SI: 2.55 mmol/L [2.1-2.6 mmol/L])
PTH = 101 pg/mL (10-65 pg/mL) (SI: 101 ng/L [10-65 ng/L])
25-Hydroxyvitamin D = 32 ng/mL (30-80 ng/mL [optimal]) (SI: 79.9 nmol/L [74.9-199.7 nmol/L])
1,25-Dihydroxyvitamin D = 82 pg/mL (16-65 pg/mL) (SI: 213.2 pmol/L [41.6-169.0 pmol/L])
Creatinine = 1.0 mg/dL (0.7-1.3 mg/dL) (SI: 88.4 μmol/L [61.9-114.9 μmol/L])
Albumin = 4.1 g/dL (3.5-5.0 g/dL) (SI: 41 g/L [35-50 g/L])
Magnesium = 1.8 mg/dL (1.5-2.3 mg/dL) (SI: 0.74 mmol/L [0.6-0.9 mmol/L])
Phosphate = 2.4 mg/dL (2.3-4.7 mg/dL) (SI: 0.8 mmol/L [0.7-1.5 mmol/L])
24-Hour urinary calcium clearance-to-creatinine clearance ratio = 0.01

Which of the following is the most likely etiology of his laboratory results?

A. Excess vitamin D supplementation
B. Familial hypercalcemic hypocalciuria
C. Incipient primary hyperparathyroidism
D. Reversible lithium effect
E. Sarcoidosis

6 A 65-year-old woman with a history of osteoporosis is starting alendronate therapy.

Which of the following represents the approximate expected changes to her lumbar spine bone density and vertebral fracture risk at 36 months based on the pivotal clinical trials leading to drug approval?

Answer	Lumbar spine bone density	Vertebral fracture risk reduction
A.	+4%	50%
B.	+4%	70%
C.	+8%	50%
D.	+8%	70%
E.	+12%	70%

7 A 40-year-old woman with end-stage kidney disease from systemic lupus erythematosus develops severe, diffuse bone pain and fractures. She has been undergoing hemodialysis 3 times per week for more than 10 years. Over the past several years, her serum calcium and PTH levels have increased dramatically and have been resistant to high dosages of cinacalcet.

Initial laboratory test results:

Serum calcium = 12.5 mg/dL (8.2-10.2 mg/dL) (SI: 3.1 mmol/L [2.1-2.6 mmol/L])
Serum albumin = 3.5 g/dL (3.5-5.0 g/dL) (SI: 35 g/L [35-50 g/L])
Serum phosphate = 4.7 mg/dL (2.3-4.7 mg/dL) (SI: 1.5 mmol/L [0.7-1.5 mmol/L])
Serum 25-hydroxyvitamin D = 18 ng/mL (30-80 ng/mL [optimal]) (SI: 44.9 nmol/L [74.9-199.7 nmol/L])
Intact PTH = 5300 pg/mL (10-65 pg/mL) (SI: 5300 ng/L [10-65 ng/L])
Alkaline phosphatase = 842 U/L (50-120 U/L) (SI: 14.1 µkat/L) ([0.84-2.00 µkat/L])
Magnesium = 2.0 mg/dL (1.5-2.3 mg/dL) (SI: 0.8 mmol/L [0.6-0.9 mmol/L])

Because of worsening bone pain and uncontrolled hyperparathyroidism, she undergoes a 3.5-gland parathyroidectomy. A few hours after surgery, she presents to the emergency department with severe muscle spasms and paresthesias. Her weight is 154 lb (70 kg).

Interim laboratory test results:

Serum calcium = 7.8 mg/dL (SI: 2.0 mmol/L)
Serum albumin = 3.8 g/dL (SI: 38 g/L)
Serum phosphate = 2.0 mg/dL (SI: 0.6 mmol/L)

In addition to calcitriol therapy, which of the following is the best next step?

Answer	Initial therapy	Subsequent therapy
A.	Oral calcium carbonate, 500 mg 3 times daily	None
B.	Intravenous bolus of 100 mg calcium chloride	Continuous calcium chloride infusion of 0.5 mg/kg per h
C.	Intravenous bolus of 1 g calcium chloride	Continuous calcium chloride infusion of 2 mg/kg per h
D.	Intravenous bolus of 150 mg calcium gluconate	Continuous calcium gluconate infusion of 1 mg/kg per h
E.	Intravenous bolus of 500 mg calcium gluconate	Continuous calcium gluconate infusion to achieve a total dose of 2000 mg calcium over 24 hours

8 A 64-year-old man with benign prostatic hypertrophy presents with right ankle pain while running. He brings a copy of radiographs that demonstrate periosteal thickening of the distal tibial diaphysis and a possible cyst vs lytic lesion (*figure 1*).

Laboratory test results:

Calcium = 8.9 mg/dL (8.2-10.2 mg/dL) (SI: 2.2 mmol/L [2.1-2.6 mmol/L])
Albumin = 4.3 g/dL (3.5-5.0 g/dL) (SI: 43 g/L [35-50 g/L])
PTH = 45 pg/mL (10-65 pg/mL) (SI: 45 ng/L [10-65 ng/L])
Alkaline phosphatase = 125 U/L (50-120 U/L) (SI: 2.09 µkat/L [0.84-2.00 µkat/L])
Bone-specific alkaline phosphatase = 42 mg/L (≤22 mg/L)
Phosphate = 3.0 mg/dL (2.3-4.7 mg/dL) (SI: 1.0 mmol/L [0.7-1.5 mmol/L])
25-Hydroxyvitamin D = 28 ng/mL (30-80 ng/mL [optimal]) (SI: 69.9 nmol/L [62.4-199.7 nmol/L])
PSA = 7.5 ng/mL (<5.3 ng/mL) (SI: 7.5 µg/L [<5.3 µg/L])

MRI demonstrates a diffuse periosteal reaction along the anterior and medial aspect of the distal tibia; chronic osteomyelitis is not excluded, although no definitive sinus tract is identified. The lytic lesion on radiograph corresponds to an area of periosteal thickening. A nuclear medicine bone scan demonstrates increased activity in the distal right tibia (*figure 2*) without other abnormal uptake. Findings on bone biopsy are significant for active osteoclasts, reactive woven bone, peritrabecular fibrosis, and prominent reverse cement lines.

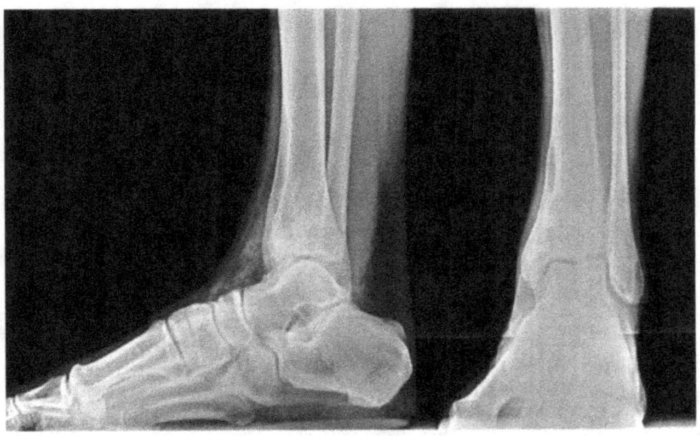

Figure 1. Radiographs of the right ankle.

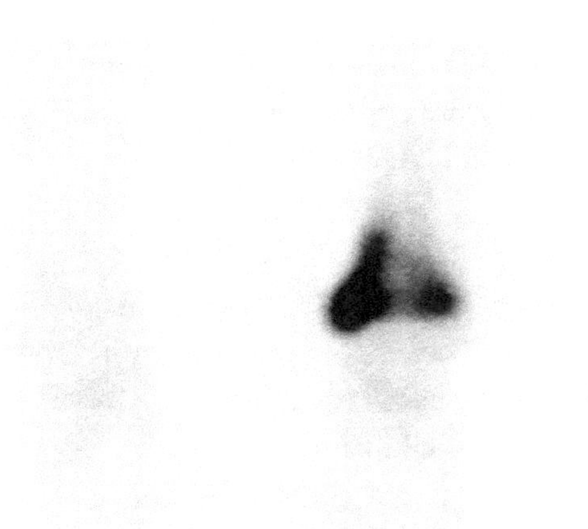

Figure 2. Nuclear medicine bone scan demonstrating increased uptake in the right ankle.

Which of the following is this patient's most likely diagnosis?

A. Fibrous dysplasia
B. Metastatic prostate cancer
C. Multiple myeloma
D. Osteomyelitis
E. Paget disease

9 A 65-year-old woman presents for follow-up of osteoporosis diagnosed last year before initiation of aromatase inhibitor therapy. She has a diagnosis of ductal carcinoma in situ status post lumpectomy and radiation therapy. She takes anastrozole, with a plan to complete a 5-year course. She received a dose of zoledronic acid, 5 mg intravenously, last year. Her bone density prior to treatment was significant for T-scores of –2.9 at the lumbar spine, –2.2 at the femoral neck, and –2.4 at the total hip. Her bone density report this year performed on the same machine has demonstrated significant improvements, with T-scores of –2.1 at the lumbar spine (+15% from previous), –1.6 at the femoral neck, and –1.9 at the total hip (+10% from previous) (*see figure 1*).

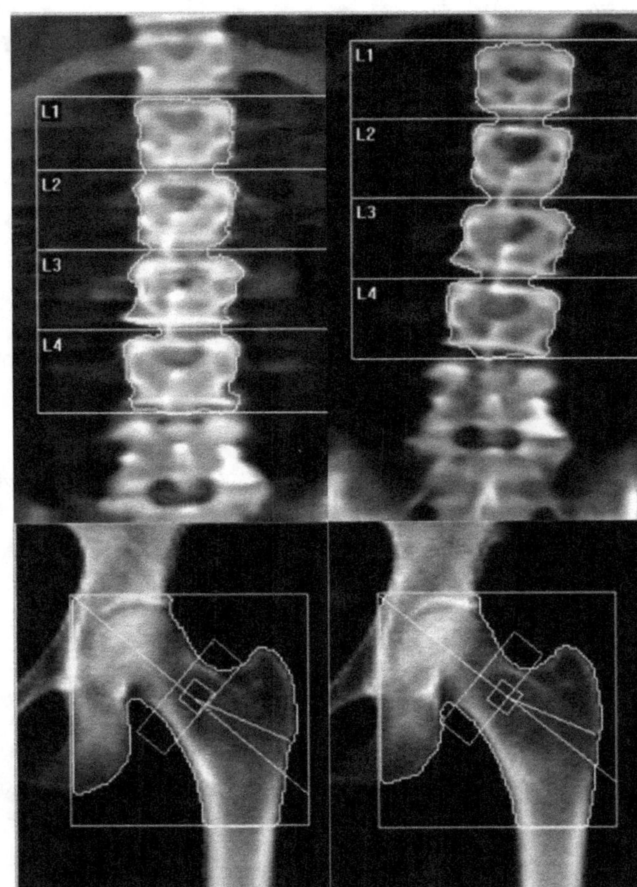

Figure 1.

Which of the following is the best next step?

A. Inquire about the calibration of the densitometer
B. Request PET/CT imaging due to concern for metastatic disease
C. Request reevaluation of the lumbar spine bone density measurement
D. Request reevaluation of the total hip bone density measurement
E. Start a "drug holiday" since her bone density is in the osteopenic range

10 A 67-year-old woman presents to establish care for osteoporosis. Osteoporosis was diagnosed at age 62 years on routine bone density testing. She has no history of fragility fracture. Metabolic evaluation for secondary causes of bone loss was previously negative. She has received therapy with denosumab, 60 mg subcutaneously every 6 months, for the past 5 years, and her last injection was 6 months ago. Her most recent bone density measurement demonstrates T-scores of −2.2 at the lumbar spine (+12% from baseline), −1.9 at the femoral neck (+6.0% from baseline), −1.1 at the total hip (+7.0% from baseline), and −1.8 at the one-third radius (+2.1% from baseline). Her insurance will no longer cover denosumab because her bone density is within the osteopenic range.

Which of the following is the best next step to preserve bone density and reduce risk of adverse effects based on the available literature?

A. Alendronate, 70 mg weekly for 1 year
B. "Drug holiday" from antiresorptive therapy
C. Ibandronate, 150 mg monthly indefinitely
D. Raloxifene, 60 mg daily for 1 year
E. Zoledronic acid, 5 mg intravenously, once in 6 months

11 A 65-year-old woman is referred to the emergency department by her primary care provider for hypercalcemia. She was recently evaluated for fatigue that she had been experiencing for the past 3 months. She has hypertension treated with amlodipine but otherwise has no notable medical history. She is not taking any additional medications or supplements. She has had no anorexia, nausea, vomiting, abdominal pain, polyuria, polydipsia, or other new symptoms.

Physical examination demonstrates pallor of the mucus membranes. She is alert and oriented to person, place, and time.

Laboratory test results:

Serum calcium = 18.4 mg/dL (8.2-10.2 mg/dL) (SI: 4.6 mmol/L [2.1-2.6 mmol/L])
Ionized calcium = 4.90 (4.60-5.08 mg/dL) (SI: 1.23 mmol/L [1.2-1.3 mmol/L])
PTH = 23 pg/mL (10-65 pg/mL) (SI: 23 ng/L [10-65 ng/L])
25-Hydroxyvitamin D = 22 ng/mL (30-80 ng/mL [optimal]) (SI: 54.9 nmol/L [74.9-199.7 nmol/L])
Albumin = 3.9 g/dL (3.5-5.0 g/dL) (SI: 39 g/L [35-50 g/L])
Hemoglobin = 9.9 g/dL (13.8-17.2 g/dL) (SI: 99 g/L [138-172 g/L])
Creatinine = 1.5 mg/dL (0.6-1.1 mg/dL) (SI: 132.6 μmol/L [53.0-97.2 μmol/L])
Serum protein electrophoresis, positive for monoclonal protein

Which of the following is the best next step for treatment of this patient's elevated calcium?

A. Cinacalcet, 30 mg orally 3 times daily
B. Emergency plasmapheresis
C. Normal saline intravenously
D. No treatment necessary
E. Pamidronate, 60 mg intravenously

12 A 25-year-old man presents for follow-up of hypoparathyroidism. He initially presented at age 3 years with a seizure and severe hypocalcemia. Since then, he has taken calcium and calcitriol. He has also been treated for intermittent oral candidiasis and fungal infections of his fingernails and toenails since childhood. He otherwise feels well.

On physical examination, he has some tinea of the nails and negative Chvostek and Trousseau signs.

In addition to measuring calcium, phosphate, and kidney function, which of the following should be measured now?

A. Antiphospholipid antibodies
B. Glutamic acid decarboxylase (GAD-65) antibodies
C. 21-Hydroxylase antibodies
D. Tissue transglutaminase antibodies
E. TPO antibodies

13 A 59-year-old woman with osteoporosis has been on daily calcium plus vitamin D and alendronate, 70 mg orally weekly, for the past 2 years. She entered menopause 5 years ago and did not take hormone therapy. Despite excellent adherence to the regimen, her repeated DXA shows significant declines in bone mineral density at both the spine (4% decline) and hip (6% decline). On review of systems, she notes an 8-lb (3.6-kg) weight loss and mild fatigue.

Laboratory test results:
Calcium = 8.9 mg/dL (8.2-10.2 mg/dL) (SI: 2.2 mmol/L [2.1-2.6 mmol/L])
Albumin = 3.8 g/dL (3.5-5.0 g/dL) (SI: 38 g/L [35-50 g/L])
Creatinine = 0.8 mg/dL (0.6-1.1 mg/dL) (SI: 70.2 µmol/L [53.0-97.2 µmol/L])
Intact PTH = 90 pg/mL (10-65 pg/mL) (SI: 90 ng/L [10-65 ng/L])
25-Hydroxyvitamin D = 20 ng/mL (30-80 ng/mL [optimal]) (SI: 49.9 nmol/L [74.9-199.7 nmol/L])
Hemoglobin = 11.5 g/dL (12.1-15.1 g/dL) (SI: 115 g/L [121-151 g/L])

Which of the following laboratory studies would be most useful for diagnosing the cause of this patient's poor response to therapy?

A. Cosyntropin-stimulation test
B. Fasting serum C-telopeptide measurement
C. Measurement of urinary calcium excretion (24-hour urine collection)
D. Serum protein electrophoresis
E. Tissue transglutaminase antibody assessment

14 A 37-year-old woman is admitted to the hospital with hypercalcemia. She moved 6 months ago from New York where she pursued an acting career. She has a 2-month history of progressive anorexia, 15-lb (6.8-kg) weight loss, nausea, fatigue, polyuria, and polydipsia. She has had no fevers or night sweats. She has no notable medical history and has never had kidney stones, bone pain, or fractures. She takes no medications and states that she has not recently used alcohol, tobacco, or illicit drugs.

On physical examination, she is afebrile, oriented but lethargic, and dehydrated. Findings on breast examination are normal. There is no palpable lymphadenopathy. Nodularity in both buttocks is noted.

Laboratory test results:
Calcium = 14.5 mg/dL (8.2-10.2 mg/dL) (SI: 3.63 mmol/L [2.1-2.6 mmol/L])
Albumin = 4.1 g/dL (3.5-5.0 g/dL) (SI: 41 g/L [35-50 g/L])
Creatinine = 2.0 mg/dL (0.6-1.1 mg/dL) (SI: 176.8 µmol/L [53.0-97.2 µmol/L])
Phosphate = 4.9 mg/dL (2.3-4.7 mg/dL) (SI: 1.6 mmol/L [0.7-1.5 mmol/L])
PTH = <10 pg/mL (10-65 pg/mL) (SI: <10 ng/L [10-65 ng/L])
25-Hydroxyvitamin D = 15 ng/mL (25-80 ng/mL [optimal]) (SI: 37.4 nmol/L [62.4-199.7 nmol/L])
1,25-Dihydroxyvitamin D = 82 pg/mL (16-65 pg/mL) (SI: 213.2 pmol/L [41.6-169.0 pmol/L])

CT of the buttocks is shown (*see image*).

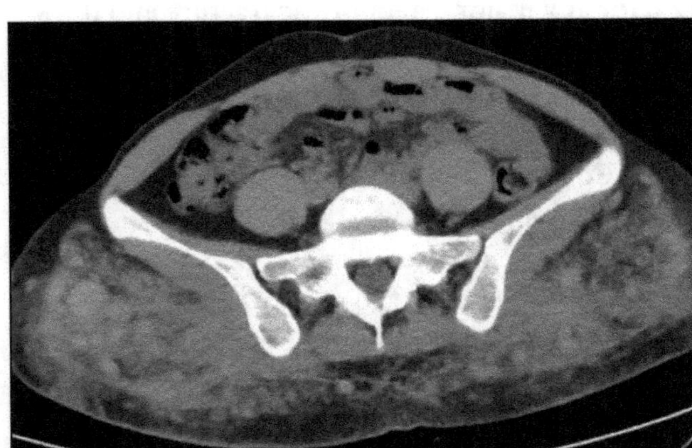

Reprinted from Leyva A et al. Cureus 2018;10(9) © The Authors.

Which of the following is the most likely diagnosis?

A. Calciphylaxis
B. Fibrodysplasia ossificans progressiva
C. Foreign-body granulomas
D. Sarcoidosis
E. T-cell lymphoma

15 A 55-year-old woman is referred after results of a screening DXA. Her last menstrual period was 3 years ago, and she has occasional mild hot flashes that do not interfere with her quality of life. Her BMI is 20 kg/m^2. She is generally healthy, but she fractured 2 ribs last year after missing 2 steps going down stairs. She does not smoke cigarettes, she drinks 1 glass of wine nightly, and she takes no medications. Her daily intake provides 1200 mg of calcium and 800 IU (20 mcg) of vitamin D. Her mother fractured a hip.

The patient's DXA documents the following:

Site	BMD, g/cm^2	T-score
Total hip	0.698	−1.5
Femoral neck	0.658	−1.7
L1-L4	0.983	−0.3

Vertebral fracture assessment is negative for spinal compression fractures. Her FRAX 10-year risk is 12% for any major osteoporotic fracture and 0.7% for hip fracture.

Which of the following is the correct management plan?

A. Continue calcium and vitamin D and repeat DXA in 2 years
B. Start alendronate and repeat DXA in 1 year
C. Start denosumab and repeat DXA in 1 year
D. Start estrogen replacement therapy
E. Start raloxifene and perform DXA in 1 year

16 A 58-year-old man is taken to the emergency department after a minor motorcycle crash. He is awake and alert, but he sustained trauma to his pelvis. Findings on radiographs are shown (*see image*). A radionuclide total body scan shows increased activity throughout the pelvis and left femur.

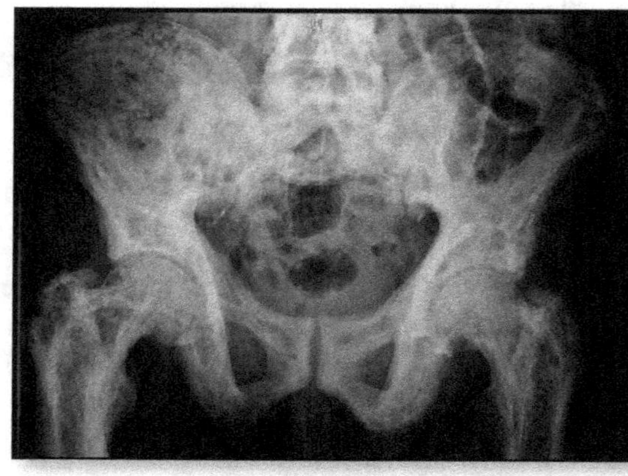

Laboratory test results document normal concentrations of serum calcium, phosphate, creatinine, 25-hydroxyvitamin D, PTH, and liver transaminases. The alkaline phosphatase concentration is 324 U/L (50-120 U/L) (SI: 5.41 µkat/L [0.84-2.00 µkat/L]).

On further questioning, the patient notes chronic pain in his left hip and pelvis, which has been getting worse over time.

Which of the following would you recommend for this patient?

A. Alendronate, 70 mg orally weekly
B. Calcitonin nasal spray, 200 IU daily
C. Physical therapy
D. Risedronate, 35 mg orally weekly
E. Zoledronate, 5 mg intravenously

17 An 18-year-old male refugee presents with a history of bone pain, joint deformities, and severe dental problems since childhood. On physical examination, he has short stature, severe genu varum (bow-leggedness), and very poor dentition, but no abnormal skin pigmentation. Family history is unavailable because he was separated from his family and grew up in an orphanage.

Laboratory blood test results:

Calcium = 8.8 mg/dL (8.2-10.2 mg/dL) (SI: 2.2 mmol/L [2.1-2.6 mmol/L])
Albumin = 4.0 g/dL (3.5-5.0 g/dL) (SI: 40 g/L [35-50 g/L])
Phosphate = 1.3 mg/dL (2.3-4.7 mg/dL) (SI: 0.4 mmol/L [0.7-1.5 mmol/L])
25-Hydroxyvitamin D = 24 ng/mL (30-80 ng/mL [optimal]) (SI: 59.9 nmol/L [74.9-199.7 nmol/L])
1,25-Dihydroxyvitamin D = 30 pg/mL (16-65 pg/mL) (SI: 78 pmol/L [41.6-169.0 pmol/L])
Intact PTH = 110 pg/mL (10-65 pg/mL) (SI: 110 ng/L [10-65 ng/L])

Which of the following is this patient's most likely diagnosis?

A. McCune-Albright syndrome
B. Tumor-induced osteomalacia
C. Vitamin D–deficient rickets
D. Vitamin D–resistant rickets
E. X-linked hypophosphatemic rickets

18 A 74-year-old man is admitted to the hospital with altered mental status, nausea, vomiting, and dehydration. His medical history is notable for chronic obstructive pulmonary disease, coronary artery disease, and an 80 pack-year smoking history.

On physical examination, he is barely arousable. His blood pressure is 96/65 mm Hg, and pulse rate is 120 beats/min. He has dry mucus membranes, and there is no lymphadenopathy.

Chest x-ray in the emergency department reveals a 3-cm spiculated mass in the right upper lung lobe with destruction of an adjacent rib.

Laboratory tests results:

Calcium = 16.8 mg/dL (8.2-10.2 mg/dL) (SI: 4.2 mmol/L [2.1-2.6 mmol/L])
Ionized calcium = 7.25 mg/dL (4.60-5.08 mg/dL) (SI: 1.8 mmol/L [1.2-1.3 mmol/L])
Serum urea nitrogen = 50 mg/dL (8-23 mg/dL) (SI: 17.9 mmol/L [2.9-8.2 mmol/L])
Creatinine = 2.5 mg/dL (0.7-1.3 mg/dL) (SI: 221.0 µmol/L [61.9-114.9 µmol/L])
Serum protein electrophoresis, normal
Urine protein electrophoresis, normal
Intact PTH = <10 pg/mL (10-65 pg/mL) (SI: <10 ng/L [10-65 ng/L])

The patient receives vigorous intravenous saline hydration (2 L in the first 4 hours followed by 150 cc/h) with subsequent improvement in creatinine. He also receives calcitonin, 4 units/kg every 6 hours; and zoledronic acid, 4 mg intravenously (1 dose). Forty-eight hours after admission, he is more alert and responsive. His blood pressure is 140/85 mm Hg, and pulse rate is 90 beats/min. His serum calcium concentration is now 13.8 mg/dL (3.5 mmol/L), and his creatinine concentration is 1.4 mg/dL (123.8 µmol/L).

Which of the following is the best next step?

A. Administer another dose of zoledronic acid, 4 mg intravenously
B. Administer denosumab, 60 mg subcutaneously
C. Begin hydrocortisone, 50 mg intravenously every 6 hours
D. Increase the rate of intravenous saline to 200 cc/h and add furosemide
E. Stop calcitonin and continue current hydration and monitoring

19 A 43-year-old man has had 2 episodes of calcium-containing kidney stones. His workup reveals normal serum calcium and PTH levels, with a 24-hour urinary calcium excretion of 335 mg/24 h (100-300 mg/24 h) (SI: 8.4 mmol/d [2.5-7.5 mmol/d]), but normal 24-hour urinary oxalate, uric acid, sodium, and citrate levels. His urine volume is 2650 mL/24 h. Kidney stone analysis reveals calcium oxalate.

Which of the following recommendations would provide the greatest reduction in his risk of future calcium oxalate stone disease?

A. Allopurinol, 300 mg daily
B. Hydrochlorothiazide, 25 mg once daily
C. Reduced dietary oxalate
D. Reduced dietary sodium
E. Sodium citrate, 500 mg 4 times daily

20 A 54-year-old woman is brought to the emergency department with seizures. She has had previous emergency department visits for alcohol intoxication. Her medical history and medications are otherwise unknown.

Physical examination demonstrates tongue biting and positive Chvostek sign. She has no neck scars, mucocutaneous candidiasis, or vitiligo.

Laboratory test results:

- Serum calcium = 5.4 mg/dL (8.2-10.2 mg/dL) (SI: 1.4 mmol/L [2.1-2.6 mmol/L])
- PTH = <3 pg/mL (10-65 pg/mL) (SI: <3 ng/L [10-65 ng/L])
- 25-Hydroxyvitamin D = 6 ng/mL (30-80 ng/mL [optimal]) (SI: 15.0 nmol/L [74.9-199.7 nmol/L])
- Magnesium = 0.6 mg/dL (1.5-2.3 mg/dL) (SI: 0.25 mmol/L [0.6-0.9 mmol/L])
- Phosphate = 1.8 mg/dL (2.3-4.7 mg/dL) (SI: 0.6 mmol/L [0.7-1.5 mmol/L])
- Albumin = 2.8 g/dL (3.5-5.0 g/dL) (SI: 28 g/dL [35-50 g/L])
- Amylase = 105 U/L (26-102 U/L) (SI: 1.75 μkat/L [0.43-1.70 μkat/L])
- Lipase = 75 U/L (10-73 U/L) (SI: 1.25 μkat/L [0.17-1.22 μkat/L])

Which of the following is the primary cause of this patient's hypocalcemia?

A. Alcohol withdrawal
B. Chronic hypoparathyroidism
C. Hypomagnesemia
D. Pancreatitis
E. Vitamin D deficiency

21 A 30-year-old woman is seeking continued management of osteogenesis imperfecta. She was diagnosed in childhood and until several years ago, her care was managed by a pediatric endocrinologist in another city. During childhood, she sustained several long-bone fractures that were initially attributed to an active lifestyle. After mild osteogenesis imperfecta was eventually diagnosed, she was treated with intravenous pamidronate for a few years. Her last fracture was at age 15 years. Currently, she has regular menses and a healthy lifestyle.

On physical examination, she is a well-appearing woman without any dysmorphic features. Her height is 65 in (165.1 cm). Sclerae appear bluish. She has no joint deformities or laxity. Her dentition appears normal.

Laboratory test results are normal, including complete blood cell count, complete chemistry panel, TSH, 25-hydroxyvitamin D, and PTH. DXA documents Z-scores of −2.0 at the lumbar spine, −1.5 at the femoral neck, and −1.4 at the total hip.

Which of the following is the best recommendation now?

A. Complete dental examination
B. Echocardiography
C. Formal hearing test
D. Kidney ultrasonography
E. Restarting of bisphosphonate therapy

22 A 28-year-old man presents with fatigue, and primary hyperparathyroidism is subsequently diagnosed.

Laboratory test results:

- Serum calcium = 11.9 mg/dL (8.2-10.2 mg/dL) (SI: 3.0 mmol/L [2.1-2.6 mmol/L])
- Serum PTH = 120 pg/mL (10-65 pg/mL) (SI: 120 ng/L [10-65 ng/L])
- Urinary calcium = 400 mg/24 h (100-300 mg/24 h) (SI: 10 mmol/d [2.5-7.5 mmol/d])

His family history is positive for recurrent hyperparathyroidism in his father, as well as kidney stones and peptic ulcers in 1 of his 3 siblings. There is no history of hypertension, spells, or medullary thyroid cancer in affected family members.

Which of the following is the most likely underlying diagnosis in this case?

A. Autoimmune polyglandular syndrome type 1
B. Hereditary activation of the calcium-sensing receptor
C. Multiple endocrine neoplasia type 1
D. Multiple endocrine neoplasia type 2A
E. Multiple endocrine neoplasia type 2B

23 A 57-year-old woman with osteoporosis has been on risedronate, 35 mg orally weekly, for the past 2 years. Her diet provides more than 1000 mg of elemental calcium each day, and she takes 1000 IU (25 mcg) of cholecalciferol daily. Her last menstrual period occurred 5 years ago, and she has never taken hormone therapy. A follow-up DXA on the same machine now shows significant declines in bone mineral density at both the spine (6% decline) and hip (5% decline) compared with values obtained 2 years ago. On review of systems, she feels well and has no new symptoms.

Her BMI is 23 kg/m^2, and physical examination findings are unchanged.

Laboratory test results, including serum calcium, albumin, creatinine, intact PTH, 25-hydroxyvitamin D, electrolytes, ferritin, and 24-hour urinary calcium excretion, are normal.

Which of the following is the most likely reason for her poor response to therapy?

A. Lack of potency of risedronate to stop rapid postmenopausal bone loss
B. Malabsorption
C. Nonadherence to treatment
D. Positioning error by the DXA technician
E. Undiagnosed eating disorder

24 A 56-year-old woman with end-stage kidney disease due to hypertension has been on hemodialysis for 8 years. She is referred due to a pelvic fracture and a femoral neck T-score of −2.2. Medications for the past 6 years include calcitriol, 0.5 mcg twice daily, and cinacalcet, 90 mg twice daily.

Laboratory test results:
Serum calcium = 8.1 mg/dL (8.2-10.2 mg/dL) (SI: 2.0 mmol/L [2.1-2.6 mmol/L])
Phosphate = 5.2 mg/dL (2.3-4.7 mg/dL) (SI: 1.7 mmol/L [0.7-1.5 mmol/L])
25-Hydroxyvitamin D = 24 ng/mL (25-80 ng/mL [optimal]) (SI: 59.9 nmol/L [62.4-199.7 nmol/L])
PTH = 78 pg/mL (10-65 pg/mL) (SI: 78 ng/L [10-65 ng/L])
Total alkaline phosphatase = 48 U/L (50-120 U/L) (SI: 0.80 µkat/L [0.84-2.00 µkat/L])

An iliac crest biopsy is performed after double-tetracycline labeling.

Which of the following is most likely to be found on the bone biopsy?

A. Adynamic bone disease
B. Mixed renal osteodystrophy
C. Osteomalacia
D. Osteoporosis
E. Osteitis fibrosa cystica

25 An 82-year-old woman is admitted to the hospital with diffuse bony pain and a pathologic, atraumatic fracture of her left distal radius. She has not had regular medical care. Radiographs reveal widespread lytic and mixed (lytic/sclerotic) lesions throughout the appendicular and axial skeleton. On physical examination, a large breast mass is palpated, and needle biopsy confirms adenocarcinoma of the breast.

Laboratory test results:
Serum calcium = 12.3 mg/dL (8.2-10.2 mg/dL) (SI: 3.1 mmol/L [2.1-2.6 mmol/L])
Albumin = 2.8 g/dL (3.5-5.0 g/dL) (SI: 28 g/L [35-50 g/L])
Creatinine = 6.2 mg/dL (0.6-1.1 mg/dL) (SI: 548.1 µmol/L [53.0-97.2 µmol/L])
Intact PTH = <10 pg/mL (10-65 pg/mL) (SI: <10 ng/L [10-65 ng/L])
25-Hydroxyvitamin D = 8 ng/mL (30-80 ng/mL [optimal]) (SI: 20.0 nmol/L [74.9-199.7 nmol/L])
Alkaline phosphatase = 320 U/L (50-120 U/L) (SI: 5.34 µkat/L [0.84-2.00 µkat/L])

After 24 hours of vigorous intravenous saline hydration, the following laboratory results are documented:
Serum calcium = 11.0 mg/dL (SI: 2.8 mmol/L)
Creatinine = 4.2 mg/dL (SI: 371.3 µmol/L)

The oncology team decides to treat her with a subcutaneous injection of denosumab, 120 mg.

In this patient, which of the following is the most likely adverse effect of this therapy?

A. Impaired fracture healing
B. Osteonecrosis of the jaw
C. Severe flulike syndrome
D. Severe hypocalcemia
E. Worsening kidney function

26 A 75-year-old man with primary hyperparathyroidism is referred for management. He is asymptomatic and generally feels well. He has not experienced kidney stones, fractures, or loss of height. His BMI is 22 kg/m^2. DXA shows T-scores of −1.8 at the lumbar spine, −1.6 at the femoral neck, and −2.2 at the one-third distal radius.

Laboratory test results:

- Serum calcium = 10.8 mg/dL (8.2-10.2 mg/dL) (SI: 2.7 mmol/L [2.1-2.6 mmol/L])
- Albumin = 4.0 g/dL (3.5-5.0 g/dL) (SI: 40 g/L [35-50 g/L])
- Intact PTH = 88 pg/mL (10-65 pg/mL) (SI: 88 ng/L [10-65 ng/L])
- 25-Hydroxyvitamin D = 22 ng/mL (30-80 ng/mL [optimal]) (SI: 54.9 nmol/L [74.9-199.7 nmol/L])
- 1,25-Dihydroxyvitamin D = 50 pg/mL (16-65 pg/mL) (SI: 130 pmol/L [41.6-169.0 pmol/L])
- Urinary calcium = 180 mg/24 h (100-300 mg/24 h) (SI: 4.5 mmol/d [2.5-7.5 mmol/d])

Which of the following is the best recommendation with respect to oral vitamin D_3 (cholecalciferol) therapy in this patient?

A. 400 IU (10 mcg) daily
B. 1000 IU (25 mcg) daily
C. 4000 IU (100 mcg) daily
D. 50,000 IU (1250 mcg) weekly
E. No supplementation

27 An 18-year-old man is referred to endocrinology. He recently immigrated, established medical care, and was noted to have abnormalities on routine blood tests. He has no known relevant medical history and is not taking any medications. Review of systems is positive for perioral and extremity numbness/tingling.

On physical examination, his height is 64 in (162.5 cm) and weight is 180 lb (81.8 kg) (BMI = 30.9 kg/m^2). He has round facies and mild cognitive impairment. His hand is shown in the photograph (*see image*). He states his mother has a similar height and physical phenotype.

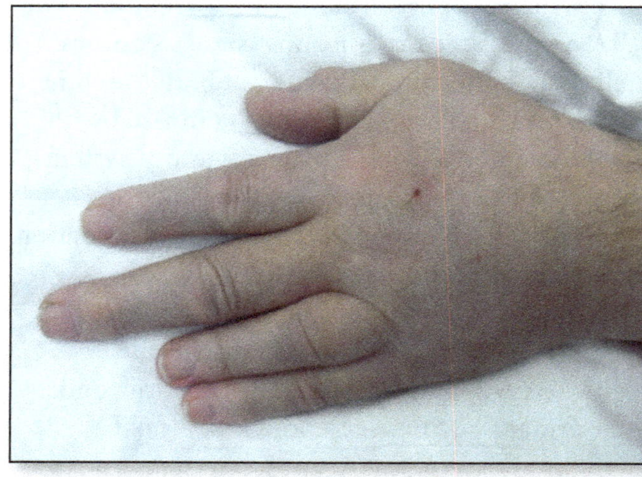

Which of the following patterns would be expected from the results of his laboratory testing?

Answer	Calcium	PTH	Phosphate
A.	Low	Low	Low
B.	Low	Low	High
C.	Low	High	Low
D.	Low	High	High
E.	Normal	Normal	Normal

28 A 55-year-old man is referred because of vitamin D deficiency and secondary hyperparathyroidism that were discovered after ankle fracture. His medical history is positive for class 3 obesity and hypertension. Lisinopril is his only medication.

On physical examination, his BMI is 48 kg/m^2 and blood pressure is 120/70 mm Hg. Examination findings are otherwise normal.

Laboratory test results (baseline):

- Serum calcium = 8.9 mg/dL (8.2-10.2 mg/dL) (SI: 2.2 mmol/L [2.1-2.6 mmol/L])
- Albumin = 4.0 g/dL (3.5-5.0 g/dL) (SI: 40 g/L [35-50 g/L])

Intact PTH = 88 pg/mL (10-65 pg/mL) (SI: 88 ng/L [10-65 ng/L])
25-Hydroxyvitamin D = 8 ng/mL (30-80 ng/mL [optimal]) (SI: 20.0 nmol/L [74.9-199.7 nmol/L])
Urinary calcium = 70 mg/24 h (100-300 mg/24 h) (SI: 1.8 mmol/d [2.5-7.5 mmol/d])
Tissue transglutaminase antibodies, negative

Which of the following treatments should be recommended for this patient?

A. Calcitriol, 0.5 mcg daily
B. Cholecalciferol, 400 IU (20 mcg) daily
C. Cholecalciferol, 1000 IU (25 mcg) daily
D. Cholecalciferol, 10,000 IU (250 mcg) weekly
E. Cholecalciferol, 50,000 IU (1250 mcg) weekly

29 A 48-year-old man is referred for evaluation and management of muscle pain, fatigue, and weakness. On physical examination, he has proximal muscle weakness. His lumbar spine T-score is −3.3.

Laboratory test results:

Chemistry panel, normal
25-Hydroxyvitamin D = 28 ng/mL (30-80 ng/mL [optimal]) (SI: 69.9 nmol/L [74.9-199.7 nmol/L])
1,25-Dihydroxyvitamin D = 12 pg/mL (16-65 pg/mL) (SI: 31.2 pmol/L [41.6-169.0 pmol/L])
PTH = 98 pg/mL (10-65 pg/mL) (SI: 98 ng/L [10-65 ng/L])
Serum and urine protein electrophoresis, free kappa and lambda light chains, normal
Serum phosphate = 1.1 to 1.3 mg/dL (2.3-4.7 mg/dL) [SI: 0.36 to 0.41 mmol/L [0.72-1.52 mmol/L])
Serum FGF-23 = 350 RU/mL (<180 RU/mL)

Which of the following treatments should be recommended now?

A. Alendronate
B. Cholecalciferol and calcitriol
C. Potassium phosphate alone
D. Potassium phosphate and calcitriol
E. Zoledronic acid

30 A 55-year-old woman is referred for management of primary hyperparathyroidism. She was noted to have serum calcium concentration of 10.7 mg/dL (8.2-10.2 mg/dL) (SI: 2.7 mmol/L [2.1-2.6 mmol/L]) on a routine chemistry panel. A previous serum calcium measurement from 2 years ago was 10.0 mg/dL (2.5 mmol/L). She feels well and has no symptoms of hypercalcemia. She has no history of fractures or kidney stones.

Her medical history is notable for mild hypertension. Current medications are hydrochlorothiazide, 12.5 mg daily (for the last 4 years), and cholecalciferol, 1000 IU (25 mcg) daily. Her family history is noncontributory. She feels well today and has no acute issues.

On physical examination, her blood pressure is 120/72 mm Hg.

Laboratory test results:

Serum calcium = 11.0 mg/dL (8.2-10.2 mg/dL) (SI: 2.8 mmol/L [2.1-2.6 mmol/L])
Albumin, normal
Creatinine, normal
Phosphate = 3.0 mg/dL (2.3-4.7 mg/dL) (SI: 10.0 mmol/L [0.7-1.5 mmol/L])
Intact PTH = 30 pg/mL (10-65 pg/mL) (SI: 30 ng/L [10-65 ng/L])
25-Hydroxyvitamin D = 35 ng/mL (30-80 ng/mL [optimal]) (SI: 87.4 nmol/L [74.9-199.7 nmol/L])
Urinary calcium (adequate collection) = 105 mg/24 h (100-300 mg/24 h) (SI: 2.6 mmol/d [2.5-7.5 mmol/d])

Which of the following is the best next step?

A. Calculate the calcium-to-creatinine clearance ratio
B. Measure calcium and PTH after stopping hydrochlorothiazide for 3 months
C. Measure 1,25-dihydroxyvitamin D
D. Order an octreotide scan
E. Start cinacalcet

31 A 70-year-old woman with type 2 diabetes mellitus presents for follow-up after screening bone density testing. She has been taking metformin, 1000 mg twice daily, and pioglitazone, 45 mg daily, for many years. She has 2 servings of dairy per day and takes supplements with 600 mg of calcium and 800 IU (20 mcg) vitamin D daily. She has no personal history of fracture, no parental history of hip fracture, and no other known risk factors for osteoporosis.

On physical examination, her height is 62 in (157.5 cm) and weight is 140 lb (63.6 kg) (BMI = 25.6 kg/m^2).

Laboratory test results:

- Complete blood count, normal
- Comprehensive metabolic panel, normal
- Hemoglobin A_{1c} = 7.9% (4.0%-5.6%) (63 mmol/mol [20-38 mmol/mol])
- 25-Hydroxyvitamin D = 31 ng/mL (30-80 ng/mL [optimal]) (SI: 77.4 nmol/L [74.9-199.7 nmol/L])

Recent bone density testing is notable for T-scores of −1.8 at the lumbar spine, −2.0 at the femoral neck, and −2.1 at the total hip. Her 10-year risk of fracture calculated by FRAX is 12% for major osteoporotic fracture and 2.5% for hip fracture. Trabecular bone score is 1.150 (degraded).

Which of the following is the best next step for management of her bone health?

A. Add dulaglutide to her regimen
B. Adjust FRAX score for trabecular bone score
C. Change pioglitazone to canagliflozin
D. Increase vitamin D supplementation
E. Repeat bone density testing in 2 years

32 A 41-year-old pregnant woman with a history of postoperative hypoparathyroidism presents at 39 weeks' gestation with headache, nausea, and vomiting. She developed hypoparathyroidism after parathyroid surgery for primary hyperparathyroidism at age 35 years. Genetic evaluation at that time was negative for pathogenic variants in the *MEN1* and *RET* genes. Her treatment regimen for hypoparathyroidism before pregnancy consisted of calcium, 600 mg 4 times daily; calcitriol, 0.75 mcg twice daily; and vitamin D, 1000 IU (25 mcg) daily. On this regimen, her serum calcium concentration was 8.4 mg/dL (2.1 mmol/L) before pregnancy. She is currently taking calcium, 600 mg 3 times daily; calcitriol, 0.5 mcg twice daily; and vitamin D, 1000 IU (25 mcg) daily. Because of gastroesophageal reflux, she has been substituting several chewable calcium carbonate tablets per day instead of her usual calcium supplement.

Laboratory test results:

- Serum calcium = 10.8 mg/dL (8.2-10.2 mg/dL) (SI: 2.7 mmol/L [2.1-2.6 mmol/L])
- 25-Hydroxyvitamin D = 34 ng/mL (30-80 ng/mL [optimal]) (SI: 84.9 nmol/L [74.9-199.7 nmol/L])
- 1,25-Dihydroxyvitamin D = 82 pg/mL (16-65 pg/mL) (SI: 213.2 pmol/L [41.6-169.0 pmol/L])
- PTHrP = 4.0 pmol/L (<2.0 pmol/L)
- Bicarbonate = 24 mEq/L (21-28 mEq/L) (SI: 24 mmol/L [21-28 mmol/L])
- Albumin = 3.3 g/dL (3.5-5.0 g/dL) (SI: 33 g/L [35-50 g/L])
- Phosphate = 5.0 mg/dL (2.3-4.7 mg/dL) (SI: 1.6 mmol/L [0.7-1.5 mmol/L])
- Creatinine = 0.6 mg/dL (0.6-1.1 mg/dL) (SI: 53.0 μmol/L [53.0-97.2 μmol/L])

Which of the following is the most likely cause of this patient's hypercalcemia?

A. Granulomatous disease
B. Humoral hypercalcemia of malignancy
C. Milk-alkali syndrome
D. Recurrence of primary hyperparathyroidism
E. Reduced calcium and calcitriol requirements during pregnancy

33 An 80-year-old White woman presents for a second opinion regarding management of osteoporosis. Osteoporosis was diagnosed after bone density assessment documented a T-score of −3.3 at the femoral neck. She has no personal or family history of fracture and has never been treated with glucocorticoids. Her primary care provider recommended bisphosphonate therapy, but the patient declined due to concern for adverse effects, stating, "Don't those medications just make the bone stiffer and actually cause hip fractures?"

How should this patient be counseled regarding the estimated benefits of antiresorptive therapy vs risks of atypical femoral fracture and osteonecrosis of the jaw?

Answer	Fracture risk reduction	Atypical femoral fracture risk	Osteonecrosis of the jaw risk
A.	75%	1/100,000	5/10,000
B.	50%	1/100,000	5/10,000
C.	50%	5/10,000	1/100,000
D.	25%	1/100,000	5/10,000
E.	25%	5/10,000	1/100,000

Diabetes Mellitus, Section 1 Board Review

Anne L. Peters, MD

1 A 40-year-old man presents for evaluation of type 2 diabetes mellitus. Diabetes was diagnosed approximately 5 years ago after a hemoglobin A_{1c} value of 6.8% (51 mmol/mol) was documented on routine blood testing. At diagnosis, his BMI was 26.4 kg/m^2. He was very motivated to improve his hemoglobin A_{1c}, and his target was less than 6.5% (<48 mmol/mol). He dedicated himself to a lifestyle approach, started cycling for 1 to 2 hours 5 days per week, and he lost 10 lb (5.0 kg). After 3 months, his hemoglobin A_{1c} measurement was 6.7% (50 mmol/mol). A variety of antidiabetes medications were tried, including metformin, a sulfonylurea, and pioglitazone without significant improvement in his hemoglobin A_{1c}. He has a strong family history of both type 1 and type 2 diabetes.

Laboratory test results:

Uric acid = 5.0 mg/dL (3.5-7.0 mg/dL)
(SI: 297.4 μmol/L [208.2-416.4 μmol/L])
Magnesium = 1.9 mg/dL (1.5-2.3 m/dL)
(SI: 0.8 mmol/L [0.6-0.9 mmol/L])

His continuous glucose monitoring data on no medication are shown (*see figure*).

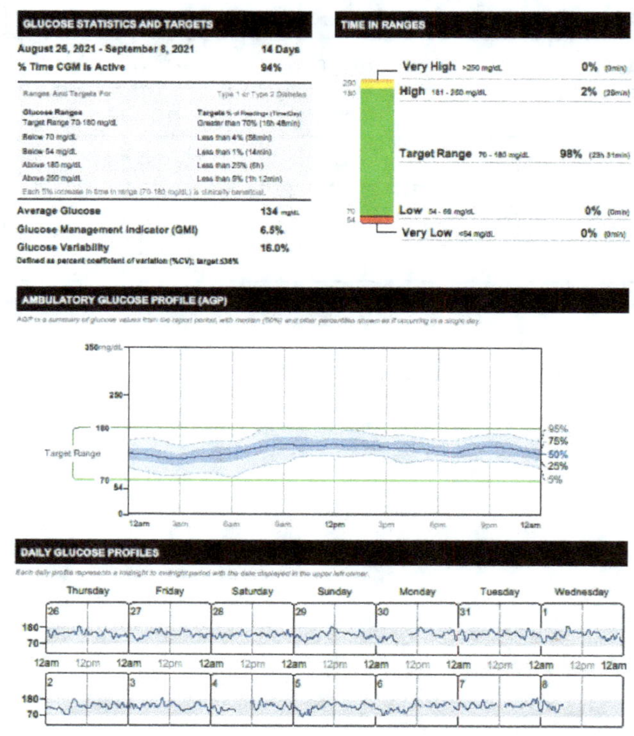

Which of the following types of maturity-onset diabetes of the young (MODY) is the most likely diagnosis?

A. *GCK*
B. *HNF1A*
C. *HNF1B*
D. *HNF4A*
E. *KCNJ11*

2 A 32-year-old woman is referred for evaluation by the emergency department. Type 2 diabetes mellitus was diagnosed 1 year ago when she was incidentally found to have elevated glucose. She was treated with metformin with minimal improvement. She now has symptoms of weight loss, polyuria, and polydipsia. She has no family history of diabetes, although there is a history of thyroid disease in her mother.

Laboratory test results:

Hemoglobin A_{1c} = 13.4% (4.0%-5.6%) (123 mmol/mol [20-38 mmol/mol])
TSH = 8.5 mIU/L (0.5-5.0 mIU/L)
Random blood glucose = 346 mg/dL (SI: 19.2 mmol/L)
Urine ketones, trace positive

Her BMI is 23.4 kg/m^2.

Which of the following tests would be most helpful in guiding her therapy?

A. Genetic testing for maturity-onset diabetes of the young (MODY)
B. Glutamic acid decarboxylase antibody assessment
C. Islet-cell antibody assessment
D. Serum insulin measurement

3 A 48-year-old woman presents with new-onset type 2 diabetes mellitus. Her hemoglobin A_{1c} value is 8.7% (72 mmol/mol), and she is mildly symptomatic. Her BMI is 26.2 kg/m^2. She is coached on lifestyle changes and is prescribed metformin. She has no family history of type 2 diabetes, but her sister has celiac disease.

After 3 months of metformin treatment, her hemoglobin A_{1c} level is 8.5% (69 mmol/mol). Due to her weight, family history, and lack of response to type 2 diabetes treatment, laboratory testing is ordered to rule out type 1 diabetes:

Glutamic acid decarboxylase antibodies = 105 U/mL
C-peptide (postprandial) = 0.7 ng/mL (SI: 0.23 nmol/L)
Glucose = 245 mg/dL (SI: 13.6 mmol/L)
Urine ketones, negative

Her therapeutic goal is to decrease her glucose levels without weight gain. She works full time, is a single mother, and is often not able to focus on her own health. Therefore, she would like a simple treatment plan.

In light of her goals, which of the following is the best patient-centered treatment plan?

A. Add a DPP-4 inhibitor
B. Add an SGLT-2 inhibitor
C. Add basal insulin and a GLP-1 receptor agonist
D. Start a multiple daily injection insulin regimen

4 On a blood test done as part of a life insurance evaluation, a 30-year-old lean man is found to have new-onset diabetes with minimal symptoms and a hemoglobin A_{1c} value of 7.6% (60 mmol/mol). Islet-cell antibodies are negative.

Which of the following would be the most helpful next step in determining his type of diabetes?

A. Measure fasting C-peptide
B. Measure postprandial C-peptide
C. Obtain a family history
D. Order genetic testing for maturity-onset diabetes of the young

5 A 65-year-old man with a 4-year history of stage 4 melanoma develops diabetes ketoacidosis approximately 9 months after he was treated with pembrolizumab. Multiple daily injection insulin therapy is initiated, and he wants to know what to expect regarding diabetes.

Which of the following is the most likely scenario?

A. He will gradually wean off insulin and will no longer need treatment for diabetes
B. He will be able to change to oral medication for diabetes
C. He will need to stay on multiple daily insulin injections or use an insulin pump
D. He will be able to be switch from multiple daily injection to basal insulin alone

6 A 26-year-old man was hospitalized for diabetic ketoacidosis 8 years ago and was diagnosed with type 1 diabetes mellitus. Laboratory testing documented negative autoantibodies and a C-peptide concentration of 0.9 ng/mL (0.3 nmol/L). His BMI was 21.2 kg/m^2. He was discharged on insulin therapy. However, after discharge he slowly weaned himself off insulin and was able to maintain good glycemic control, with a hemoglobin A_{1c} value of approximately 6.2% (44 mmol/mol). His mother, brother, and maternal first cousin have diabetes.

At age 27 years, the patient is diagnosed with sensorineural hearing loss. When he is 30 years old, his mother is diagnosed with a pathogenic variant in the *MT-TL1* gene (maternally inherited diabetes and deafness [MIDD]), and he is found to have the same variant. He is lost to follow-up for 6 years. He returns to clinic and says that he is "in trouble" and has a hemoglobin A_{1c} value of 11.2% (99 mmol/mol). He says he has tried every treatment, including insulin, which "didn't work." He is a runner and is training for a marathon. His current BMI is 18.1 kg/m^2. He prefers to treat his diabetes with lifestyle modifications.

His continuous glucose monitor tracing while on insulin glargine, 10 units twice daily, is shown (*see image*).

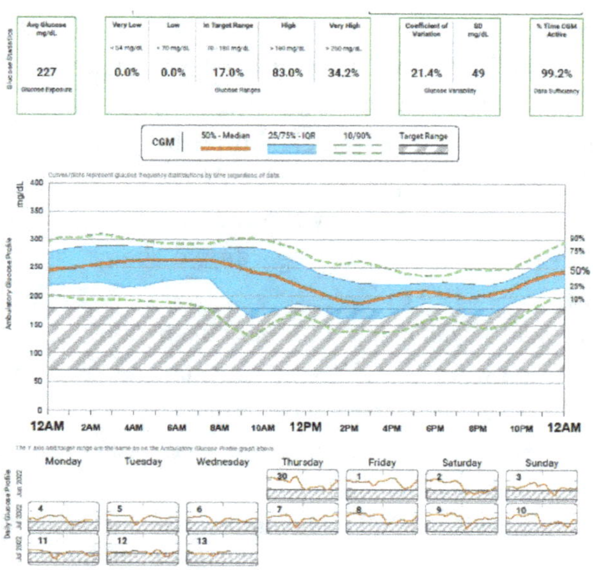

Based on his diagnosis, clinical scenario, and personal wishes for treatment, which of the following is the best recommendation?

A. Add a GLP-1 receptor agonist
B. Add a sulfonylurea
C. Add metformin
D. Increase the insulin dosage
E. Intensify lifestyle efforts

7 A 46-year-old woman has recently started continuous glucose monitoring. She has had type 1 diabetes mellitus since age 17 years. While in college, her hemoglobin A_{1c} values ranged from 9.0% to 11.0% (75-97 mmol/mol) and she had several episodes of diabetic ketoacidosis. She has been pregnant twice, and during both pregnancies, her hemoglobin A_{1c} values ranged from 6.0% to 7.0% (42-53 mmol/mol) on insulin pump therapy. Her infants weighed 8.2 and 8.6 lb (3719 and 3900 g). Aside from insulin pump use during pregnancy, she has been on a regimen of multiple daily insulin injections, with hemoglobin A_{1c} ranging from 8.0% to 8.5% (64-69 mmol/mol). She has been reluctant to wear a sensor or a pump, but a recent diagnosis of macular edema and moderate retinopathy in both eyes has motivated her to wear a continuous glucose monitor. Her ambulatory glucose profile is shown (*see image*), while on long-acting insulin plus rapid-acting insulin given before and after meals, depending on her glucose values.

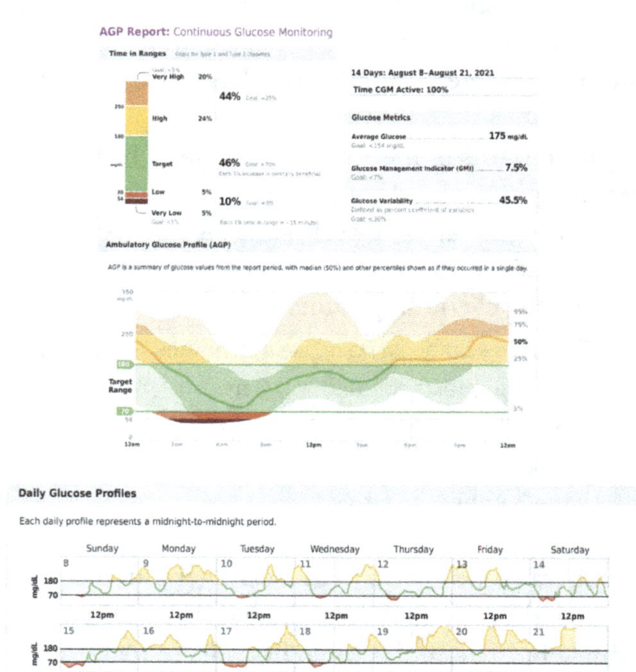

Reprinted from Holt RIG, DeVries JH, Hess-Fischl A, et al. The management of type 1 diabetes in adults. A consensus report by the American Diabetes Association (ADA) and the European Association for the Study of Diabetes (EASD). *Diabetes Care*. 2021;44(11):2589-2625.

After analyzing her data, which of the following is the best recommendation?

A. Decrease her long-acting insulin dose
B. Increase her daytime carbohydrate dose
C. Increase her long-acting insulin dose
D. Reduce her correction dose at bedtime
E. Start insulin pump therapy

8 A 32-year-old man is referred for evaluation of prediabetes. His paternal great grandmother, paternal grandmother, father, and identical twin brother had/have diabetes. His family members were all diagnosed with type 2 diabetes, but all of them eventually required insulin. They are of Eastern-European Jewish descent. The patient's twin developed diabetes at age 30 years and was found to have positive glutamic acid decarboxylase antibodies. His current treatment regimen consists of insulin and a GLP-1 receptor agonist.

The patient's fasting plasma glucose concentration is 120 mg/dL (6.7 mmol/L), and his hemoglobin A_{1c} measurement is 6.2% (44 mmol/mol). He has positive glutamic acid decarboxylase antibodies and zinc transporter antibodies. His BMI is 22.3 kg/m^2. Stage 2 type 1 diabetes is diagnosed. He would like to stop progression to overt diabetes.

Which of the following would be the most effective therapy considering his goal?

A. Golimumab
B. Insulin therapy
C. Intensive lifestyle regimen
D. Teplizumab

9 A 26-year-old woman with an 8-year history of type 1 diabetes mellitus is 6 weeks pregnant. Her most recent hemoglobin A_{1c} measurement is 6.6% (49 mmol/mol). She is self-monitoring her blood glucose before meals, 1 hour after meals, and at bedtime. She takes insulin detemir, 10 units twice daily, and insulin aspart immediately before meals based on an insulin-to-carbohydrate ratio of 1:12 and a sensitivity (or correction) factor of 1:30, with a target glucose value of 90 mg/dL (5.0 mmol/L). Her blood glucose log for the past few days is shown (*see table*).

Which of the following changes should be recommended?

A. Allow 15 minutes between the bolus and the meal
B. Change the insulin-to-carbohydrate ratio to 1:15
C. Change the sensitivity factor to 1:20
D. Continue the same regimen
E. Increase the dosage of insulin detemir to 12 units twice daily

10 A 24-year-old woman without diabetes whose husband has had type 1 diabetes mellitus since age 5 years is contemplating pregnancy and is inquiring about the risk of type 1 diabetes developing in her child. None of her family members has type 1 diabetes.

Which of the following characterizes the risk of type 1 diabetes developing in this patient's offspring?

A. 0.1%
B. 1.0%
C. 6.0%
D. 20.0%
E. 30.0%

Table for Question 9

Day	Before breakfast	After breakfast	Before lunch	After lunch	Before dinner	After dinner	Bedtime
Day 1	89 mg/dL (SI: 4.9 mmol/L)	187 mg/dL (SI: 10.4 mmol/L)	111 mg/dL (SI: 6.2 mmol/L)	174 mg/dL (SI: 9.7 mmol/L)	85 mg/dL (SI: 4.7 mmol/L)	137 mg/dL (SI: 7.6 mmol/L)	118 mg/dL (SI: 6.5 mmol/L)
Day 2	72 mg/dL (SI: 4.0 mmol/L)	182 mg/dL (SI: 10.1 mmol/L)	68 mg/dL (SI: 3.8 mmol/L)	153 mg/dL (SI: 8.5 mmol/L)	82 mg/dL (SI: 4.6 mmol/L)	149 mg/dL (SI: 8.3 mmol/L)	96 mg/dL (SI: 5.3 mmol/L)
Day 3	89 mg/dL (SI: 4.9 mmol/L)	201 mg/dL (SI: 11.2 mmol/L)	84 mg/dL (SI: 4.7 mmol/L)	181 mg/dL (SI: 10.0 mmol/L)	85 mg/dL (SI: 4.7 mmol/L)	202 mg/dL (SI: 11.2 mmol/L)	88 mg/dL (SI: 4.9 mmol/L)

11 A 56-year-old man with a 28-year history of type 1 diabetes mellitus has been using an insulin pump for 11 years with a rapid-acting insulin analogue. He has recently been experiencing recurrent high fasting blood glucose values. His diabetes is complicated by proliferative retinopathy, microalbuminuria with a stable creatinine concentration of 1.1 mg/dL (97.2 μmol/L), and peripheral sensory neuropathy. Examination of his logbook documents self-monitored blood glucose measurements 4 to 5 times daily before meals. He has a bedtime snack most days. Most mornings, fasting glucose levels are in the high 100s to low 200s (10.0-12.2 mmol/L). He is seeking guidance about achieving better glycemic control. His current hemoglobin A_{1c} level is 7.8% (62 mmol/mol). He is reluctant to wear a continuous glucose monitor because he does not want another device attached to his body.

Which of the following is the best recommendation?

A. Change the method of insulin delivery to multiple daily injections
B. Eliminate the bedtime snack
C. Increase the basal insulin rate 2 hours before the time fasting hyperglycemia is occurring
D. Increase the basal insulin rate overnight
E. Recommend overnight basal testing

12 A 68-year-old man with longstanding type 2 diabetes mellitus and peripheral neuropathy presents for a follow-up visit. He has had a right plantar ulcer in the past. His hemoglobin A_{1c} level is 7.6% (60 mmol/mol) on oral antidiabetes agents.

On foot examination, he has absent sensation to a 10-g monofilament, absent ankle reflexes, callus formation on the plantar aspect of the second and third metatarsal heads, and absent pedal pulses.

Which of the following is the strongest predictor of the development of future foot ulcers in this patient?

A. Abnormal monofilament testing
A. Absent ankle reflexes
B. Absent pedal pulses
C. Callus formation
D. History of previous ulceration

13 A 34-year-old man with type 1 diabetes mellitus is in the clinic waiting room when the receptionist notes he seems confused when his name is called, speaks with slurred words, and is unable to follow commands. He is found to have a fingerstick blood glucose value of 39 mg/dL (2.2 mmol/L). After recovery with oral glucose, he reports that despite careful monitoring, including use of his real-time continuous glucose monitor, he has been losing his sensing of lows and has had 5 or 6 episodes of hypoglycemia with blood glucose values between 40 and 50 mg/dL (2.2-2.8 mmol/L). During one of the episodes, a co-worker had to call the paramedics for treatment. His current hemoglobin A_{1c} level is 5.9% (41 mmol/mol), and his treatment regimen consists of multiple daily insulin injections and daily exercise in the evening. He lives alone and has worked hard to achieve a hemoglobin A_{1c} level less than 6.0% (<42 mmol/mol) out of a fear of developing diabetes-related complications.

Which of the following is the most important immediate next step in this patient's care?

A. Begin using an automated insulin delivery system for insulin administration
B. Instruct him to always carry a glucagon emergency kit
C. Recommend attending a diabetes education class focused on hypoglycemia avoidance
D. Suggest he stop exercising
E. Temporarily relax his tight glucose targets

14 A 21-year-old woman with a 2-year history of type 1 diabetes mellitus comes to the emergency department after experiencing 1 week of polyuria, weight loss, and blurred vision. For several days, her blood glucose values have ranged between 200 and 300 mg/dL

(11.1-16.7 mmol/L), and she states she has been administering more correction doses of insulin lispro than usual despite reduced food intake. She had onset of nausea and vomiting this morning and came to the emergency department because she is unable to hold fluids down.

She is following a multiple daily insulin injection regimen. She has gained 25 lb (11.4 kg) since her diabetes diagnosis, mostly in the past 6 months. She is very upset by this. She has depression, which has been treated with a selective serotonin reuptake inhibitor for the past year. She takes an oral contraceptive pill and is feeling extremely stressed due to preparation for final exams at her university next month.

On physical examination, her BMI is 27 kg/m^2. She has moderate midepigastric tenderness to palpation and appears to be acutely ill and dehydrated. She has no localized signs or symptoms of infection.

Initial laboratory test results:

Serum glucose = 594 mg/dL (70-99 mg/dL) (SI: 33.0 mmol/L [3.9-5.5 mmol/L])
Hemoglobin A_{1c} = 9.2% (4.0%-5.6%) (77 mmol/mol [20-38 mmol/mol])
Bicarbonate = 14 mEq/L (21-28 mEq/L) (SI: 14 mmol/L [21-28 mmol/L])
Serum pH = 7.2 (7.35-7.45)
Serum urea nitrogen = 34 mg/dL (8-23 mg/dL) (SI: 12.1 mmol/L [2.9-8.2 mmol/L])
Serum creatinine = 1.9 mg/dL (0.6-1.1 mg/dL) (SI: 168.0 µmol/L [53.0-97.2 µmol/L])
Serum potassium = 5.3 mEq/L (3.5-5.0 mEq/L) (SI: 5.3 mmol/L [3.5-5.0 mmol/L])
Urinalysis = 4+ glucose, large ketones, few white blood cells, no red blood cells, no blood

On the basis of her clinical history, which of the following is the most likely cause of diabetic ketoacidosis in this patient?

A. Acute kidney injury
B. Early pregnancy
C. Infection
D. Nonadherence to insulin therapy

15 A 19-year-old woman with type 1 diabetes mellitus who uses an insulin pump wants to train for an endurance event. She is planning to do cross-training, including jogging, weight-lifting, and stair training. She is concerned about her risk of hypoglycemia and asks for advice on how to minimize this possibility.

Which of the following should this patient do in addition to monitoring blood glucose before, during, and after exercise?

A. Consume 30 to 45 g of simple carbohydrates for every 30 minutes of aerobic exercise
B. Plan to do anerobic exercise prior to aerobic exercise
C. Reduce her basal rate immediately before exercise begins
D. Start exercising when her glucose concentration is above 100 mg/dL (>5.6 mmol/L)

16 A 31-year-old woman with a 22-year history of type 1 diabetes mellitus was recently told by her ophthalmologist that she has early nonproliferative diabetic retinopathy. She is concerned about losing her vision and asks what she can do to help prevent progression of this complication.

In addressing her concern, you explain that the amount of vision loss due to diabetic retinopathy that can be prevented at this early nonproliferative stage with targeted glycemic, blood pressure, and lipid control is expected to be:

A. <10%
B. 20%-30%
C. 50%
D. 75%
E. >90%

17 A 33-year-old woman with a 20-year history of type 1 diabetes mellitus presents for a follow-up visit. She starts to cry because of major stress due to recent divorce. She reports having intermittent nausea for the last few days. She feels unwell and attributes it to stress. She uses insulin pump therapy with insulin aspart at a basal rate of 1.2 units/h, an insulin-to-carbohydrate ratio of 1:15, and a sensitivity factor of 1:40. She has not been doing glucose fingerstick readings at home on a regular basis, but when she does, the values range between 70 and 250 mg/dL (3.9-13.9 mmol/L) without a real pattern. She had declined the use of a continuous glucose sensor in the past. A glucose fingerstick measurement in the office today is 385 mg/dL (21.4 mmol/L).

Laboratory tests from 2 weeks ago show a hemoglobin A_{1c} value of 9.3% (78 mmol/mol) with normal results on a basic metabolic panel. A pregnancy test is negative.

Which of the following is the best immediate next step?

A. Assessment for ketones
B. Basal rate testing
C. Diabetes education
D. Initiation of a continuous glucose sensor
E. Therapy for stress management

18 A 19-year-old man with type 1 diabetes mellitus reports a 6-month history of diarrhea, unintentional weight loss, suboptimal glycemic control, and a rash. On physical examination, he has no abdominal tenderness, normal sensation to 1-g monofilament testing, and a rash that is characterized by erythematous, papular, small and large blisters that burn and itch intensely (*see image*).

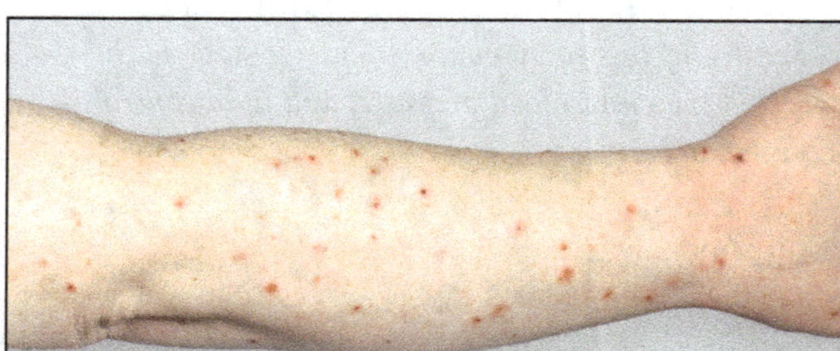

Which of the following is the best initial approach to evaluate his symptoms and rash?

A. Colonoscopy
B. Measurement of tissue transglutaminase antibodies
C. Measurement of TPO antibodies
D. Skin biopsy
E. Upper gastrointestinal series with small-bowel follow-through

19 A colleague in primary care calls with a question about the diagnosis of diabetes mellitus. She screened an overweight (BMI = 28 kg/m^2) 44-year-old man who has a grandmother and sister with diabetes. Neither of his parents has diabetes. Because the patient has sickle-cell disease, hemoglobin A_{1c} was not measured. Instead, a 75-g oral glucose tolerance test was performed and the following results were obtained:

Fasting glucose = 116 mg/dL (SI: 6.4 mmol/L)
1-hour glucose = 224 mg/dL (SI: 12.4 mmol/L)
2-hour glucose = 188 mg/dL (SI: 10.4 mmol/L)

On the basis of these results, which of the following should be recommended now?

A. Another measurement of fasting glucose to exclude type 2 diabetes
B. Another oral glucose tolerance test with measurements of serum insulin to assess insulin resistance
C. Genetic screening for pathogenic variants known to cause maturity-onset diabetes of the young
D. Initiation of metformin to treat early type 2 diabetes
E. Weight loss and exercise to prevent type 2 diabetes

20 A 31-year-old man with type 2 diabetes has a hemoglobin A_{1c} value of 9.2% (77 mmol/mol) on therapy with triple oral agents. Initiation of insulin is recommended. After some discussion, he agrees to start once-daily basal insulin. His job requires frequent travel across time zones, and he wonders if it will be a problem to time the basal insulin injections when he travels to Australia or Latin America. He is concerned about the risk of hypoglycemia while traveling.

Formulary issues aside, which of the following regimens should be recommended for this patient?

A. Insulin degludec; take it at his convenience once daily
B. Insulin detemir at bedtime; decrease the insulin dose by half when traveling
C. NPH insulin at bedtime; give it at the same time when traveling
D. U300 insulin glargine; give at the same time as he would take it at home

21 A 54-year-old man is referred for management of diabetes. He has had diabetes for 4 years and is treated with metformin, 1000 mg twice daily, and glimepiride, 2 mg twice daily. He also has hypertension treated with ramipril, 10 mg daily, and dyslipidemia treated with atorvastatin, 20 mg daily. Proliferative diabetic retinopathy was diagnosed at his last eye examination 6 months ago, and he underwent panretinal photocoagulation. He has a history of multinodular goiter and benign findings on FNA biopsy 2 years ago. He has no concerns except that he has been unable to lose weight despite trying various diets.

On physical examination, his blood pressure is 130/80 mm Hg and BMI is 32 kg/m^2. He has a goiter with a left dominant nodule of approximately 2 cm that is unchanged from ultrasonography done 1 year ago.

Laboratory test results:

Hemoglobin A_{1c} = 10.2% (4.0%-5.6%) (88 mmol/mol [20-38 mmol/mol])
Creatinine = 0.7 mg/dL (0.7-1.3 mg/dL) (SI: 61.9 µmol/L [61.9-114.9 µmol/L])
TSH, normal

Once-weekly semaglutide is added, and a follow-up visit is scheduled for 3 months after the semaglutide is started.

At this visit, which of the following should be done, assuming he remains asymptomatic?

A. Amylase and lipase measurement
B. Calcitonin measurement
C. Creatinine measurement
D. Referral for retinal examination
E. Thyroid ultrasonography

22 A 63-year-old woman with a 10-year history of type 2 diabetes mellitus presents for follow-up. Her medical history is notable for hypertension, dyslipidemia, nonproliferative diabetic retinopathy, toe amputation, and congestive heart failure.

Her current medications are metformin, 500 mg twice daily; long-acting insulin, 20 units at bedtime; ramipril, 10 mg daily; metoprolol, 50 mg daily; spironolactone, 25 mg daily; furosemide, 40 mg daily; atorvastatin, 40 mg daily; and aspirin.

On physical examination, her blood pressure is 138/85 mm Hg and BMI is 36 kg/m^2. She has a 2/6 systolic ejection murmur, weak dorsalis pedis pulses bilaterally, and absence of the left great toe with no active foot ulcers. Her lungs are clear to auscultation.

Laboratory test results:

Hemoglobin A_{1c} = 8.2% (4.0%-5.6%) (66 mmol/mol [20-38 mmol/mol])
Estimated glomerular filtration rate = 53 mL/min per 1.73 m^2 (>60 mL/min per 1.73 m^2)
Albumin-to-creatinine ratio = 356 mg/g creat
Complete blood cell count, normal
Electrolytes, normal
Liver function tests, normal
TSH, normal

Which of the following agents would be best to add next?

A. Bexagliflozin
B. Canagliflozin
C. Empagliflozin
D. Ertugliflozin
E. Saxagliptin

23 A 20-year-old previously well man with type 1 diabetes mellitus is found vomiting and disoriented after attending a party with his friends. He moved out of his family's home 4 months ago to live on his own. He manages his diabetes with multiple daily insulin injections. Five months ago, his hemoglobin A_{1c} level was 6.9% (52 mmol/mol).

His roommate calls the paramedics who transport him to the emergency department. In the emergency department, he appears somewhat confused and lethargic. He admits to having consumed an unusual amount of cannabis, as well as 2 beers, that evening. He describes vaping cannabis frequently since moving away from home. He recalls giving himself insulin earlier in the day.

On physical examination, he is afebrile. His blood pressure is 110/72 mm Hg, pulse rate is 90 beats/min, and respiratory rate is 30 breaths/min.

Laboratory test results:

- Plasma glucose = 280 mg/dL (70-99 mg/dL) (SI: 15.4 mmol/L [3.9-5.5 mmol/L])
- Serum sodium = 146 mg/dL (136-142 mEq/L) (SI: 146 mmol/L [136-142 mmol/L])
- Bicarbonate = 18 mEq/L (21-28 mEq/L) (SI: 18 mmol/L [21-28 mmol/L])
- β-Hydroxybutyrate = 2.1 mmol/L
- Hemoglobin A_{1c} = 7.1% (4.0%-5.6%) (54 mmol/mol [20-38 mmol/mol])
- Serum pH = 7.45 (7.35-7.45)
- Serum urea nitrogen = 34 mg/dL (8-23 mg/dL) (SI: 12.1 mmol/L [2.9-8.2 mmol/L])
- Serum creatinine = 1.4 mg/dL (0.7-1.3 mg/dL) (SI: 123.8 μmol/L [61.9-114.9 μmol/L])
- Serum potassium = 5.0 mEq/L (3.5-5.0 mEq/L) (SI: 5.0 mmol/L [3.5-5.0 mmol/L])
- Urinalysis = 4+ glucose, large ketones, few white blood cells, no red blood cells

Which of the following most likely precipitated his condition?

A. Adrenal insufficiency
B. Alcohol intoxication
C. Cannabis
D. Infection
E. Insulin rationing

24 A 31-year-old woman with a history of type 1 diabetes mellitus since age 2 years and Hashimoto thyroiditis is concerned about the sudden onset of a rash on her upper extremities. It started at 8:30 AM, at which point her hands became swollen, red, painful, and burning with a pruritic rash covering both of her arms. She had not yet given her morning insulin injection. She had a similar episode 2 years ago. At that time, her physician changed her brands of insulin and the type of thyroid hormone replacement. The lesions resolved over the course of 3 months with symptomatic improvement with cetirizine HCl and diphenhydramine. When she administers her insulin injections, there is no redness or itching at the shot site. She has not made any changes in soaps, lotions, or laundry detergent. She has a house cat that is on flea prevention therapy. The appearance of the rash is shown (*see image).*

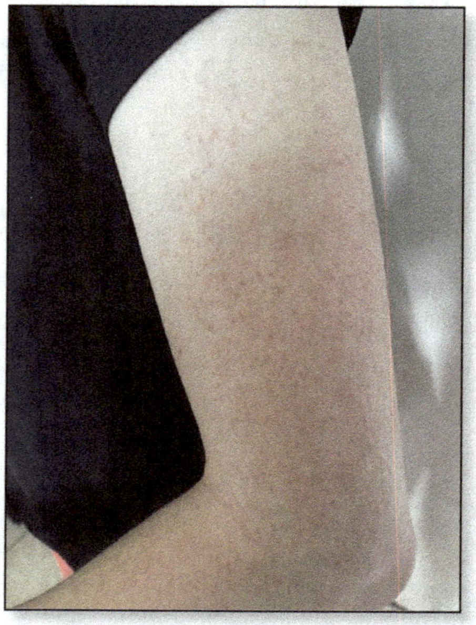

Which of the following is the diabetes-associated cause of the patient's pruritic skin condition?

A. Chronic autoimmune urticaria
B. Hypersensitivity reaction to flea bites
C. Insulin allergy
D. Necrobiosis lipoidica diabeticorum
E. Perforating collagenosis

25 A 33-year-old woman presents to her primary care physician for an annual visit. She feels well and has no concerns. She has a history of gestational diabetes during a pregnancy 5 years ago. She has no history of hypertension, dyslipidemia, or cardiovascular disease. Her only medication is a daily multivitamin. She has no known family history of diabetes and does not smoke cigarettes or drink alcohol. She exercises regularly.

On physical examination, her blood pressure is 120/70 mm Hg and BMI is 23.0 kg/m^2. The rest of her examination findings are unremarkable.

Her current hemoglobin A_{1c} level is 5.4% (36 mmol/mol).

Regarding lifelong screening with respect to her prediabetes/diabetes risk, how often should she be screened?

A. No screening needed
B. At least every year
C. At least every 3 years
D. At least every 5 years
E. At least every 10 years

26 A 53-year-old woman with an 18-year history of type 2 diabetes mellitus, hypertension complicated by chronic kidney disease, proliferative retinopathy, peripheral neuropathy, and peripheral vascular disease has been admitted to the hospital following several syncopal episodes. An endocrine consult is requested to assess whether dysautonomia could have a role in her presentation and, if so, to recommend how to manage her supine hypertension.

She is recovering from a recent viral syndrome and describes 2 episodes before hospital admission that occurred after she attempted to get up and ambulate. She became lightheaded, had palpitations, and fell to the ground. For several years, she has been having lightheadedness if she gets up quickly, especially in the morning. She has blunted hypoglycemia awareness. She has not noticed early satiety. She has a tendency to be constipated. She reports often eating fast food, and home meals include processed and canned foods. She does not exercise.

Medications include long-acting insulin once daily, rapid-acting insulin with meals, metoprolol extended release, losartan, atorvastatin, and aspirin.

On physical examination, she is in no acute distress. She has obesity (BMI = 30 kg/m^2). Her temperature is 98.2°F (36.8°C), pulse rate is 92 beats/min, and blood pressure is 176/84 mm Hg supine. When standing, her blood pressure drops 49 mm Hg systolic and 22 mm Hg diastolic. Her heart rate does not increase concomitantly with the fall in blood pressure. Findings on head and neck examination are normal. Findings on cardiorespiratory examination are normal. There is markedly decreased sensation in both feet to 10 g monofilament.

Laboratory test results:

- Blood glucose levels in the hospital = range from 101-140 mg/dL (70-99 mg/dL) (SI: ranges from 5.6-7.8 mmol/L [3.9-5.5 mmol/L])
- Hemoglobin A_{1c} = 8.3% (4.0%-5.6%) (89 mmol/mol [20-38 mmol/mol])
- Creatinine (at admission) = 2.1 mg/dL (0.6-1.1 mg/dL) (SI: 185.6 µmol/L [53.0-97.2 µmol/L])
- Creatinine (current) = 1.4 mg/dL (SI: 123.8 µmol/L)
- Urinary albumin-to-creatinine ratio = 1654.7 mg/g (<30 mg/g creat)
- Hemoglobin = 9.8 g/dL (12.1-15.1 g/dL) (SI: 98 g/L [121-151 g/L])
- Hematocrit = 32.3% (35%-45%) (SI: 0.323 [0.35-0.45])

Despite requiring fluids and discontinuing all antihypertensive agents upon hospital admission, systolic blood pressure measurements are around 180 mm Hg while recumbent, coupled with overt orthostatic hypotension with persistent drop in systolic blood pressure greater than 20 mm Hg and drop in diastolic blood pressure greater than 10 mm Hg upon standing. Echocardiography demonstrates normal left ventricular ejection fraction and evidence of diastolic dysfunction. Autonomic neuropathy with orthostatic hypotension and marked supine hypertension are diagnosed.

In addition to avoiding the supine position during the day and raising the head of her bed, which pharmacologic intervention should be recommended at bedtime to treat her supine hypertension?

A. Clonidine
B. Hydralazine
C. Ibuprofen
D. Midodrine
E. Propranolol

Diabetes Mellitus, Section 2 Board Review

Marie E. McDonnell, MD

27 A 24-year-old woman who is 3 weeks post partum presents for evaluation following hospitalization for an episode of unconsciousness witnessed by her husband. Upon arrival by ambulance, she was arousable but lethargic with a glucose concentration of 28 mg/dL (1.6 mmol/L). Following treatment with intravenous 50% dextrose in the emergency department, her glucose value was 102 mg/dL (5.7 mmol/L). After a meal and 4 hours observation without hypoglycemia, she was discharged and advised to follow-up with her obstetrician.

Since the initial episode, she has been using her father's glucose monitor and notes she has glucose values as low as 38 mg/dL (2.1 mmol/L) accompanied by mild tremulousness and sweating that she has been attributing to postpartum hormonal changes. She believes the episodes are mostly after meals, but she has not observed a clear pattern. She is nursing her baby on demand and reports an erratic sleep and eating schedule.

Eighteen months ago, she underwent Roux-en-Y gastric bypass surgery for treatment of obesity complicated by hypertension. She reports that her hunger was not well controlled after bariatric surgery. Despite losing 52 lb (23.6 kg) in the first 6 months, she regained approximately 50% of her lost weight before her pregnancy.

Laboratory test results (after fasting for 6 hours at home):

Glucose = 54 mg/dL (70-99 mg/dL) (SI: 3.0 mmol/L [3.9-5.5 mmol/L])
Insulin = 5.5 µIU/mL (1.4-14.0 µIU/mL) (SI: 38.2 pmol/L [9.7-97.2 pmol/L])
C-peptide = 1.9 ng/mL (0.5-2.0 ng/mL) (SI: 0.63 nmol/L [0.17-0.66 nmol/L])
β-Hydroxybutyrate = 1.0 mg/dL (<3.0 mg/dL) (SI: 100 µmol/L [SI: <288.2 µmol/L])
Cortisol = 21 µg/dL (2-14 µg/dL) (SI: 579.2 nmol/L [55.2-386.2 nmol/L])
Blood screening for sulfonlyurea/meglitinides, negative
TSH = 1.2 mIU/L (0.5-5.0 mIU/L)
Sodium = 142 mEq/L (136-142 mEq/L) (SI: 142 mmol/L [136-142 mmol/L])
Potassium = 4.2 mEq/L (3.5-5.0 mEq/L) (SI: 4.2 mmol/L [3.5-5.0 mmol/L])
Serum urea nitrogen = 42 mg/dL (8-23 mg/dL) (SI: 15.0 mmol/L [2.9-8.2 mmol/L])
Creatinine = 1.4 mg/dL (0.6-1.1 mg/dL) (SI: 123.8 µmol/L [53.0-97.2 µmol/L])
Albumin = 3.9 g/dL (3.5-5.0 g/dL) (SI: 39 g/L [35-50 g/L])
Calcium = 11.1 mg/dL (8.2-10.2 mg/dL) (SI: 2.8 mmol/L [2.1-2.6 mmol/L])
Phosphate = 2.0 mg/dL (2.3-4.7 mg/dL) (SI: 0.6 mmol/L [0.7-1.5 mmol/L])

Which of the following is the best next diagnostic test?

A. 72-Hour fast
B. Endoscopic ultrasonography
C. Genetic testing
D. Mixed-meal tolerance test
E. Selective intraarterial calcium-stimulation test

28 A 58-year-old woman presents for evaluation of type 2 diabetes mellitus. Diabetes was diagnosed at age 34 years in the setting of class 3 obesity. Since being diagnosed, she has struggled to maintain good disease control. Most of her hemoglobin A1c values are between 9.0% and 10.0% (75-86 mmol/mol). She has moderate to severe nonproliferative retinopathy in both eyes and distal polyneuropathy affecting her feet.

Her current medications include dulaglutide, 1.5 mg weekly; losartan, 25 mg daily; and rosuvastatin, 40 mg daily.

Five months ago, she underwent Roux-en-Y gastric bypass and lost 30% of her body weight. She continues to lose weight, feels well, and bikes 30 minutes daily. She has smoked one-half pack cigarettes per day for 20 years and has been unable to quit despite numerous attempts. Her hope today is, given her excellent progress, that she might be able to discontinue 1 or more medications.

On physical examination, she appears well. Her blood pressure is 146/88 mm Hg, pulse rate is 84 beats/min, and BMI is 32 kg/m^2. Mucous membranes are moist. There are palpable distal pulses in the feet and no peripheral edema.

Laboratory test results:

- Point-of-care hemoglobin A_{1c} = 6.4% (4.0%-5.6%) (46 mmol/mol [20-38 mmol/mol])
- Creatinine = 1.68 mg/dL (0.6-1.1 mg/dL) (SI: 148.5 µmol/L [53.0-97.2 µmol/L])
- Estimated glomerular filtration rate = 52 mL/min per 1.73 m^2 (>60 mL/min per 1.73 m^2)
- Potassium = 4.8 mEq/L (3.5-5.0 mEq/L) (SI: 4.8 mmol/L [3.5-5.0 mmol/L])
- Glucose = 180 mg/dL (70-99 mg/dL) (SI: 10.0 mmol/L [3.9-5.5 mmol/L])
- Urinary albumin-to-creatinine ratio = 480 mg/g creat (<30 mg/g creat)
- LDL cholesterol = 72 mg/dL (<100 mg/dL [optimal]) (SI: 1.86 mmol/L [<2.59 mmol/L])
- HDL cholesterol = 36 mg/dL (>60 mg/dL [optimal]) (SI: 0.93 mmol/L [>1.55 mmol/L])

In addition to referring her to a smoking cessation program, which of the following is the best next step in this patient's management?

A. Add empagliflozin, 10 mg daily
B. Add finerenone, 10 mg daily
C. Increase the dulaglutide dosage to 3.0 mg weekly
D. Increase the losartan dosage to 50 mg daily
E. Switch dulaglutide to semaglutide

29 A 67-year-old man with type 2 diabetes mellitus, obesity, and hypertension presents to follow-up after starting an SGLT-2 inhibitor (empagliflozin) 4 weeks ago. He has a history of HIV with an undetectable viral load on combination antiviral therapy and was treated for hepatitis C in the past. One year ago, he presented to the emergency department with polyuria, polydipsia, and 5-lb (2.3-kg) weight loss. His glucose concentration was 486 mg/dL (27.0 mmol/L), and he did not have evidence of ketoacidosis. After 2 to 3 months on combination basal insulin and metformin therapy, he was then able to maintain good glycemic control on metformin alone for the subsequent 3 to 4 months.

After discussion, he agreed to start SGLT-2 inhibitor therapy due to the combined scenario of a hemoglobin A_{1c} value of 7.1% (54 mmol/mol) (goal <7.0% [<53 mmol/mol]), chronic kidney disease, and suboptimally controlled blood pressure.

His other medications include metformin, 500 mg twice daily; lisinopril, 20 mg twice daily; simvastatin, 40 mg daily; and biketgravir 50 mg/emtricitabine 200 mg/tenofovir alafenamide 25 mg daily.

Baseline evaluation 4 weeks ago included the following data:

- Blood pressure = 138/78 mm Hg
- Serum creatinine = 1.91 mg/dL (0.7-1.3 mg/dL) (SI: 168.8 µmol/L [61.9-114.9 µmol/L])
- Estimated glomerular filtration rate = 35 mL/min per 1.73 m^2 (>60 mL/min per 1.73 m^2)

Today's evaluation 4 weeks after initiation of empagliflozin, 10 mg daily:

- Blood pressure = 134/72 mm Hg
- Serum creatinine = 2.35 mg/dL (SI: 207.7 µmol/L)
- Estimated glomerular filtration rate = 29 mL/min per 1.73 m^2

Which of the following is the best next management step?

A. Advise increased hydration
B. Refer for urgent kidney biopsy
C. Stop metformin
D. Stop empagliflozin
E. Stop metformin and empagliflozin

30 An 83-year-old woman presents with her daughter for routine follow-up. She has had type 2 diabetes mellitus for approximately 25 years, with a recent hemoglobin A_{1c} measurement of 8.9% (74 mmol/mol). She has well-controlled hypertension, and her condition has been stable following 3-vessel coronary artery bypass grafting at age 72 years. Her BMI is 32 kg/m^2.

Approximately 4 months ago, she fell at home and has been evaluated for problems with slow gait and increased pain with walking. Hip replacement has been recommended due to severe osteoarthritis, but she has been informed that her diabetes would need to be better controlled to undergo surgery. Recently, she has had more difficulty with memory and now lives with her daughter due to safety concerns.

Her current diabetes regimen consists of insulin glargine, 24 units at bedtime; insulin aspart, 4 units before breakfast and 10 units before dinner; and metformin, 1000 mg daily. Her fasting blood glucose measurements from the last 30 days show a mean value of 152 mg/dL (8.4 mmol/L) and a range of 105-172 mg/dL [5.8-9.5 mmol/L]). Professional continuous glucose monitoring is performed, and the ambulatory glucose profile from 14 days of glucose data shows the following:

Average glucose = 210 mg/dL (11.7 mmol/L)
Percentage of time very high (>250 mg/dL [>13.9 mmol/L]) = 16%
Percentage of time high (180-250 mg/dL [10.0-13.9 mmol/L]) = 25%
Percentage of time in target range (70-180 mg/dL [3.9-10.0 mmol/L]) = 54%
Percentage of time below range (55-70 mg/dL [3.1-3.9 mmol/L]) = 4%
Percentage of time very low range (<55 mg/dL [<3.1 mmol/L]) = 1%

Which of the following is the most appropriate next step?

A. Add semaglutide and discontinue insulin aspart
B. Increase meal insulin doses by 20%
C. Measure hemoglobin A_{1c} and hemoglobin and perform iron studies
D. Recommend no change
E. Increase the insulin glargine dosage by 20%

31 A 58-year-old man with recent-onset type 2 diabetes mellitus and childhood-onset obesity presents for follow-up after a recent emergency department visit for severe lower abdominal pain. After several hours of intravenous fluid, he passes a kidney stone without intervention.

In the final report from a noncontrast CT, the radiologist noted, "fatty infiltration of the liver in a patchy distribution...clinical correlation required."

He reports drinking alcohol on rare occasions (approximately 2 drinks per month) and does not take acetaminophen or herbal supplements on a regular basis.

On physical examination, he appears well. His blood pressure is 138/72 mm Hg, and BMI is 43 kg/m^2. There is diffuse adiposity distributed mostly in the abdomen and no appreciable precervical fat deposition. He has mildly reduced vibration sensation in his toes bilaterally but intact sensation to monofilament testing throughout. The rest of his examination findings are normal and unchanged from prior visits.

Laboratory test results (sample drawn in the emergency department):

Creatinine = 1.18 mg/dL (0.7-1.3 mg/dL) (SI: 104.3 µmol/L [61.9-114.9 µmol/L])
Glucose = 180 mg/dL (70-99 mg/dL) (SI: 10.0 mmol/L [3.9-5.5 mmol/L])
Triglycerides = 220 mg/dL (<150 mg/dL [optimal]) (SI: 2.49 mmol/L [<1.70 mmol/L])
Lipase = 40 U/L (10-73 U/L) (SI: 0.67 µkat/L [0.17-1.22 µkat/L])
AST = 18 U/L (20-48 U/L) (SI: 0.30 µkat/L [0.33-0.80 µkat/L])
ALT = 10 U/L (10-40 U/L) (SI: 0.17 µkat/L [0.17-0.67 µkat/L])

Which of the following is the best diagnostic test to determine this patient's risk of cirrhosis?

A. DXA
B. Hemoglobin measurement
C. Liver biopsy
D. Platelet count
E. Transient elastography

32 A 38-year-old woman with a 25-year history of type 1 diabetes mellitus presents with her husband and her mother for follow-up to determine candidacy for pancreas transplant. Since starting a hybrid closed-loop insulin pump, her glycemic control is much improved with rare episodes of severe hypoglycemia, although she finds dealing with the technology to be a daily struggle.

Her diabetes is complicated by retinopathy, neuropathy, and nephropathy, and she just started hemodialysis 3 months ago. She walks 2 miles every other day. She was activated on the kidney transplant list 6 months ago and would like to be considered for a pancreas transplant either at the same time or following kidney transplant.

During her assessment, an altruistic kidney donor was recently identified who is an ideal match for her.

She is advised that the average wait time for deceased donors for simultaneous pancreas-kidney transplant at the site is 15 months.

Which of the following should this patient be told is the best transplant strategy for optimal overall survival?

A. Cadaveric islet transplant followed by live donor kidney transplant

B. Live donor kidney transplant and simultaneous cadaveric islet transplant

C. Live donor kidney transplant followed by pancreas transplant as a second surgery

D. Pancreas transplant as soon as available followed by live donor kidney transplant

E. Simultaneous kidney and pancreas transplant from the same deceased donor

33 A 72-year-old woman presents for follow-up. She has a 35-history of type 2 diabetes mellitus and lifelong obesity complicated by osteoarthritis and obstructive sleep apnea. Two years ago, in response to a hemoglobin A_{1c} value of 7.8% (62 mmol/mol), dulaglutide (a GLP-1 receptor agonist) was added to her regimen of metformin and glipizide, 5 mg twice daily. Over 3 months, glipizide was stopped. The patient was able to lower her average fasting blood glucose and reduce her hemoglobin A_{1c} to 7.0% (53 mmol/mol). She also lost 5% of her body weight.

She brings a report downloaded from her glucose meter, which she uses to check her fingerstick glucose before eating breakfast daily. She reports increased thirst on some days and new-onset nocturia most nights of the week.

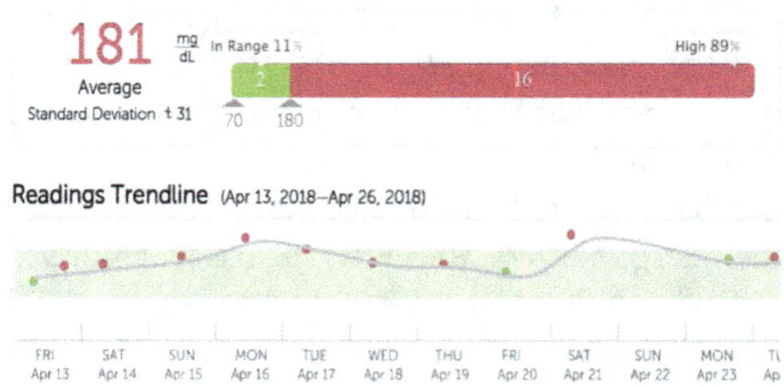

Her current medications include dulaglutide, 4.5 mg once weekly; metformin, 1000 mg twice daily; lisinopril, 30 mg once daily; and rosuvastatin, 20 mg once daily.

Laboratory test results:

Hemoglobin A_{1c} = 8.4% (4.0%-5.6%) (68 mmol/mol [20-38 mmol/mol])

Sodium = 142 mEq/L (136-142 mEq/L) (SI: 142 mmol/L [136-142 mmol/L])

Potassium = 3.8 mEq/L (3.5-5.0 mEq/L) (SI: 3.8 mmol/L [3.5-5.0 mmol/L])

Creatinine = 1.4 mg/dL (0.6-1.1 mg/dL) (SI: 123.8 μmol/L [53.0-97.2 μmol/L])

Estimated glomerular filtration rate = 48 mL/min per 1.73 m^2 (>60 mL/min per 1.73 m^2)

Urinary albumin-to-creatinine ratio = 24 mg/g creat (<30 mg/g creat)

LDL cholesterol = 58 mg/dL (<100 mg/dL [optimal]) (SI: 1.50 mmol/L [<2.59 mmol/L])

HDL cholesterol = 42 mg/dL (>60 mg/dL [optimal]) (SI: 1.09 mmol/L [>1.55 mmol/L])

Triglycerides = 180 mg/dL (<150 mg/dL [optimal]) (SI: 2.03 mmol/L [<1.70 mmol/L])

Which of the following is the best next step for this patient's glycemic management?

A. Add basal insulin
B. Add linagliptin
C. Add pioglitazone
D. Add rapid-acting insulin prior to largest meal
E. Stop dulaglutide and add basal insulin once daily and rapid-acting insulin prior to largest meal

34 A 32-year-old pregnant woman (G3P2) with type 2 diabetes mellitus diagnosed during her prior pregnancy presents for routine follow-up at 28 weeks' gestation for management of diabetes. She expresses concern because the growth assessment by ultrasonography today is notable for an estimated fetal weight in the fourth percentile. Other features of the scan and the recent biophysical profile are normal.

Her first baby, born 24 months ago, weighed 10 lb 2 oz. Her own birth weight was 5 lb 2oz, and her husband's birth weight was more than 10 lb.

She had difficulty controlling her blood glucose during her last pregnancy. In the last 2 years, she has been successful in comprehensive behavioral lifestyle change, including exercising daily and following a time-restricted eating pattern. Prior to this pregnancy, she lost 15 lb (6.8 kg) and her prepregnancy BMI was 28 kg/m^2.

On physical examination, she appears well. She has gained approximately 15 lb (6.8 kg) during the pregnancy. Her blood pressure is 98/62 mm Hg. There is no pedal edema.

Current medications include a prenatal vitamin; aspirin, 81 mg daily; metformin, 1000 mg twice daily; and insulin levemir, 42 units at bedtime.

She monitors fingerstick blood glucose before and after meals. Approximately 90% of her fasting glucose values and 85% of her postmeal glucose values are in target range. She detects glucose values between 60 and 70 mg/dL (3.3-3.9 mmol/L) approximately 4 times weekly.

Which of the following maternal factors increases her risk of delivering a small-for-gestational-age baby?

A. Age
B. Current blood pressure
C. Current glycemic control
D. Metformin therapy
E. Weight gain in pregnancy

35 A 78-year-old man with type 2 diabetes mellitus was recently seen by an orthopedic surgeon for severe osteoarthritis of the left knee that has limited his ability to exercise. The surgeon has informed him that that she will schedule knee replacement once he is able to bring his hemoglobin A_{1c} below 7.0% (<53 mmol/mol). The patient has been referred to improve his glycemic control. His current diabetes medications are U300 insulin glargine, metformin, and sitagliptin.

On physical examination, he appears well. His BMI is 30.1 kg/m^2.

His most recent hemoglobin A_{1c} measurement is 7.7% (61 mmol/mol). Home glucose monitoring documents fasting glucose values ranging from 109 to 186 mg/dL (6.0-10.3 mmol/L) and bedtime glucose values ranging from 138 to 282 mg/dL (7.7-15.7 mmol/L) with an overall average value of 178 mg/dL (9.9 mmol/L). He reports occasional sweatiness relieved by juice while working in his garden.

Which of the following is the best next step in this patient's management?

A. Add once-daily glimepiride
B. Add rapid-acting insulin prior to the largest meal of the day
C. Advise the surgeon that the patient's current hemoglobin A_{1c} is acceptable for the planned surgical procedure
D. Increase dosage of U300 insulin glargine by 20%

36 A 48-year-old man was admitted to the hospital 2 days ago after a non–ST-elevation myocardial infarction. He has required insulin throughout his stay. He has had excellent glycemic control in the hospital, and the care team asks for advice on the best treatment plan after hospital discharge.

He has been treated with metformin for 4 years after an elevated blood glucose concentration was detected on routine screening. His glycemic control has varied, and a sulfonylurea was added last year when his hemoglobin A_{1c} level increased to greater than 8.0% (>64 mmol/mol). However, he gained 11 lb (5 kg) with this treatment and stopped the drug after 6 months. He is otherwise healthy and his only medications before hospitalization were metformin and lisinopril.

On physical examination, his blood pressure is 122/74 mm Hg and BMI is 36 kg/m^2. His ejection fraction is 42%.

Laboratory test results (sample drawn at hospital admission):

- Hemoglobin A_{1c} = 7.6% (4.0%-5.6%) (60 mmol/mol [20-38 mmol/mol])
- LDL cholesterol = 142 mg/dL (<100 mg/dL [optimal]) (SI: 3.68 mmol/L [<2.59 mmol/L])
- Creatinine = 1.2 mg/dL (0.7-1.3 mg/dL) (SI: 106.1 µmol/L [61.9-114.9 µmol/L])
- Estimated glomerular filtration rate = 80 mL/min per 1.73 m^2 (>60 mL/min per 1.73 m^2)
- Urinary albumin-to-creatinine ratio = 108 mg/g creat (<30 mg/g creat)

In addition to metformin, current medications include aspirin, 325 mg daily; atorvastatin, 80 mg daily; lisinopril, 40 mg daily; and metoprolol, 100 mg daily.

Which of the following medications is the best option to add to metformin at hospital discharge?

A. Dapagliflozin
B. Glargine
C. Pioglitazone
D. Semaglutide
E. Sitagliptin

37 Consultation is requested to provide insulin management recommendations for a 49-year-old man who presented to the hospital 3 days ago after sustaining multiple injuries in a car accident. There are no records available regarding his medical history or prior medication. His vital signs are now stable, and he is ready to transfer out of intensive care.

Diabetes management has included an insulin infusion, which was initiated in response to glucose levels between 221 and 326 mg/dL (12.3-18.1 mmol/L) in the first 6 hours of his evaluation. The insulin infusion rate over 6 hours during the last overnight period has been stable at 1.5 units per hour. As he has not been able to demonstrate safe swallowing, and he has just started "trickle" enteral feeding this morning, which will advance as tolerated.

On physical examination, he is lethargic and has difficulty communicating. His blood pressure is 148/76 mm Hg, pulse rate is 78 beats/min, and weight is 216 lb (98 kg). He has normally distributed adiposity. Visible wounds are dressed without surrounding erythema. Foot examination reveals diffuse mild hammer toe deformity and dry skin without ulceration.

Which of the following insulin regimens would best match his physiologic basal-bolus insulin needs to enable glycemic control during continuous enteral tube feeding?

A. U100 NPH insulin, 10 units once nightly plus rapid-acting insulin every 4 hours
B. U100 insulin glargine, 10 units once nightly plus regular insulin correction scale every 6 hours
C. Scheduled regular insulin dose plus correction scale administered every 6 hours
D. U300 insulin glargine, 50 units once daily plus rapid-acting insulin correction scale administered every 4 hours
E. Insulin glargine, 30 units once daily, plus a scheduled regular insulin dose plus correction scale administered every 6 hours

38 A 52-year-old woman with a 25 pack-year cigarette smoking history presents to discuss alternative management of her type 2 diabetes mellitus. Two months ago, she experienced a transient ischemic attack involving the motor function of her left arm. She had full recovery 2 days later. She was advised that her hemoglobin A_{1c} value of 9.2% (77 mmol/mol) places her at high risk of a stroke.

On physical examination, she appears well. Her blood pressure is 128/77 mm Hg, and her BMI is 36 kg/m^2. Findings on heart and lung examination are normal. She has barely palpable peripheral pulses, but findings on foot examination are otherwise unremarkable.

Current medications are metformin and sitagliptin. Sitagliptin is replaced with semaglutide, 0.25 mg once weekly.

After 2 semaglutide injections, she starts experiencing daily nausea and foul-smelling eructations. She has also developed new symptoms of gastroesophageal reflux that have disrupted her sleep. One morning, she has an episode of vomiting at work. She reports that she "tried but gave up" on semaglutide and stopped the medication after a 6-week trial. She is adamant about not taking semaglutide again.

When measured in the office today, her blood glucose is 265 mg/dL (14.7 mmol/L) 3 hours after a meal of yogurt and berries.

Which of the following medications should be started as the most appropriate next step?

A. Dulaglutide
B. Insulin degludec/liraglutide combination injectable
C. Insulin glargine
D. Pioglitazone
E. Tirzepatide

39 A 57-year-old woman with class 3 obesity and a 5-year history of type 2 diabetes mellitus underwent sleeve gastrectomy 12 months ago. Six months before surgery, her hemoglobin A_{1c} level was 9.2% (77 mmol/mol) on a treatment regimen of metformin, glipizide, and maximum-tolerated dosage of dulaglutide. She was able to reduce her hemoglobin A_{1c} to 7.9% (63 mmol/mol) on a preparatory liquid diet in the weeks before surgery. She is extremely pleased to learn that her hemoglobin A_{1c} level today is 5.9% (41 mmol/mol) despite stopping all of her antidiabetes medications.

She wonders what her future holds and expresses fear that her success will be short-lived, like so many of her prior weight-loss attempts.

In advising her on her diabetes health moving forward, which of the following statements is correct?

A. Her risk of future microvascular complications has been reduced by 40%
B. She has a 50% chance of having a hemoglobin A_{1c} level <7.0% (<53 mmol/mol) on no medications in 3 years
C. She has a 10% chance of having a hemoglobin A_{1c} level <6.5% (<48 mmol/mol) on no medications in 5 years
D. In 5 years, her quality of life will likely be the same as it would have been if she did not have surgery

40 A 64-year-old woman with an 18-year history of suboptimally controlled type 2 diabetes mellitus presents to the emergency department with a 1-week history of left-sided flank pain. She has no fever, chills, dysuria, nausea, postprandial pain, or change in bowel habit. Her medical history is notable for retinopathy requiring laser photocoagulation and distal somatosensory neuropathy. She has had 2 toe amputations, coronary artery bypass surgery, and right femoral popliteal bypass surgery.

On physical examination, she is afebrile. The left flank and left upper quadrant are exquisitely tender to superficial palpation. Muscle strength in the legs is normal; sensation is reduced below the knees and absent in the feet. There is no rash.

Laboratory test results:

Fecal occult blood screening, negative
Urinalysis, 2+ protein and 3 to 5 red blood cells per high-power field
White blood cell count = 7200/μL (4500-11,000) (SI: 7.2 × 10^9/L [4.5-11.0 × 10^9/L]), with normal differential

Chemistry panel, normal
Liver function tests, normal
Amylase and lipase, normal

Abdominal CT is negative for urinary or biliary calcification, and there are no abnormalities of the pancreas, intestine, or kidneys.

Which of the following is the most likely cause of this patient's pain?

A. Diabetic autonomic neuropathy
B. Diabetic radiculopathy
C. Herpes zoster
D. Pancreatitis
E. Passed kidney stone

41 A 57-year-old woman is referred by her primary care physician because of uncontrolled diabetes. The patient has a long history of severe asthma requiring multiple hospital admissions in the past and several episodes of respiratory failure. She has been treated with 40 to 60 mg of prednisone for up to 6 months at a time over the past 3 years. On this regimen, she has been able to avoid hospital stays, but she has developed diabetes that requires insulin therapy. After an initial favorable response to insulin, her hemoglobin A_{1c} level has climbed to greater than 9.0% (>75 mmol/mol) over the past year and time-in-range on her continuous glucose monitor has dropped to only 25%.

Her insulin requirements have escalated, and she is now taking 100 units of insulin glargine in the morning, 75 to 80 units of insulin aspart before meals, and occasional coverage of snacks with 20 to 30 units. She also takes metformin extended release, 1000 mg twice daily. She is adherent to her injection regimen and misses only 2 to 3 doses per month, although she reports it is becoming more discouraging to inject insulin without results. Recently, she has noticed fatigue and decreased appetite, with nocturia 2 to 3 times per night.

Two years ago, she tried to combine insulin therapy with a GLP-1 receptor agonist but could not tolerate it after many attempts over nearly a year, including very low daily dosed liraglutide while off metformin.

On physical examination, her BMI is 30 kg/m^2. She has acanthosis on the back of her neck and under her arms. There is no hepatomegaly or evidence of diabetic neuropathy.

Which of the following therapeutic interventions would lower this patient's blood glucose most effectively?

A. Add canagliflozin
B. Add insulin glargine, 100 units in the evening
C. Add pioglitazone
D. Change the insulin delivery to an insulin pump
E. Switch to U500 insulin, 300 units in divided doses

42 A 63-year-old man has had type 2 diabetes mellitus for 16 years complicated by stage 2 chronic kidney disease, mild nonproliferative retinopathy, and mild peripheral neuropathy. His current therapy consists of insulin glargine, 65 units in the morning; metformin, 1000 mg twice daily; and repaglinide, 2 mg before meals. Recent laboratory evaluation included a hemoglobin A_{1c} measurement of 8.4% (68 mmol/mol) and a fasting plasma glucose value of 111 mg/dL (6.2 mmol/L). Fingerstick blood glucose monitoring daily before breakfast shows an average of 116 mg/dL (6.4 mmol/L), with a range of 84 to 132 mg/dL (4.7 to 7.3 mmol/L) on 26 readings taken over the past 30 days. Over the past 2 to 3 weeks, he has experienced 2 episodes of nocturnal hypoglycemia based on classic symptoms (he was too groggy to check his fingerstick).

Which of the following is the best test to help inform next steps in management?

A. C-peptide measurement
B. Diagnostic continuous glucose monitoring
C. Glycosylated albumin measurement
D. Insulin antibody assessment

43 A 42-year-old woman with a 33-year history of type 1 diabetes mellitus presents for routine follow-up. She has nonproliferative retinopathy. She takes lisinopril, 5 mg daily, for proteinuria. She has been feeling fatigued.

Her insulin regimen includes insulin detemir twice daily and insulin glulisine with meals. She is having frequent episodes of hypoglycemia that are sometimes, but not always, related to skipped meals. She is not sleeping well and sometimes awakens with low blood glucose levels. She has adjusted her basal insulin dosage down in 10% decrements several times, but she is still having frequent hypoglycemia. Her lifestyle regimen has not changed. She also reports becoming lightheaded when she stands up quickly.

On physical examination, her weight is 139 lb (63.2 kg) (BMI = 22 kg/m^2). When supine, her blood pressure is 124/74 mm Hg and pulse rate is 84 beats/min; when standing, her blood pressure is 91/68 mm Hg and pulse rate is 106 beats/min. Findings on cardiorespiratory examination are otherwise unremarkable. Neurologic examination reveals hyperesthesia at the foot compared with the knee on 1-g monofilament testing and mild delayed ankle reflex recovery.

Pertinent nonfasting laboratory test results:

- Serum sodium = 133 mg/dL (136-142 mEq/L) (SI: 133 mmol/L [136-142 mmol/L])
- Potassium = 4.7 mEq/L (3.5-5.0 mEq/L) (SI: 4.7 mmol/L [3.5-5.0 mmol/L])
- Creatinine = 0.9 mg/dL (0.6-1.1 mg/dL) (SI: 79.6 μmol/L [53.0-97.2 μmol/L])
- Urinary albumin-to-creatinine ratio = 35 mg/g creat (<30 mg/g creat)
- TSH = 8.2 mIU/L (0.5-5.0 mIU/L)
- Hemoglobin A_{1c} = 7.8% (4.0%-5.6%) (62 mmol/mol [20-38 mmol/mol])

Which of the following is the most likely cause of her orthostatic hypotension?

A. Adrenal insufficiency
B. Cardiovascular autonomic neuropathy
C. Hypothyroidism
D. Gitelman syndrome
E. Sensorimotor neuropathy

44 A 76-year-old woman with a 29-year history of type 2 diabetes mellitus is referred for glycemic management. She has no microvascular complications, but she had a myocardial infarction 8 years ago. Her hemoglobin A_{1c} levels in the past 6 years have ranged from 8.5% to 9.0% (69-75 mmol/mol). She is not bothered by nocturia.

Over the years, her medication regimen has been adjusted several times mainly due to high out-of-pocket costs and she has settled on twice-daily NPH insulin. She takes NPH insulin, 24 units twice daily, before breakfast and her evening meal. Once-daily glucose monitoring shows fasting values ranging from 97 to 257 mg/dL (5.4-14.3 mmol/L). She reports waking overnight several times monthly with nightmares and wanting to snack. Based on her age and comorbidities, a hemoglobin A_{1c} target of 7.5% (58 mmol/mol) is recommended if achievable without significant hypoglycemia.

Which of the following adjustments to her regimen is most likely to enable attainment of the glycemic control goals?

A. Add 6 units of regular insulin before meals and stop glipizide
B. Add a bedtime snack to her regimen
C. Decrease the evening dose of NPH insulin to 20 units and give it at bedtime
D. Increase the morning and evening insulin doses to 28 units
E. Increase the predinner NPH insulin dose to 28 units

45 A 57-year-old woman was diagnosed with type 2 diabetes mellitus 6 months ago. Other conditions include hypertension, hyperlipidemia, hypothyroidism, and atherosclerotic heart disease that required single-vessel stent placement 2 years ago. Since her diagnosis, she has taken metformin, 500 mg twice daily, without significant adverse effects. She is concerned that metformin may have a negative effect on her kidneys. Other medications include lisinopril, 30 mg daily; metoprolol, 100 mg daily; aspirin, 325 mg daily; rosuvastatin, 20 mg daily; and levothyroxine, 112 mcg daily.

She is comfortable at rest and can do her daily walk, although on occasion she feels fatigued after 10 minutes and needs to stop. Recent echocardiography shows an ejection fraction of 42%.

On physical examination, her blood pressure is 122/78 mm Hg and pulse rate is 78 beats/min. Her BMI is 27 kg/m^2. She appears comfortable. Her heart rhythm is normal, and lungs are clear to auscultation. The rest of the examination findings are unremarkable.

Laboratory test results:

Hemoglobin A_{1c} = 6.7% (4.0%-5.6%) (50 mmol/mol [20-38 mmol/mol])
Creatinine = 1.2 mg/dL (0.6-1.1 mg/dL) (SI: 106.1 μmol/L [53.0-97.2 μmol/L])
Estimated glomerular filtration rate = 58 mL/min per 1.73 m^2 (>60 mL/min per 1.73 m^2)
Urinary albumin-to-creatinine ratio = 12 mg/g creat (<30 mg/g creat)

Which of the following should be recommended for antidiabetes management?

A. Add empagliflozin, 10 mg daily
B. Add tirzepatide, 2.5 mg once weekly
C. Increase the metformin dosage to 1000 mg twice daily
D. Replace metformin with semaglutide, 3 mg once daily
E. Recommend no change

46 A 34-year-old man with a history of Graves disease reports episodes of diaphoresis, tachycardia, and tremor over the past 6 months. These episodes typically occur during exercise and are reversed with ingestion of sugary beverages. He is brought to the emergency department after losing consciousness while out jogging. His hyperthyroidism has been treated with methimazole, and his TSH levels have been normal over the past year. He has no other notable medical history. He has no family members with diabetes or hypoglycemia.

On physical examination, he is lethargic and diaphoretic. His blood pressure is 148/92 mm Hg, and his pulse rate is 108 beats/min. Vitiligo is noted. His thyroid is nonpalpable. The rest of the examination findings are normal.

A blood glucose measurement is documented to be 37 mg/dL (2.1 mmol/L). Results of other routine laboratory tests are normal, including those assessing kidney and hepatic function.

Although all of the following tests may appropriately be part of the evaluation for hypoglycemia, which test is most likely to demonstrate the cause of this patient's hypoglycemic syndrome?

A. Cortisol measurement
B. IGF-2 measurement
C. Insulin autoantibody assessment
D. Metanephrine measurement
E. Urinary sulfonylurea screen

47 A 42-year-old woman has sickle-cell disease and type 2 diabetes. On point-of-care testing, her hemoglobin A_{1c} level is consistently 4.8% (29 mmol/mol) despite suboptimal control of blood glucose levels on metformin, 1000 mg twice daily, and insulin detemir, 40 units at bedtime. Fasting values on home glucose monitoring are 160 to 190 mg/dL (8.9-10.5 mmol/L).

Which of the following tests should be used to assess the adequacy of her glycemic control?

A. 2-Hour postprandial glucose measurement
B. C-peptide measurement
C. Fructosamine measurement
D. Laboratory-based hemoglobin A_{1c} measurement
E. Urinary glucose testing

48 A 48-year-old man is self-referred because of concern for metabolic complications due to his progressive weight gain. He has gained a total of 20 lb (9.1 kg) over the past 5 years since he started antiretroviral therapy for HIV infection. He has a history of hypertension and dyslipidemia. His medications include rosuvastatin, amlodipine, and a combined antiretroviral regimen.

On physical examination, his BMI is 32 kg/m^2 and blood pressure is 135/86 mm Hg. He has truncal obesity and no cushingoid features.

In addition to checking his lipid profile and ordering other pertinent tests, which of the following should be measured as the best method to screen him for diabetes?

A. C-peptide
B. Fasting glucose
C. Fructosamine
D. Glutamic acid decarboxylase 65 antibodies
E. Hemoglobin A_{1c}

49 A 65-year-old woman presents for follow-up regarding diabetes management. She is accompanied by her daughter who is concerned about the patient's worsening gait problem. Type 2 diabetes was diagnosed 15 years ago. She was initially treated with metformin but more antidiabetes agents were added over the years, including basal insulin 4 months ago. Her glucose fingerstick values at home range between 180 and 250 mg/dL (10.0-13.9 mmol/L). She also has a history of hypertension, dyslipidemia, hypothyroidism, and acid reflux.

Her medications include metformin, 1000 mg twice daily; canagliflozin, 300 mg daily; dulaglutide, 3.0 mg weekly; insulin detemir, 20 units at bedtime; desiccated thyroid, 90 mg daily; atorvastatin, 40 mg daily; losartan, 50 mg daily; esomeprazole, 40 mg daily; and biotin, 10 mg daily.

Her review of systems is significant for gait imbalance for the past 6 months. She describes it as unsteadiness leading to several near falls when she gets up at night. She also has numbness and weakness in both lower extremities. She has gained 6 lb (2.7 kg) in the past few months.

On physical examination, her blood pressure is 135/85 mm Hg and BMI is 33 kg/m^2. She has a mildly enlarged, firm, and asymmetric thyroid gland with a slightly bigger left lobe. She has muscle atrophy and loss of pinprick sensation in both feet and loss of Achilles reflexes.

Laboratory test results:

Hemoglobin A_{1c} = 7.6% (4.0%-5.6%) (60 mmol/mol [20-38 mmol/mol])
Estimated glomerular filtration rate = 62 mL/min per 1.73 m^2 (>60 mL/min per 1.73 m^2)
TSH = 8.5 mIU/L (0.5-5.0 mIU/L)
ALT = 33 U/L (10-40 U/L) (SI: 0.55 µkat/L [0.17-0.67 µkat/L])
Hemoglobin = 12.2 g/dL (12.1-15.1 g/dL) (SI: 122 g/L [121-151 g/L])
Serum sodium = 140 mEq/L (136-142 mEq/L) (SI: 140 mmol/L [136-142 mmol/L])
Serum potassium = 4.2 mEq/L (3.5-5.0 mEq/L) (SI: 4.2 mmol/L [3.5-5.0 mmol/L])
Serum calcium = 9.4 mg/dL (8.2-10.2 mg/dL) (SI: 2.4 mmol/L [2.1-2.6 mmol/L])
25-Hydroxyvitamin D = 24 ng/mL (30-80 ng/mL [optimal]) (SI: 59.9 nmol/L [74.9-199.7 nmol/L])

Measuring which of the following would provide a diagnosis to explain her gait imbalance?

A. 8-AM serum cortisol
B. Serum magnesium
C. Serum vitamin B_{12}
D. Time-below-range using continuous glucose monitoring
E. TSH after stopping biotin

50 A 72-year-old homeless man is admitted to the hospital with severe hypoglycemia. He was found unconscious on the street. When brought to the emergency department, his glucose fingerstick concentration was 36 mg/dL (2.0 mmol/L). Blood was drawn, and intravenous dextrose was administered immediately.

His medical history is unknown, and it is not clear whether he is taking any medications.

Laboratory results:

Plasma glucose = 42 mg/dL (70-99 mg/dL) (SI: 2.3 mmol/L [3.9-5.5 mmol/L])
Plasma insulin = 35 µIU/mL (1.4-14.0 µIU/mL) (SI: 243.1 pmol/L [9.7-97.2 pmol/L])
Plasma C-peptide = 1.2 ng/mL (0.9-4.3 ng/mL) (SI: 0.40 nmol/L [0.30-1.42 nmol/L])
Plasma proinsulin = 88.2 pg/mL (26.5-176.4 pg/mL) (SI: 10.0 pmol/L [3.0-20.0 pmol/L])
Plasma β-hydroxybutyrate = 12.5 mg/dL (<3.0 mg/dL) (SI: 1201 µmol/L [<288 µmol/L])
Insulin antibodies, negative
Estimated glomerular filtration rate = 85 mL/min per 1.73 m^2 (>60 mL/min per 1.73 m^2)
TSH = 2.5 mIU/L (0.5-5.0 mIU/L)

Which of the following most likely explains the laboratory findings?

A. Adrenal insufficiency
B. Glipizide
C. Hepatic failure
D. IGF-2–secreting tumor
E. NPH insulin

51 An 82-year-old woman with a 6-year history of type 2 diabetes mellitus is referred for recurrent hypoglycemic events. She has not been able to tolerate metformin, SGLT-2 inhibitors, or GLP-1 receptor agonists. Her current diabetes treatment regimen consists of insulin degludec, 30 units at bedtime; alogliptin, 25 mg daily; and nateglinide, 120 mg before meals. She measures her blood glucose 3 times daily. Over the past few weeks, she has documented several blood glucose values less than 50 mg/dL (<2.8 mmol/L) before and after meals, but she has not felt any symptoms of hypoglycemia. Her hemoglobin A_{1c} level is 6.2% (44 mmol/mol).

Results from blood chemistries, urinalysis, and liver function tests are within normal limits.

Which of the following is the best next step in this patient's care?

Answer	Insulin degludec	Nateglinide	Alogliptin
A.	Decrease to 20 units at bedtime	Continue	Discontinue
B.	Decrease to 20 units at bedtime	Discontinue	Continue
C.	Replace with 30 units of insulin detemir	Discontinue	Discontinue
D.	Replace with 10 units of twice-daily NPH insulin	Discontinue	Continue

52 A 32-year-old man has a 20-year history of type 1 diabetes mellitus and is concerned about his risk for developing long-term complications, particularly nephropathy, because his father died of end-stage diabetic kidney disease in the setting of type 2 diabetes. There are multiple family members with type 2 diabetes and heart disease. A recent fundoscopic exam documented absence of retinopathy. He uses insulin pump therapy integrated with continuous glucose monitoring. Over the last 90 days, his time-in-range (70-180 mg/dL [3.9-10.0 mmol/L]) was 78%. He maintains a healthy lifestyle, including daily exercise, and follows a Mediterranean diet with minimal to no simple sugars or processed foods.

On physical examination, his blood pressure is 124/82 mm Hg (was 119/78 mm Hg last visit) and pulse rate is 68 beats/min. His BMI is 24 kg/m^2. On foot exam, he has early extinguished sensation of vibration using a 128-Hz tuning fork, and sensation to monofilament is normal in 3 locations on each foot.

Laboratory test results:

Hemoglobin A_{1c} = 6.8% (4.0%-5.6%) (51 mmol/mol [20-38 mmol/mol])
Creatinine = 0.8 mg/dL (0.7-1.3 mg/dL) (SI: 70.7 μmol/L [61.9-114.9 μmol/L])
Estimated glomerular filtration rate = 79 mL/min per 1.73 m^2 (>60 mL/min per 1.73 m^2)
Urinary albumin-to-creatinine ratio = 28 mg/g creat (<30 mg/g creat) (4 months ago = 34 mg/g creat)
LDL cholesterol = 168 mg/dL (<100 mg/dL [optimal]) (SI: 4.35 mmol/L [<2.59 mmol/L])
HDL cholesterol = 34 mg/dL (>60 mg/dL [optimal]) (SI: 0.88 mmol/L [>1.55 mmol/L])
Triglycerides = 172 mg/dL (<150 mg/dL [optimal]) (SI: 2.03 mmol/L [<1.94 mmol/L])
Vitamin B_{12} = 140 pg/mL (180-914 pg/mL)

Which of the following medications should be considered to reduce his overall risk of diabetes-related complications?

A. ACE inhibitor
B. Atorvastatin
C. SGLT-2 inhibitor
D. Valsartan
E. Vitamin B_{12}

Female Reproduction Board Review

Margaret Flynn Lippincott, MD

1 A 28-year-old woman with a history of depression presents for evaluation of possible hormonal contribution to her mood. Menarche was at age 12 years, and her cycles are regular. She sees a therapist for mild depression, which started after menarche. She describes bloating, breast tenderness, increased irritability, headache, and worsening mood in the week prior to her period, and she finds these symptoms interfere with her work and personal life. The symptoms resolve with the onset of her period. She does not feel depressed during other times of the month. She has no family history of clotting disorders.

Which of the following is the first-line treatment recommendation?

A. Acupuncture
B. Continuous low-dose oral contraceptive pill
C. Exercise at least 30 minutes 3 days a week
D. GnRH agonist, such as leuprolide
E. Selective serotonin reuptake inhibitor

2 A 39-year-old woman with a fragile X premutation seeks advice regarding treatment of hot flushes. She underwent normal menarche and had regular menses until 1 year ago when she noted some irregularity. Her last menstrual period was 3 months ago. She reports intractable hot flushes at night, as well as during the day. Her sleep is poor, and she is having trouble functioning at work. She has no personal or family history of breast cancer or venous thromboembolism. She and her husband have a son with fragile X syndrome and have completed family building. Findings on physical examination are normal, and her BMI is 24 kg/m^2.

Which of the following regimens would be best for managing her perimenopausal symptoms?

A. Continuous low-dose oral contraceptive pill
B. Gabapentin, 300 mg nightly
C. Low-dose transdermal estradiol patch
D. Oral 17β-estradiol, 2 mg daily, and cyclic micronized progesterone, 200 mg
E. Transdermal estradiol patch (100 mcg) and daily micronized progesterone (100 mcg)

3 A 23-year-old woman with a history of polycystic ovary syndrome presents to discuss management. Menarche was at age 11 years, and she initially presented for evaluation at age 13 years for hirsutism, acne, and irregular menstrual cycles. She has a family history of hypertension and type 2 diabetes mellitus. She has been on a combined estrogen-progestin contraceptive for the past 5 years. She thinks that acne and hair growth are well controlled. On review of systems, she reports fatigue. On review of her medical record, her weight has increased from 160 to 192 lb (73 to 87 kg) over the past year. Six months ago, her hemoglobin A_{1c} value was 5.6% (38 mmol/mol).

On physical examination, her BMI is 32 kg/m^2, waist circumference is 31 in (78.7 cm), and blood pressure is 125/80 mm Hg. She has terminal hair on her upper lip and mild acne. She has white striae on her thighs.

Laboratory test results:

Triglycerides = 142 mg/dL (<150 mg/dL [optimal] (SI: 1.60 mmol/L [<1.70 mmol/L])
HDL cholesterol = 90 mg/dL (>60 mg/dL [optimal]) (SI: 2.33 mmol/L [>1.55 mmol/L])
Hematocrit = 45% (35%-45%) (SI: 0.45 [0.35-0.45])
FIB-4 score = 1.2

In addition to recommending lifestyle changes for weight loss, which of the following is the most important next step?

A. AST and ALT measurement
B. Late-night salivary cortisol measurement
C. Metformin initiation
D. Sleep study
E. Spironolactone initiation

4 A 43-year-old woman presents for follow-up of premenstrual dysphoric disorder. Her symptoms have not been relieved from continuous oral contraceptive pills, estradiol therapy, or selective serotonin reuptake inhibitors. She continues to experience severe premenstrual dysphoric disorder. In the week preceding her menses, she reports mood swings, increased irritability, increased crying, feelings of worthlessness, fatigue, episodes of binge eating, and trouble concentrating. She often calls in sick to work for at least 1 day leading up to her menses. She has also experienced suicidal ideation without a plan during this period. Given that multiple therapies have been unsuccessful and she does not desire future fertility, she asks whether there are surgical options.

Which of the following strategies would be best help this patient manage her symptoms?

A. GnRH agonist and low-dose continuous estradiol patch
B. GnRH agonist, continuous estradiol patch, and continuous micronized progesterone
C. GnRH agonist, continuous estradiol patch, and cyclic micronized progesterone
D. Surgical oophorectomy and hysterectomy, followed by continuous estradiol patch
E. Surgical oophorectomy and hysterectomy, followed by continuous estradiol patch and micronized progesterone

5 A 58-year-old Black woman presents to discuss management of menopausal symptoms. She reports menopause at age 54 years. She has no history of diabetes, breast cancer, liver disease, blood clots, stroke, or myocardial infarction. She has a remote history of migraine without aura. From age 52 to 57 years, she was on hormone therapy for bothersome vasomotor symptoms. She stopped this treatment 1 year ago because she heard from a friend that hormone therapy should only be taken for 5 years. Since stopping, she reports hot flushes 3 to 5 times per day and night sweats 3 nights per week. She does not sleep well. On review of systems, she endorses dyspareunia and urge incontinence.

On physical examination, her is BMI 29 kg/m^2 and blood pressure is 130/85 mm Hg.

Her American College of Cardiology/American Heart Association 10-year risk of cardiovascular disease is 7.5%. Breast cancer risk assessment indicates that her 5-year National Cancer Institute risk for breast cancer is low.

She wants to know if she can restart hormone therapy (17β-estradiol [1 mg] and progesterone [100 mg] daily).

Which of the following is the best treatment recommendation for this patient?

A. Estradiol patch (50 mcg)
B. Estradiol patch (50 mcg) and progesterone (100 mg) daily
C. Estradiol tablet, 10 mg twice weekly vaginally
D. Gabapentin, 300 mg nightly
E. Oral 17β-estradiol (1 mg) and progesterone (100 mg) daily

6 A 50-year-old perimenopausal woman presents for follow-up regarding menopausal hormone therapy. At her initial visit 4 months ago, she described irregular menses occurring every 45 to 60 days, hot flushes during the day, and night sweats that were disrupting sleep. Menopausal hormone therapy (transdermal estradiol, 0.0375 mg, with micronized progesterone, 200 mg daily, for 12 days a month) was prescribed for relief of her vasomotor symptoms. Although her night sweats have resolved, she continues to have trouble sleeping (difficulty falling asleep, midcycle awakenings). Her only other medication is metformin, 1000 mg daily, with dinner, which was prescribed by her family physician for weight loss.

Which of the following is the most likely contributor to her unresolved sleep disturbance?

A. Anxiety and depression
B. Insufficient hormone therapy
C. Metformin therapy
D. Normal aging
E. Progestin therapy

7 A 20-year-old Hispanic woman presents for evaluation of irregular periods and hirsutism. She had early development of pubic hair at age 7 years. Menarche was at age 11 years. Her cycles have been irregular since then, and she has been treated intermittently with combined oral contraceptives but has been off this treatment for the past year. She is currently having periods every 2 to 3 months. Her last menstrual period was 60 days ago.

On physical examination, her BMI is 29 kg/m^2. She has terminal hair on her chin, upper lip, neck, midsternal region, and upper abdomen. Her Ferriman-Gallwey score is 12. She has no clitoromegaly, acne, or alopecia.

Laboratory test results on day 60 of her menstrual cycle:

LH = 5.0 mIU/mL (1.0-18.0 mIU/mL) (SI: 5.0 IU/L [1.0-18.0 IU/L])
FSH = 4.0 mIU/mL (2.0-12.0 mIU/mL) (SI: 4.0 IU/L [2.0-12.0 IU/L])
Testosterone = 50 ng/dL (8-60 ng/dL) (SI: 1.7 nmol/L [0.3-2.1 nmol/L])
17-Hydroxyprogesterone = 470 ng/dL (<80 ng/dL) (SI: 14.2 nmol/L [<2.42 nmol/L])
DHEA-S = 360 μg/dL (44-332 μg/dL) (SI: 9.76 μmol/L [1.19-9.00 μmol/L])
Prolactin = 18 ng/mL (4-30 ng/mL) (SI: 0.78 nmol/L [0.17-1.30 nmol/L])
TSH = 2.1 mU/L (0.5-5.0 mIU/L)
β-hCG = 2.0 mIU/mL (SI: 2.0 IU/L)

Which of the following is the best treatment for this patient?

A. Dexamethasone
B. Hydrocortisone
C. Metformin
D. Oral contraceptive
E. Spironolactone

8 A 60-year-old woman presents with worsening hirsutism since menopause 5 years earlier. Menarche was at age 12 years, and she always had regular menses. She had 2 uncomplicated pregnancies. She has gained weight over the years, and her BMI is now 35 kg/m^2. She has had increasing hair growth since menopause. More recently, she has noticed some deepening of her voice and enlargement of her clitoris.

On physical examination, she has increased facial hair and hair on her upper abdomen, midsternal area, and upper back (modified Ferriman-Gallwey score is 12 [>8 = hirsutism]). She has female-pattern balding and clitoromegaly (clitoral index 8 × 5 mm = 40 mm^2 [upper limit of normal = 35 mm^2]). Acanthosis nigricans is seen on her elbows, axillae, and neck.

Laboratory test results:

LH = 28.0 mIU/mL (>30.0 mIU/mL [postmenopausal]) (SI: 28.0 IU/L [>30.0 IU/L])
FSH = 32.0 mIU/mL (>30.0 mIU/mL [postmenopausal]) (SI: 32.0 IU/L [>30.0 IU/L])
Testosterone = 300 ng/dL (8-60 ng/dL) (SI: 10.4 nmol/L [0.3-2.1 nmol/L])
DHEA-S = 102 μg/dL (15-157 μg/dL) (SI: 2.77 μmol/L [0.41-4.25 μmol/L])

Which of the following is this patient's most likely diagnosis?

A. Adrenal virilizing tumor
B. Granulosa tumor of the ovary
C. Obesity-induced hyperandrogenism
D. Ovarian hyperthecosis
E. Sertoli-Leydig–cell tumor of the ovary

9 A 32-year-old woman presents with a 6-month history of amenorrhea. She has been in excellent health except for a history of type 1 diabetes mellitus diagnosed at age 28 years. Her glycemic control has been good, with a recent hemoglobin A_{1c} value of 7.0% (53 mmol/mol).

Recently, she has experienced hot flushes and night sweats. Both her mother and maternal aunt had early menopause at age 39 years and 40 years, respectively.

Laboratory test results:

FSH = 90.0 mIU/mL (2.0-12.0 mIU/mL) (SI: 90.0 IU/L [2.0-12.0 IU/L])
Estradiol = <20 pg/mL (10-180 pg/mL) (SI: <73.4 pmol/L [36.7-660.8 pmol/L])
TSH = 3.0 mIU/L (0.5-5.0 mIU/L)
Prolactin = 7 ng/mL (4-30 ng/mL) (SI: 0.30 nmol/L [0.17-1.30 nmol/L])

Which of the following tests is most likely to identify this patient's diagnosis?

A. Antimullerian hormone measurement
B. *FMR1* genetic testing
C. 21-Hydroxylase antibody measurement
D. Karyotype analysis
E. TPO antibody measurement

10 A 28-year-old woman presents with infertility. Menarche was at age 13 years, and she had regular menses during high school and college except for amenorrhea when she ran cross-country. She took an oral contraceptive pill from age 22 to 27 years but stopped 18 months ago to try and conceive. She has Hashimoto thyroiditis and takes a stable dosage of levothyroxine. She has menses every 24 to 25 days. She exercises 3 times per week for 1.5 hours each session. She has mild acne, no hot flushes, and no galactorrhea. Her BMI is 20 kg/m^2.

Laboratory test results from blood samples drawn on cycle day 3:

FSH = 20.0 mIU/mL (2.0-12.0 mIU/mL) (SI: 20.0 IU/L [2.0-12.0 IU/L])
LH = 10.0 mIU/mL (1.0-18.0 mIU/mL) (SI: 10.0 IU/L [1.0-18.0 IU/L])
Estradiol = 28 pg/mL (10-180 pg/mL) (SI: 102.8 pmol/L [36.7-660.8 pmol/L])
Antimullerian hormone = 0.8 ng/mL (0.9-9.5 ng/mL) (SI: 3.6 pmol/L [6.4-67.9 pmol/L])
TSH = 2.1 mIU/L (0.5-5.0 mIU/L)

Which of the following is this patient's most likely diagnosis?

A. Autoimmune oophoritis
B. FSH-secreting pituitary adenoma
C. Functional hypothalamic amenorrhea
D. Polycystic ovary syndrome
E. Primary ovarian insufficiency

11 A 23-year-old woman with an ongoing diagnosis of functional hypothalamic amenorrhea would like to discuss her recent DXA. Her last menstrual period was 2 years ago. Her bone mineral density continues to decline, and her femoral neck Z-score is now −2.2, decreased from −1.9 two years ago. She has no history of fractures. Since her last DXA, she improved her lifestyle by decreasing her amount of running from 80 to 60 miles per week. Her BMI has increased from 17 to 18 kg/m^2.

Which of the following is the best management strategy for improving this patient's bone mineral density?

A. Alendronate, 70 mg orally once weekly
B. Combined oral estrogen-progestin contraceptive (20 mcg ethinyl estradiol with norethindrone acetate 1 mg)
C. Estradiol, 100 mcg twice weekly, with oral micronized progesterone, 200 mg (first 12 days of the month)
D. Improved nutrition and weight gain

12 A 20-year-old woman with Turner syndrome is transitioning care from her pediatrician to an adult provider. She has a history of primary amenorrhea and short stature.

On physical examination, her blood pressure is 140/90 mm Hg. Her height is 56 in (142.2 cm) (BMI = 28 kg/m^2). She is on a combined estrogen-progestin regimen and has been seeing her pediatrician on a yearly basis. Last year, cardiac MRI showed no evidence of aortic dilatation and no significant cardiovascular anomalies.

Past laboratory test results:

FSH = 35.0 mIU/mL (2.0-12.0 mIU/mL)
(SI: 35.0 IU/L [2.0-12.0 IU/L])
LH = 28.0 mIU/mL (1.0-18.0 mIU/mL)
(SI: 28.0 IU/L [1.0-18.0 IU/L])
Estradiol = <10 pg/mL (10-180 pg/mL)
(SI: <36.7 pmol/L [36.7-660.8 pmol/L])
Karyotype = 45,X

Which of the following tests should be ordered today (and at each yearly visit)?

A. Antimullerian hormone measurement, transvaginal ultrasonography
B. Celiac disease screening, electrocardiography, hemoglobin A_{1c} measurement
C. Complete blood cell count, echocardiography, thyroid function tests
D. Hemoglobin A_{1c} measurement, liver enzymes, thyroid function tests
E. Hemoglobin A_{1c} measurement, kidney ultrasonography, liver enzymes

13 A 19-year-old woman seeks evaluation because she has still not had a period. She experienced normal growth and development, similar to that of her peers. She recalls developing axillary and pubic hair at about age 10 years and breast development at age 12 years. She has never been sexually active and has no other medical problems. She sometimes experiences cyclic mood changes, but she has never had pelvic pain. She has had minimal facial acne in the past and no hirsutism. A physical examination done by her pediatrician documented normal external genitalia, normal axillary and pubic hair, and Tanner stage 5 breast development. Her height is 69 in (175.3 cm), and weight is 135 lb (61.2 kg) (BMI = 19.9 kg/m^2).

Laboratory test results:

LH = 6.0 mIU/mL (SI: 6.0 IU/L)
FSH = 7.0 mIU/mL (SI: 7.0 IU/L)
Estradiol = 55 pg/mL (SI: 202 pmol/L)
Prolactin = 14 ng/mL (4-30 ng/mL)
(SI: 0.61 nmol/L [0.17-1.30 nmol/L])
Testosterone = 30 ng/dL (8-60 ng/dL)
(SI: 1.0 nmol/L [0.3-2.1 nmol/L])

After 10 days of micronized progesterone, 200 mg daily, she has no withdrawal bleed. A course of estrogen followed by progestin still does not result in a withdrawal bleed. Pelvic ultrasonography is ordered.

Which of the following is the most likely finding on pelvic ultrasonography?

A. Absent uterus
B. Absent uterus and ovaries
C. Intrauterine adhesions
D. Streak ovaries
E. Transverse vaginal septum

14 A 35-year-old woman with polycystic ovary syndrome presents for follow-up. She has a history of oligomenorrhea with heavy bleeding, severe hirsutism, and obesity. She has been on a combined estrogen-progestin oral contraceptive containing 35 mcg ethinyl estradiol. During a ski trip 9 months ago, she sustained a traumatic femur fracture that required surgical repair. Her recovery was complicated by a deep venous thrombosis. Her combined oral contraceptive was discontinued during hospitalization, and she notes that her facial hair has become much worse, which she finds very distressing. This is her second provoked deep venous thrombosis, but she has no family history of deep venous thrombosis, pulmonary embolism, or stroke. A hypercoagulability panel done during hospitalization showed no evidence of a thrombophilia. She is worried about her future risk of deep venous thrombosis.

On physical examination, her BMI is 30 kg/m^2. She has moderate to severe facial hirsutism. Her modified Ferriman-Gallwey score is 16 (hirsutism defined by a score >8).

Which of the following is the best next step in this patient's management?

A. Continue oral contraceptive, but decrease the ethinyl estradiol dose to 20 mcg
B. Recommend nonhormonal form of contraception and metformin
C. Recommend oral progestin-only contraceptive
D. Recommend progestin intrauterine device and spironolactone
E. Switch to estrogen-progestin contraceptive patch

15 A 35-year-old transgender woman is admitted to the hospital with acute pancreatitis. Hypertriglyceridemia was diagnosed when she was in her late teens. She was prescribed rosuvastatin and fenofibrate, but she has not taken her medications consistently. She has been treated with conjugated equine estrogens, 1.25 mg daily, and spironolactone, 100 mg twice daily, since age 18 years when she started living as a woman. In her late 20s, she had breast augmentation and facial feminization surgery. She does not smoke cigarettes.

Laboratory test results (sample drawn while fasting):

Total testosterone = 125 ng/dL (SI: 4.3 nmol/L)
Estradiol = 25 pg/mL (SI: 91.8 pmol/L)
Triglycerides = 1050 mg/dL (<150 mg/dL [optimal]) (SI: 11.87 mmol/L [<1.70 mmol/L])
Glucose = 90 mg/dL (70-99 mg/dL) (SI: 5.0 mmol/L [3.9-5.5 mmol/L])
Lipase = 640 IU/L (<160 IU/L) (SI: 10.7 μkat/L [<2.7 μkat/L])

Following discontinuation of hormone therapy, her triglyceride concentration decreased to 380 mg/dL (4.29 mmol/L). During the consultation, the patient expresses a keen desire to resume gender-affirming hormone therapy.

Which of the following is the most appropriate management option for this patient's gender dysphoria following discharge from the hospital?

A. Resume spironolactone and add finasteride, 5 mg
B. Resume spironolactone and switch her estrogen regimen to ethinyl estradiol
C. Resume spironolactone but remain off conjugated equine estrogen
D. Switch her regimen to a GnRH agonist with a 0.05-mg estradiol patch
E. Tell the patient that she is not a candidate for any further hormone therapy

16 A 21-year-old transgender woman calls to discuss her hormone regimen for gender dysphoria. She started this treatment 6 months earlier, and it consists of monthly injections of the GnRH agonist leuprolide, 3.75 mg intramuscularly, and a 17β-estradiol patch, 0.1 mg twice weekly. Her estrogen dosage was increased from 0.075 mg 6 weeks ago. Her estradiol concentration is now 150 pg/mL (551 pmol/L) with a testosterone concentration of 22 ng/dL (0.76 nmol/L). She has noticed a significant decrease in facial and body hair but would like to see more breast development. At her last physical examination, her BMI was 30 kg/m^2 and she had Tanner stage 3 breast development.

Which of the following is the best next step in this patient's management?

A. Continue current regimen
B. Continue current regimen and add spironolactone, 50 mg twice daily
C. Continue leuprolide but increase the dosage of estradiol patch to 0.2 mg twice weekly
D. Continue leuprolide but switch from the estradiol patch to an oral contraceptive pill containing 35 mcg of ethinyl estradiol
E. Refer for breast augmentation

Male Reproduction Board Review

Stephanie Page, MD, PhD

1 A 24-year-old transgender man states that he consistently administers biweekly testosterone injections (150 mg testosterone cypionate every 2 weeks) and yet he is continuing to menstruate after 5 months of gender-affirming therapy. He finds this troubling, and he is also not yet satisfied with the physical changes he is experiencing, which include acne and increased facial, chest, and leg hair. He is sexually active with his cis-male partner.

Laboratory test results obtained just prior to his scheduled testosterone dose:

Hemoglobin = 17.1 g/dL (13.8-17.2 g/dL) (SI: 171 g/L [138-172 g/L])
Hematocrit = 50% (41%-51%) (SI: 0.50 [0.41-0.51])
Total testosterone = 330 ng/dL (300-900 ng/dL) (SI: 11.5 nmol/L [10.4-31.2 nmol/L])
Free testosterone = 12.0 ng/dL (9.0-30.0 ng/dL) (SI: 0.42 nmol/L [0.31-1.04 nmol/L])

On physical examination, he has mild acne on his forehead at the midline and over his back, scant facial hair at the chin line and above his upper lip, and acne at the midline of his anterior chest. His voice seems unchanged.

Which of the following is the most appropriate next step to address his concerns?

A. Add anastrozole, 1 mg daily
B. Add medroxyprogesterone, 5 mg daily
C. Decrease testosterone dosage to 125 mg every 2 weeks
D. Increase testosterone dosage to 200 mg every 2 weeks
E. Initiate once-monthly phlebotomy

2 A 68-year-old man is referred by his primary care physician for concerns regarding erectile function and libido. He has noted these changes gradually over the last few years. He no longer has morning erections and now is noting erectile dysfunction sometimes during intercourse. His referring provider measured serum total testosterone, which was 175 ng/dL (6.1 nmol/L).

His medical history is noteworthy for a myocardial infarction 4 years ago with 3 stents placed after which he was started on a high-dosage atorvastatin, 80 mg daily; lisinopril, 20 mg daily for hypertension; and metformin, 1000 mg twice daily for insulin resistance; and nitroglycerin as needed. Since his cardiac event, he has lost 20 lb (9.1 kg), improved his diet, and increased his exercise capacity. He fractured his wrist a year ago when he slipped on ice, and he has since been using an exercise bike 30 to 45 minutes 5 times per week. He has no history of blood clots.

On physical examination, his blood pressure is 130/80 mm Hg and pulse rate is 80 beats/min. His BMI is 32 kg/m^2. He has a normal male hair pattern. There is central adiposity and 2-cm gynecomastia bilaterally. Findings on genitourinary exam are normal, and testes are 15 mL bilaterally.

Laboratory test results (sample drawn in the morning while fasting):

LH = 11.0 mIU/mL (1.0-9.0 mIU/mL) (SI: 11.0 IU/L [1.0-9.0 IU/L])
FSH = 14.0 mIU/mL (1.0-13.0 mIU/mL) (SI: 14.0 IU/L [1.0-13.0 IU/L])
Total testosterone = 185 ng/dL (300-900 ng/dL) (SI: 6.4 nmol/L [10.4-31.2 nmol/L])
Calculated free testosterone = 8.2 ng/dL (9.0-30.0 ng/dL) (SI: 0.28 nmol/L [0.31-1.04 nmol/L])

Total cholesterol = 150 mg/dL (<200 mg/dL [optimal]) (SI: 3.89 mmol/L [<5.18 mmol/L])
LDL cholesterol = 48 mg/dL (<100 mg/dL [optimal]) (SI: 1.24 mmol/L [<2.59 mmol/L])
HDL cholesterol = 32 mg/dL (>60 mg/dL [optimal]) (SI: 0.83 mmol/L [>1.55 mmol/L])
Triglycerides = 180 mg/dL (<150 mg/dL [optimal]) (SI: 2.03 mmol/L [<1.70 mmol/L])
Hemoglobin A_{1c} = 7.2% (4.0%-5.6%) (55 mmol/mol [20-38 mmol/mol])

Which of the following is the best next step in this patient's management?

A. Council regarding the importance of exercise and weight loss and see him back for evaluation in 3 months
B. Initiate phosphodiesterase inhibitor therapy for erectile dysfunction
C. Initiate transdermal testosterone gel plus anastrozole, 1 mg daily
D. Initiate testosterone transdermal gel
E. Switch statin to a PCSK9 inhibitor and re-measure testosterone in 2 months

3 A couple is referred for infertility with failure to conceive over 18 months. The female partner, age 36 years, is cycling regularly and has undergone a complete evaluation by her obstetrician/gynecologist and is healthy and fertile. The male partner, age 50 years, is in good health and takes only hydrochlorothiazide for essential hypertension and duloxetine for depression (a serotonin and norepinephrine reuptake inhibitor). He has had no surgeries and has no sexual concerns; he has not fathered a pregnancy that he is aware of. The couple has regular intercourse timed to her cycle.

The male partner reports normal puberty at age 15 years, no history of genitourinary trauma, normal sexual development, and no current or previous use of androgens.

On physical examination, he has normal male-pattern hair. His BMI is 26 kg/m^2. He has no gynecomastia, a normal phallus, testicular volume of 18 mL bilaterally, and no varicocele.

Laboratory test results:
LH = 4.0 mIU/mL (1.0-9.0 mIU/mL) (SI: 4.0 IU/L [1.0-9.0 IU/L])
FSH = 6.0 mIU/mL (1.0-13.0 mIU/mL) (SI: 6.0 IU/L [1.0-13.0 IU/L])
Total testosterone = 380 ng/dL (300-900 ng/dL) (SI: 13.2 nmol/L [10.4-31.2 nmol/L])
Calculated free testosterone = 12 ng/dL (9.0-30.0 ng/dL) (SI: 0.42 nmol/L [0.31-1.04 nmol/L])
Comprehensive metabolic panel, normal

Semen analysis:
Volume = 2.4 mL (≥ 1.5 mL)
Sperm concentration = 25 million/mL of ejaculate (≥15 million/mL)
Morphology = 4% normal forms (≥4%)
Motility = 5% total motility (≥40%)

Which of the following is the best next step for this couple pursuing fertility?

A. Refer to assisted reproductive endocrinologist for intracytoplasmic sperm injection
B. Refer to assisted reproductive endocrinologist for testicular sperm extraction followed by intracytoplasmic sperm injection
C. Treat with subcutaneous hCG 1000 units 3 times weekly and repeat semen analysis in 3 months
D. Treat with testosterone gel for 3 months and repeat semen analysis
E. Work with his mental health team to discontinue duloxetine and repeat semen analysis in 3 months

4 A 34-year-old man is referred for consideration of testosterone therapy. He states that he has been regularly engaged in strength training at his local gym for 5 years and has noted in the last year that he has plateaued in his musculature and weight maximums in comparison with his peers. He also has noted mild breast tenderness. He has normal sexual function and morning erections but a mild decrease in libido that he attributes to changes in his body image. He has a normal reproductive history. He eats a high-protein, mostly plant-based diet. He lives with his wife of 10 years and their 2 children aged 9 and 7 years. He takes no medications.

On physical examination, his blood pressure is 150/90 mm Hg and pulse rate is 80 beats/min. His BMI is 26 kg/m^2. He is muscular with 1-cm gynecomastia bilaterally and normal male-pattern hair on his face and chest. He has mild acne on his chest. Testicular volume is 20 mL bilaterally with no masses, and his phallus is normal.

Laboratory test results:

- Hematocrit = 50% (41%-51%) (SI: 0.50 [0.41-0.51])
- Total testosterone = 600 ng/dL (300-900 ng/dL) (SI: 20.8 nmol/L [10.4-31.2 nmol/L])
- Calculated free testosterone = 26 ng/dL (9.0-30.0 ng/dL) (SI: 0.90 nmol/L [0.31-1.04 nmol/L])
- LH = 0.1 mIU/mL (1.0-9.0 mIU/mL) (SI: 0.1 IU/L [1.0-9.0 IU/L])
- Prolactin = 5 ng/mL (4-23 ng/mL) (SI: 0.22 nmol/L [0.17-1.00 nmol/L])
- TSH = 0.9 mIU/L (0.5-5.0 mIU/L)
- Ferritin, normal
- Total cholesterol = 220 mg/dL (<200 mg/dL [optimal]) (SI: 5.70 mmol/L [<5.18 mmol/L])
- LDL cholesterol = 180 mg/dL (<100 mg/dL [optimal]) (SI: 4.66 mmol/L [<2.59 mmol/L])
- HDL cholesterol = 50 mg/dL (>60 mg/dL [optimal]) (SI: 1.30 mmol/L [>1.55 mmol/L])
- Triglycerides = 135 mg/dL (<150 mg/dL [optimal]) (SI: 1.53 mmol/L [<1.70 mmol/L])

Which of the following is the most likely explanation for these findings?

A. Erythropoietin ("epo") abuse
B. Oral androstenedione abuse
C. Oral enclomifene abuse
D. Pituitary microadenoma
E. Subcutaneous hCG abuse

5 A 29-year-old transgender man is referred for gender-affirming hormone therapy. He meets criteria for initiation of care and has a mental health provider. He currently takes no medications and is having regular menses. He is up to date on health care maintenance (last Papanicolaou test 2 years ago, vaccinated), has no history of fracture, and has a family history of breast cancer (aunt). He is currently sexually active with a cis-male partner.

Testosterone enanthate, 200 mg intramuscular injections every 2 weeks, is initiated, and he is counseled regarding the importance of continuing contraception since he wishes to avoid pregnancy. He returns after 6 months of therapy and is pleased that he has had cessation of menses, some male-pattern hair growth, and increases in upper body musculature. He would like his voice to deepen and does not feel this has happened. He has some acne on his back. He is taking no new medications.

Laboratory test results (1 week following his last testosterone injection):

- Hematocrit = 40% (41%-51%) (SI: 0.40 [0.41-0.51])
- Total testosterone = 400 ng/dL (300-900 ng/dL) (SI: 13.9 nmol/L [10.4-31.2 nmol/L])
- Calculated free testosterone = 13.0 ng/dL (9.0-30.0 ng/dL) (SI: 0.45 nmol/L [0.31-1.04 nmol/L])

A follow-up appointment is scheduled in 6 months. Follow-up care at that time should include which of the following?

A. DXA
B. Mammography
C. Papanicolaou test
D. Serum estradiol serum measurement
E. Serum free testosterone measurement

6 A 20-year-old college sophomore is referred because of a decrease in sex drive, difficulty getting and sustaining an erection, and low total testosterone noted on initial evaluation (200 ng/dL [6.9 nmol/L]). He reports going through puberty at the same time as his peers. He had been feeling depressed due to academic pressures and was prescribed paroxetine, 20 mg daily. He finds that exercising up to 2 hours per day helps to alleviate his stress, and he has recently lost about 8.8 lb (4 kg). He eats what he reports to be a very healthy, vegan diet.

On physical examination, he is a fit, muscular man with a BMI of 20 kg/m^2. He is normally virilized and has no gynecomastia. Testicular volume is 15 mL bilaterally, and he has a right-sided hydrocele.

Laboratory test results:

- Testosterone = 155 ng/dL (300-900 ng/dL) (SI: 5.4 nmol/L [10.4-31.2 nmol/L])
- LH = 1.2 mIU/mL (1.0-9.0 mIU/mL) (SI: 1.2 IU/L [1.0-9.0 IU/L])
- FSH = 3.0 mIU/mL (1.0-13.0 mIU/mL) (SI: 3.0 IU/L [1.0-13.0 IU/L])
- Prolactin = 12 ng/mL (4-23 ng/mL) (SI: 0.52 nmol/L [0.17-1.00 nmol/L])
- Hemoglobin = 12.8 g/dL (13.8-17.2 g/dL) (SI: 128 g/L [138-172 g/L])
- Hematocrit = 39.8% (41%-51%) (SI: 0.39 [0.41-0.51])
- Leptin = <0.6 ng/mL (0.7-5.3 ng/mL)

Findings on pituitary MRI are normal.

Which of the following is the most likely cause of this patient's hypogonadism?

A. Anabolic steroid use
B. Congenital leptin deficiency
C. Functional hypogonadotropic hypogonadism
D. Hydrocele
E. Kallmann syndrome

7 A 19-year-old man is referred for evaluation following a new diagnosis of Kallmann syndrome based on his inability to smell, lack of any secondary sex characteristics, and hypogonadotropic hypogonadism. His family history is notable for a 10-year-old brother who is also anosmic and a maternal uncle with Kallmann syndrome. Genetic testing identifies a pathogenic variant in the *ANOS1* gene (formerly known as *KAL1*).

Which of the following features is most likely to be present on this patient's physical examination?

A. Axillary freckling
B. Coloboma
C. Short fourth metacarpal
D. Syndactyly
E. Synkinesia

8 A 64-year-old man presents for evaluation of a 3-month history of fatigue. His history is notable for migraine headaches for which he has been prescribed topiramate, 50 mg twice daily. He is a former alcoholic and has been sober for 10 years. He has type 2 diabetes mellitus and takes metformin, 1000 mg twice daily.

On physical examination, his BMI is 30.5 kg/m^2. He is well virilized. His thyroid is firm to palpation. He has no stigmata of chronic liver disease.

Laboratory test results:

- Testosterone = 350 ng/dL (300-900 ng/dL) (SI: 12.1 nmol/L [10.4-31.2 nmol/L])
- SHBG = 1.8 μg/mL (1.1-6.7 μg/mL) (SI: 16 nmol/L [10-60 nmol/L])
- TSH = 25.0 mIU/mL (0.5-5.0 mIU/L)
- Free T_4 = 0.5 ng/mL (0.8-1.8 ng/dL) (SI: 6.44 pmol/L [10.30-23.17 pmol/L])
- AST = 60 U/L (20-48 U/L) (SI: 1.00 μkat/L [0.33-0.80 μkat/L])
- ALT = 58 U/L (10-40 U/L) (SI: 0.97 μkat/L [0.17-0.67 μkat/L])
- Hemoglobin A_{1c} = 7.8% (4.0%-5.6%) (62 mmol/mol [20-38 mmol/mol])

Which of the following is the most likely cause of this patient's SHBG level?

A. Hyperestrogenemia
B. Hypothyroidism
C. Liver disease
D. Obesity
E. Topiramate

9 A 39-year-old man with a 20-year history of type 1 diabetes mellitus presents for routine diabetes follow-up. On review of systems, he reports normal libido but some difficulty getting and sustaining erections. He has also noticed that he produces less semen when he ejaculates. He wishes to start a family and has been having regular, unprotected intercourse with his 36-year-old wife for the past 9 months without success.

Laboratory test results:

- Testosterone = 280 ng/dL (300-900 ng/dL) (SI: 9.7 nmol/L [10.4-31.2 nmol/L])
- LH = 3.5 mIU/mL (1.0-9.0 mIU/mL) (SI: 3.5 IU/L [1.0-9.0 IU/L])
- FSH = 6.9 mIU/mL (1.0-13.0 mIU/mL) (SI: 6.9 IU/L [1.0-13.0 IU/L])

Hemoglobin A_{1c} = 9.5% (4.0%-5.6%) (80 mmol/mol [20-38 mmol/mol])
Semen analysis shows a volume of 0.5 mL (normal >1.5 mL) and sperm concentration of 9 million/mL (similar pattern on repeated testing)

Which of the following is the most appropriate next step in this patient's management?

A. Perform a postejaculatory urine analysis for semen
B. Refer to urology for microdissection testicular sperm extraction
C. Start an α-adrenergic blocker
D. Start hCG injections
E. Start testosterone therapy

10 A 33-year-old man with Kallmann syndrome is referred by a colleague for a second opinion on fertility management. He has been treated with hCG, 1000 IU by subcutaneous injection every other day, for 9 months. On this regimen, his testes increased in size from 2 to 4 mL in the first 6 months and have now reached a plateau.

Hormone profile checked on the day his injection is due:
Testosterone = 350 ng/dL (300-900 ng/dL) (SI: 12.1 nmol/L [10.4-31.2 nmol/L])
Estradiol = 40 pg/mL (10-40 pg/mL) (SI: 146.8 pmol/L [36.7-146.8 pmol/L])
LH = 0.6 mIU/mL (1.0-9.0 mIU/mL) (SI: 0.6 IU/L [1.0-9.0 IU/L])
FSH = 1.0 mIU/mL (1.0-13.0 mIU/mL) (SI: 1.0 IU/L [1.0-13.0 IU/L])

Semen analysis shows azoospermia.

Which of the following would be most helpful in improving this patient's fertility?

A. Add FSH, 75 IU daily
B. Increase the dosage of hCG to 1500 IU every other day
C. Switch from hCG to recombinant LH injections
D. Switch his current hCG regimen from every other day to daily
E. Switch to clomiphene citrate, 50 mg daily

11 A 35-year-old man is referred for evaluation of infertility as his 32-year-old wife has not conceived after 12 months of regular, unprotected intercourse. He reports normal libido and erections. He is taking no medications and does not use recreational drugs. His wife has a 4-year-old daughter from a previous relationship and is ovulating according to basal body temperature measurements.

On physical examination, he has normal secondary sexual characteristics and no gynecomastia. Testicular volume is 25 mL bilaterally.

Evaluation shows the following:
Total testosterone = 500 ng/dL (300-900 ng/dL) (SI: 17.4 nmol/L [10.4-31.2 nmol/L])
FSH = 4.4 mIU/mL (1.0-13.0 mIU/mL) (SI: 4.4 IU/L [1.0-11.0 IU/L])
LH = 6.1 mIU/mL (1.0-9.0 mIU/mL) (SI: 6.1 IU/L [1.0-9.0 IU/L])

Seminal fluid analysis:
Volume = 1.3 mL (>1.5 mL)
pH = 6.8 (>7.2)

No sperm are present. A repeated analysis confirms azoospermia.

Which of the following is the most likely cause of this patient's infertility?

A. Anabolic steroid use
B. Congenital bilateral absence of the vas deferens
C. Mosaic Klinefelter syndrome
D. Partial androgen insensitivity syndrome
E. Y-chromosome microdeletions

12 A 37-year-old man presents with a 6-month history of increasing fatigue, loss of libido, and erectile dysfunction. He underwent normal puberty. HIV infection was diagnosed 3 years ago, and his CD4 cell count is currently stable on highly active antiretroviral therapy. He states that he does not use androgens or recreational drugs.

On physical examination, the patient is normally virilized. His BMI is 24.5 kg/m^2. Testicular volume is 15 mL bilaterally.

Laboratory test results:

- Total testosterone (8 AM) (by liquid chromatography tandem mass spectrometry) = 750 ng/dL (300-900 ng/dL) (SI: 30 nmol/L [10.4-31.2 nmol/L]) (repeated measurement = 680 ng/dL [SI: 28.0 nmol/L])
- LH = 5.6 mIU/mL (1.0-13.0 mIU/mL) (SI: 5.6 IU/L [1.0-13.0 IU/L])
- FSH = 6.1 mIU/mL (1.0-9.0 mIU/mL) (SI: 6.1 IU/L [1.0-9.0 IU/L])
- TSH = 2.2 mIU/L (0.5-5.0 mIU/L)
- Hematocrit = 42% (41%-51%) (SI: 0.42 [0.41-0.51])

Which of the following is the best next diagnostic step in this patient's evaluation?

A. Determine the urinary testosterone-to-epitestosterone ratio
B. Measure estradiol
C. Measure free testosterone by equilibrium dialysis
D. Measure serum ferritin
E. Screen for pathogenic variants in the androgen receptor gene

13 An 18-year-old high school senior is referred because of lack of secondary sex characteristics and small testes. He followed the 50th percentile for growth throughout childhood but did not experience a growth spurt in his teenage years. His height is now at the 25th percentile. He has a normal sense of smell. He does not take any prescribed medications. His father, who accompanies him, reports that he himself was also a "late bloomer" but then developed fully and had no problems with fertility.

On physical examination, his height is 66 in (168 cm), arm span is 68.9 in (175 cm), and BMI is 22 kg/m^2. He has slight axillary hair and Tanner stage 2 pubic hair but no facial or chest hair. He has no gynecomastia. His testes measure 2 mL bilaterally. His visual fields are full to confrontation.

Laboratory test results (sample drawn at 8 AM):

- Total testosterone = 50 ng/dL (300-900 ng/dL) (SI: 1.7 nmol/L [10.4-31.2 nmol/L])
- Free T_4 = 1.3 ng/dL (0.8-1.8 ng/dL) (SI: 16.7 pmol/L [10.30-23.17 pmol/L])
- LH = <0.2 mIU/mL (1.0-9.0 mIU/mL) (SI: <0.2 IU/L [1.0-9.0 IU/L])
- FSH = 0.3 mIU/mL (1.0-13.0 mIU/mL) (SI: 0.3 IU/L [1.0-13.0 IU/L])
- Prolactin = 10 ng/mL (4-18 ng/mL) (SI: 0.43 nmol/L [0.17-0.78 nmol/L])
- Cortisol (8 AM) = 20.0 μg/dL (5-25 μg/dL) (SI: 551.8 nmol/L [137.9-689.7 nmol/L])
- IGF-1, low-normal for age and sex

Which of the following is the most likely diagnosis?

A. Congenital hypogonadotropic hypogonadism
B. Constitutional delay of growth and puberty
C. Pathogenic variant in the *POU1F1* gene
D. Pathogenic variant in the *PROP1* gene

14 A 19-year-old male college student presents for evaluation of bilateral breast enlargement, which has been present for 2 years. The breast tissue is no longer growing and the tenderness he initially experienced has waned. However, he has started dating and is embarrassed by the cosmetic appearance. He takes no medications or herbal products. He drinks alcohol on the weekends only (6 drinks in one night) and uses oral edible marijuana approximately twice a month.

On physical examination, the patient is well virilized and has facial acne. Palpation of the breasts reveals rubbery, mobile subareolar tissue with chest hair. There is no nipple discharge or retraction and no palpable masses. Genital exam findings are normal with testes of 15 mL bilaterally and Tanner stage 5 pubic hair.

Laboratory test results:

- Total testosterone = 400 ng/dL (300-900 ng/dL) (SI: 13.9 nmol/L [10.4-31.2 nmol/L])
- Estradiol = 25 pg/mL (10-40 pg/mL) (SI: 91.8 pmol/L [36.7-146.8 pmol/L])
- LH = 3.5 mIU/mL (1.0-13.0 mIU/mL) (SI: 3.5 IU/L [1.0-13.0 IU/L])
- FSH = 4.0 mIU/mL (1.0-9.0 mIU/mL) (SI: 4.0 IU/L [1.0-9.0 IU/L])
- TSH = 1.0 mIU/mL (0.5-5.0 mIU/L)

Which of the following is the most likely diagnosis?

A. Inadvertent estrogen exposure
B. Leydig-cell tumor
C. Marijuana-induced gynecomastia
D. Mosaic Klinefelter syndrome
E. Persistent postpubertal gynecomastia

15 A 70-year-old man was prescribed testosterone therapy by his primary care physician to treat hypogonadism. He had several questions about the risks and benefits of his treatment that his primary care physician was not able to answer to his satisfaction, so he requested a referral to a specialist. He has a history of well-controlled hypertension but is otherwise in good health. He reports nocturia once nightly but no other lower urinary tract symptoms.

On physical examination, his blood pressure is 130/80 mm Hg and BMI is 29 kg/m^2. Rectal examination reveals a mildly enlarged, smooth prostate without nodules.

Laboratory test results:

Hematocrit = 44% (41%-50%) (SI: 0.44 [0.41-0.50])
PSA = 1.7 ng/mL (<5.3 ng/mL) (SI: 1.7 μg/L [<5.3 μg/L])

Which of the following adverse effects should the patient be counseled is most likely to occur if treated with testosterone?

A. Abnormal liver function test results
B. Acute urinary retention
C. Erythrocytosis
D. Increased aggression
E. PSA elevation above 4 ng/mL (>4 μg/L)

16 A 47-year-old man presents with a low-impact rib fracture that occurred when he was leaning on a rake. He describes progressive fatigue, exercise intolerance, trouble concentrating, irritability, weight gain of 15 lb (6.8 kg) (BMI = 28 kg/m^2), and diminished interest in sexual activity over the last year. He currently has no other medical problems and takes no medications, but he did have a kidney stone in his early 20s. There is a family history of osteoporosis in his mother but no history of fractures. He is married and has 2 children.

DXA is performed to assess bone mineral density, and it documents low bone density for age in the lumbar spine. PTH, calcium, and albumin levels are normal. His 25-hydroxyvitamin D level is low at 23 ng/mL (57.4 nmol/L), and vitamin D supplementation is prescribed. Morning testosterone levels are low (2 measurements) at 136 ng/dL (4.7 nmol/L) and 148 ng/dL (5.1 nmol/L).

Laboratory test results:

Total testosterone = 136 ng/dL (SI: 4.7 nmol/L)
LH = 1.3 mIU/mL (1.0-9.0 mIU/mL) (SI: 1.3 IU/L [1.0-9.0 IU/L])
FSH = 1.4 mIU/mL (1.0-13.0 mIU/mL) (SI: 1.4 IU/L [1.0-13.0 IU/L])

Repeated morning laboratory test results:

Total testosterone = 148 ng/dL (SI: 5.1 nmol/L)
LH = 1.5 mIU/mL (SI: 1.5 IU/L)
FSH = 1.0 mIU/mL (SI: 1.0 IU/L)
Prolactin = 12 ng/mL (SI: 0.52 nmol/L)

DXA:

Lumbar spine Z-score = −2.1
Femoral neck Z-score = −1.0
Distal one-third radius Z-score = −1.7

Which of the following tests should be ordered next to diagnose his condition?

A. No further evaluation needed; initiate testosterone therapy
B. Pituitary MRI
C. Semen analysis
D. Testicular ultrasonography
E. Testosterone-to-epitestosterone ratio

Obesity and Lipids Board Review

Sangeeta Kashyap, MD

1 A 59-year-old woman has a family history of premature atherosclerotic cardiovascular disease. Her father had a myocardial infarction at age 48 years. She is taking hydrochlorothiazide, 25 mg daily, for hypertension (average blood pressure at home is 133/68 mm Hg). Since her early 40s, she has taken methotrexate, 12.5 mg once weekly, and glucosamine/chondroitin daily for rheumatoid arthritis. She follows a low-sodium diet and exercises most days by stretching and walking for 30 minutes. She does not drink alcohol and has never smoked cigarettes. Her BMI is 29 kg/m^2.

Laboratory test results:

- Hepatic transaminases, normal
- Serum creatinine, normal
- TSH, normal
- Hemoglobin A_{1c}, normal
- High-sensitivity C-reactive protein = 3.8 mg/L (0.8-3.1 mg/L) (SI: 36.19 nmol/L [7.62-29.52 nmol/L])
- Total cholesterol = 194 mg/dL (<200 mg/dL [optimal]) (SI: 5.02 mmol/L [<5.18 mmol/L])
- HDL cholesterol = 53 mg/dL (>60 mg/dL [optimal]) (SI: 1.37 mmol/L [>1.55 mmol/L])
- Triglycerides = 135 mg/dL (<150 mg/dL [optimal]) (SI: 1.53 mmol/L [<1.70 mmol/L])
- LDL cholesterol = 114 mg/dL (<100 mg/dL [optimal]) (SI: 2.95 mmol/L [<2.59 mmol/L])
- Non–HDL cholesterol = 141 mg/dL (<130 mg/dL [optimal]) (SI: 3.65 mmol/L [<3.37 mmol/L])

Her American College of Cardiology/American Heart Association 10-year atherosclerotic cardiovascular disease risk score is 8%.

Which of the following is the best next step in this patient's management?

A. Baby aspirin daily if the coronary artery calcium score is greater than 50
B. Ezetimibe daily after checking carotid intimal thickness
C. Low-intensity statin daily after measuring LDL particle size and lipoprotein B
D. Moderate-intensity statin daily and aspirin if lipoprotein (a) is elevated

2 A 63-year-old woman takes amlodipine, 5 mg daily, for high blood pressure and has mixed dyslipidemia with the following lipid values:

- LDL cholesterol = 110 mg/dL (<100 mg/dL [optimal]) (SI: 2.85 mmol/L [<2.59 mmol/L])
- HDL cholesterol = 49 mg/dL (>60 mg/dL [optimal]) (SI: 1.27 mmol/L [>1.55 mmol/L])
- Triglycerides = 185 mg/dL (<150 mg/dL [optimal]) (SI: 2.09 mmol/L [<1.70 mmol/L])

She takes pravastatin, 20 mg daily. She "didn't feel good" while on atorvastatin, 40 mg daily, and is hesitant to try a third statin. She also states, "they can cause diabetes," and is concerned that the statin is putting her at higher risk of diabetes because of her family history. Both of her parents developed type 2 diabetes and atherosclerotic cardiovascular disease in their early 60s.

Additional laboratory test results:

- Fasting blood glucose = 101 mg/dL (70-99 mg/dL) (SI: 5.6 mmol/L [3.9-5.5 mmol/L])
- Hemoglobin A_{1c} = 5.9% (4.0%-5.6%) (41 mmol/mol [20-38 mmol/mol])
- Serum creatinine = 1.0 mg/dL (0.6-1.1 mg/dL) (SI: 88.4 μmol/L [53.0-97.2 μmol/L])

Urine analysis, normal
Hepatic transaminases, normal

On physical examination, her blood pressure is 142/86 mm Hg. Her BMI is 31 kg/m^2, and waist circumference is 36 in (91.5 cm).

She has never smoked cigarettes and drinks alcohol occasionally. She walks for an hour twice weekly. Her American College of Cardiology/American Heart Association 10-year atherosclerotic cardiovascular disease risk score is 7.8%.

Which of the following is the best next step in this patient's management?

A. Change pravastatin to fenofibrate, 160 mg daily, and monitor lipids, fasting glucose, and hemoglobin A_{1c} in 6 months
B. Change pravastatin to rosuvastatin twice weekly and monitor fasting glucose and hemoglobin A_{1c} every 6 months
C. Continue pravastatin and monitor fasting glucose and hemoglobin A_{1c} every 6 months
D. Discontinue statin therapy, intensify exercise training, and monitor her lipid profile in 6 months

3 A 56-year-old man with HIV is on antiretroviral therapy and is referred for evaluation of his lipid profile.

Laboratory test results:

Fasting blood glucose = 99 mg/dL (70-99 mg/dL) (SI: 5.5 mmol/L [3.9-5.5 mmol/L])
Hemoglobin A_{1c} = 5.8% (4.0%-5.6%) (40 mmol/mol [20-38 mmol/mol])
Serum creatinine = 1.2 mg/dL (0.7-1.3 mg/dL) (SI: 106.1 µmol/L [61.9-114.9 µmol/L])
Hepatic transaminases, normal
Urine analysis, normal
Total cholesterol = 192 mg/dL (<200 mg/dL [optimal]) (SI: 4.97 mmol/L [<5.18 mmol/L])
HDL cholesterol = 46 mg/dL (>60 mg/dL [optimal]) (SI: 1.19 mmol/L [>1.55 mmol/L])
Triglycerides = 180 mg/dL (<150 mg/dL [optimal]) (SI: 2.03 mmol/L [<1.70 mmol/L])
LDL cholesterol = 110 mg/dL (<100 mg/dL [optimal]) (SI: 2.85 mmol/L [<2.59 mmol/L])
Non–HDL cholesterol = 146 mg/dL (<130 mg/dL [optimal]) (SI: 3.78 mmol/L [<3.37 mmol/L])

The lipid values are similar to those of his last 2 lipid profiles.

He quit cigarette smoking last year (60 pack-year history), and he drinks 2 alcoholic beverages per week. He engages in no formal exercise. He reports taking simvastatin in his 40s but discontinued because of fatigue and myalgias. His American College of Cardiology/American Heart Association 10-year risk score is 7.7%. His family history is complicated by tobacco and alcohol abuse. He is aware of diabetes mellitus and atherosclerotic cardiovascular disease in his family, although details are limited.

On physical examination, his blood pressure is 148/88 mm Hg. A repeated measurement is 146/86 mm Hg (his hypertension has not been treated). His BMI is 29 kg/m^2, and waist circumference is 40 in (101.6 cm).

Which of the following is the best next step in this patient's management?

A. Cholestyramine, 4 packets daily, and once-daily ezetimibe; lipid panel in 6 months
B. Fenofibrate, 160 mg daily; lipid panel in 6 months
C. High-dosage lovastatin daily
D. Low-dosage rosuvastatin twice weekly and titrate up slowly every 6 months
E. Omega-3 fatty acids (icosapent ethyl), 4 mg daily; lipid panel in 6 months

4 A 48-year-old woman underwent gastric bypass 3 years ago for class 3 obesity complicated by obstructive sleep apnea and polycystic ovary syndrome. Her BMI before surgery was 57 kg/m^2, and it dropped to 42 kg/m^2 1 year after surgery. With diet, a structured exercise program, and semaglutide, 1 mg once weekly, she has lost an additional 30 lb (13.6 kg) (current BMI = 33 kg/m^2). She is taking a multivitamin; sublingual B_{12}; and vitamin D_3, 2000 IU (50 mcg) daily. She is experiencing increasing generalized fatigue, brittle nails, cold hands, and some hair thinning.

Which of the following biochemical parameters are the most relevant to monitor at this visit?

A. Bone density, 24-hour urinary calcium, and urinary cortisol
B. Calcium, PTH, and 25-hydroxyvitamin D
C. Complete blood cell count, liver transaminases, iron, ferritin, vitamin B_{12}, and prealbumin
D. Fasting glucose, fasting insulin, and hemoglobin A_{1c}
E. TSH, cortisol, and DHEA-S

5 A 50-year-old woman with a history of binge-eating disorder, gastroesophageal reflux disease, asthma, and iron deficiency anemia returns to the weight management clinic with the concern of weight regain 4 years after Roux-en-Y gastric bypass. Her initial body weight was 389 lb (176.4 kg) (BMI = 65 kg/m^2), and her nadir weight after surgery was 183 lb (83.0 kg) (BMI = 30.5 kg/m^2), which represented a weight loss of 53% of initial weight. During the next 2 years, she was treated with venlafaxine for mild depression. She started to notice hunger and regained 25 lb (11.3 kg) (13% over nadir). Over the next 2 years, she gained another 20 lb (9.1 kg) for a total of 45 lb (20.4 kg) over nadir despite counseling on lifestyle modification.

Now, because of concern for a gastrogastric fistula or other anatomic abnormalities, an upper gastrointestinal series is performed, and findings are normal. After fistula is ruled out, she is prescribed phentermine/topiramate. With the help of intermittent antiobesity medications over the next 3 years, she is able to maintain a stable weight of 240 lb (108.9 kg). However, her weight creeps up to 261 lb (118.4 kg) in the next 2 years, and she is still concerned about hunger and eating larger meal portions. Over the next 3 years, she loses 40 lb (18.1 kg). Her physical activity diminishes because of sciatica and fatigue from iron deficiency, and she gains 29 lb (13.2 kg) over a 6-month interval.

Which of the following factors is most likely contributing to weight regain in this patient?

A. Anemia leading to lack of physical activity
B. Antidepressant therapy
C. Dilation of gastric pouch leading to increase food intake
D. Increased alcohol use
E. Increased grazing and sweets consumption and binge-eating disorder

6 A 46-year-old woman with a 10-year history of type 2 diabetes mellitus with suboptimal glycemic control (despite taking metformin and basal-bolus insulin) comes for evaluation. She has a 10-year history of mixed hyperlipidemia treated with atorvastatin, 40 mg daily, and stable hypertension controlled with lisinopril and hydrochlorothiazide. Her BMI is 32 kg/m^2, and waist circumference is 34 in (86.4 cm). She has a remote history of cigarette smoking and drinks 6 to 8 alcoholic beverages per week. Her hemoglobin A_{1c} level is 7.7% (61 mmol/mol, serum creatinine is normal, and liver function is normal. She would like to follow a Mediterranean meal plan for weight loss and achieve better glycemic control.

Given her risk for nonalcoholic fatty liver disease, a FIB-4 score is calculated, which is 1.7.

Which of the following is the best initial approach in this patient's management?

A. Advise the patient to abstain from alcohol and perform liver ultrasonography in 8 weeks
B. Advise the patient to increase caffeine intake and start vitamin E, 800 IU daily
C. Perform liver elastography and refer her to hepatology for further workup
D. Target weight loss of 3% to 5% and recommend that she follow the DASH diet

7 A 44-year-old man with class 2 obesity, prediabetes, hyperlipidemia, and obstructive sleep apnea is interested in starting a medically supervised, protein-sparing modified meal plan consisting of less than 800 calories daily with very low carbohydrate intake, high protein intake, and low fat intake.

Which of the following are expected outcomes specific to a ketogenic meal plan for this patient?

A. Additional weight loss after refeeding of carbohydrates
B. Dehydration, depletion of potassium, and elevated uric acid levels
C. Elevation of blood pressure related to worsening of insulin sensitivity
D. Worsening of glucose and triglyceride levels

8 A 31-year-old patient with a medical history of class 3 obesity (BMI = 46 kg/m^2), gastroesophageal reflux disease, type 2 diabetes mellitus well controlled on metformin (hemoglobin A_{1c} <5.7% [<39 mmol/mol]), polycystic ovary syndrome, nonalcoholic steatohepatitis, pulmonary and neurosarcoidosis treated with infliximab and methotrexate, and worsening chronic pain presents for weight management evaluation. She has a history of opioid use disorder due to chronic pain, although this is in remission. She has been on several weight-promoting pain medications for symptom control, including gabapentin, duloxetine, and nortriptyline. Contributing factors to her weight gain over the years include antipsychotic medication–induced weight gain. She has a diagnosis of bipolar disorder (previously trialed aripiprazole, responded to lurasidone with decreasing efficiency, and now finally stable on paliperidone, although it is weight-promoting). Her highest adult weight is her current weight of 295 lb (133.8 kg); her lowest adult weight was 140 lb (63.5 kg), which predated her diagnoses of bipolar disorder and sarcoidosis several years ago. She has stable eating patterns, often chooses healthy meals, and exercises regularly at the gym. Recent stressors include her close aunt being diagnosed with cancer. The patient also has insomnia and has been evaluated closely by sleep therapists and sleep hygiene specialists. She has no sleep apnea on polysomnography.

In addition to a 3-month trial of an antiobesity agent, which of the following would be the most appropriate approach for durable weight loss in this patient?

A. Biliopancreatic diversion with duodenal switch
B. Endoscopic balloon
C. Gastric bypass
D. Laparoscopic banding
E. Sleeve gastrectomy

9 A 55-year-old man is referred for management of hyperlipidemia. He has type 2 diabetes mellitus (hemoglobin A_{1c} = 6.6% [49 mmol/mol]), hypertension, and coronary heart disease. He had a non–ST-elevation myocardial infarction 2 years ago. He most likely has heterozygous familial hyperlipidemia given his peak total cholesterol concentration of 382 mg/dL (9.89 mmol/L) and LDL-cholesterol concentration of 293 mg/dL (7.59 mmol/L). He had myalgias while taking atorvastatin, rosuvastatin, and simvastatin. He is currently tolerating pravastatin, 20 mg daily; ezetimibe, 10 mg daily; and niacin, 500 mg daily. He is very concerned about preventing a second cardiovascular disease event.

Laboratory test results:

Total cholesterol = 284 mg/dL (<200 mg/dL [optimal]) (SI: 7.36 mmol/L [<5.18 mmol/L])
LDL cholesterol = 200 mg/dL (<100 mg/dL [optimal]) (SI: 5.18 mmol/L [<2.59 mmol/L])
HDL cholesterol = 55 mg/dL (>60 mg/dL [optimal]) (SI: 1.42 mmol/L [>1.55 mmol/L])
Triglycerides = 300 mg/dL (<150 mg/dL [optimal]) (SI: 3.39 mmol/L [<1.70 mmol/L])

Which of the following is the best next step in this patient's management?

A. Add alirocumab
B. Add fenofibrate
C. Increase niacin dosage to 1 g daily
D. Increase pravastatin dosage to 80 mg daily
E. Perform lipopheresis

10 A 28-year-old woman has lipid levels drawn at a health fair. She is found to have a triglyceride concentration of 525 mg/dL (5.93 mmol/L) and an HDL-cholesterol concentration of 82 mg/dL (2.12 mmol/L). Her LDL-cholesterol level cannot be calculated. She is asymptomatic and has no personal or family history of coronary disease, pancreatitis, or known lipid disorders. She is currently taking an oral contraceptive pill.

Which of the following is the most likely explanation for her lipid levels?

A. Apolipoprotein C2 deficiency
B. Cholesteryl ester transfer protein deficiency
C. Lipoprotein lipase deficiency
D. Oral contraceptive pill use
E. Soy isoflavones

11 A 42-year-old man, who is originally from India, would like to have screening for diabetes mellitus. He is concerned because his mother and father both developed type 2 diabetes later in life. Height is 65 in (165.1 cm), and weight is 168 lb (76.4 kg) (BMI = 28 kg/m^2). His waist circumference is 36.2 in (92 cm). His hip circumference is 30.7 in (78 cm). His waist-to-hip ratio is 0.85.

Regarding his risk of metabolic diseases, on the basis of applicable guidelines, this patient is:

A. At increased risk because his waist circumference is greater than 30 in (>76 cm)
B. At increased risk because his waist circumference is greater than 35.4 in (>90 cm)
C. At increased risk because his waist-to-hip ratio is greater than 0.8
D. Not at increased risk because his BMI is less than 30 kg/m^2
E. Not at increased risk because his waist circumference is less than 40 in (102 cm)

12 A 22-year-old male college student is referred for severe hypertriglyceridemia (>1500 mg/dL [>17.0 mmol/L]). He has a history of pancreatitis. His height is 67 in (170.2 cm), and weight is 185 lb (84.1 kg) (BMI = 29 kg/m^2). He reports that much of this weight gain has occurred in the past 3 years, as he weighed 145 lb (65.9 kg) (BMI = 23 kg/m^2) when he graduated from high school. He usually eats in the school food court—pizzas, burgers, and fries. He does not take any medications or supplements.

Which of the following is the most important immediate lifestyle change to recommend?

A. Avoid alcohol
B. Avoid omega-3 saturated fats
C. Reduce intake of fried foods
D. Reduce intake of noncomplex carbohydrates
E. Substitute fruit juice for soda

13 The mother of an 18-year-old girl is concerned about her daughter's weight and long-term health risks. She tells you that her daughter was always the tallest kid in her class. She gained weight quickly as an infant and toddler and her weight was greater than the 95th percentile by the age of 2 years. She was hungry all the time as a child and struggled with obesity despite being very physically active and playing sports. She performed well academically and had many friends. She went through puberty at age 11 years and has always had regular menses. Her BMI is 36 kg/m^2.

A pathogenic variant in which of the following genes is the most likely cause of obesity in this young woman?

A. Fat mass and obesity-associated protein (*FTO*)
B. Leptin (*LEP*)
C. Leptin receptor (*LEPR*)
D. Melanocortin 4 receptor (*MC4R*)
E. Proopiomelanocortin (*POMC*)

14 A 62-year-old man is referred by his cardiologist for help with weight loss. His medical history is notable for hypertension, type 2 diabetes mellitus, familial combined hyperlipidemia, and coronary artery disease. He had a myocardial infarction 6 months ago complicated by tachyarrhythmias initially but with preserved cardiac function according to transthoracic echocardiography. He just completed a cardiac rehabilitation program. His cardiologist would like him to lose weight to reduce his risk of a second cardiovascular event.

On physical examination, his blood pressure is 156/92 mm Hg and pulse rate is 76 beats/min. His BMI is 63 kg/m². Lungs are clear to auscultation, with no rales. Cardiovascular examination reveals an increased heart rate but no murmurs. He has bilateral edema with a woody quality consistent with venous stasis.

In addition to a diet and exercise program, which of the following medications should be recommended?

A. Liraglutide
B. Naltrexone/bupropion
C. Phentermine extended-release
D. Phentermine/topiramate
E. Tirzepatide

15 A 54-year-old postmenopausal woman presents for medically supervised weight loss with a meal replacement program. Her height is 66 in (167.5 cm), and weight is 188 lb (85.5 kg) (BMI = 30 kg/m²). She has seasonal allergies treated with cetirizine, asthma treated with fluticasone, hypertension treated with atenolol, type 2 diabetes mellitus treated with metformin and glipizide, and hyperlipidemia treated with atorvastatin. Physical examination findings are notable for central adiposity. A review of her current medications reveals that she is on multiple weight-promoting medications.

Of the patient's medications, which of the following is considered weight neutral?

A. Atenolol
B. Atorvastatin
C. Cetirizine
D. Fluticasone
E. Glipizide

16 A 58-year-old man is referred for treatment of high cholesterol in the setting of progressive coronary artery disease despite lipid-lowering therapy after his first myocardial infarction at age 48 years. He has hypertension and type 2 diabetes mellitus and is a former cigarette smoker. His father had his first myocardial infarction at age 52 years, another at 58 years, and a fatal myocardial infarction at 63 years. The patient has been taking atorvastatin, 80 mg daily, but he developed anginal symptoms 3 months ago and had 2 stents placed. His last LDL-cholesterol measurement was 108 mg/dL (2.80 mmol/L). He wants to know what he can do to decrease his risk of another cardiovascular event.

Total cholesterol = 160 mg/dL (<200 mg/dL [optimal]) (SI: 4.14 mmol/L [<5.18 mmol/L])
LDL cholesterol = 95 mg/dL (<100 mg/dL [optimal]) (SI: 2.46 mmol/L [<2.59 mmol/L])
HDL cholesterol = 30 mg/dL (>60 mg/dL [optimal]) (SI: 0.78 mmol/L [>1.55 mmol/L])
Triglycerides = 98 mg/dL (<150 mg/dL [optimal]) (SI: 1.11 mmol/L [<1.70 mmol/L])

Which of the following is the best management strategy?

A. Add bempedoic acid
B. Add evolocumab
C. Add icosapent ethyl
D. Change atorvastatin to rosuvastatin
E. No further treatment

17 A 32-year-old woman is referred because of "low" blood cholesterol levels. She had a bout of abdominal pain several weeks ago and her physician ordered right upper-quadrant ultrasonography, which revealed a fatty liver. She was previously healthy and takes no medications. Her BMI is 25 kg/m². Her physical examination findings are unremarkable. Given her fatty liver disease, her physician ordered a cholesterol panel and a hemoglobin A_{1c} measurement.

Laboratory test results:

Hemoglobin A_{1c} = 5.5% (4.0%-5.6%) (37 mmol/mol [20-38 mmol/mol])
Total cholesterol = 56 mg/dL (<200 mg/dL [optimal]) (SI: 1.45 mmol/L [<5.18 mmol/L])
HDL cholesterol = 24 mg/dL (>60 mg/dL [optimal]) (SI: 0.62 mmol/L [>1.55 mmol/L])
LDL cholesterol = 24 mg/dL (<100 mg/dL [optimal]) (SI: 0.62 mmol/L [<2.59 mmol/L])
Triglycerides = 38 mg/dL (<150 mg/dL [optimal]) (SI: 0.43 mmol/L [<1.70 mmol/L])
Hepatic profile, within normal limits

Which of the following is the most likely diagnosis?

A. Abetalipoproteinemia
B. Dysbetalipoproteinemia
C. Hypoalphalipoproteinemia
D. Hypobetalipoproteinemia

18 A 43-year-old man seeks help addressing high cholesterol. After experiencing an episode of angina, he had a positive treadmill stress test. On physical examination, notable findings included a firm papulonodular rash on both elbows and orange-yellow linear xanthomas of his palmar creases.

Fasting lipid panel:

Total cholesterol = 325 mg/dL (<200 mg/dL [optimal]) (SI: 8.42 mmol/L [<5.18 mmol/L])
Triglycerides = 340 mg/dL (<150 mg/dL [optimal]) (SI: 3.84 mmol/L [<1.70 mmol/L])
HDL cholesterol = 30 mg/dL (>60 mg/dL [optimal]) (SI: 0.78 mmol/L [>1.55 mmol/L])
LDL cholesterol = 227 mg/dL (<100 mg/dL [optimal]) (SI: 5.88 mmol/L [<2.59 mmol/L])

Which of the following abnormalities does this man most likely have?

A. ABCA1 deficiency
B. Apolipoprotein CII deficiency
C. Apolipoprotein *E2/E2*
D. LDL-receptor deficiency
E. Lipoprotein lipase deficiency

19 A 64-year-old woman is referred for hyperlipidemia. She has a history of primary biliary cirrhosis, and ursodeoxycholic acid was prescribed 10 months ago. She currently has no signs or symptoms of coronary artery disease, but there is a strong history of cardiovascular disease in her family.

Laboratory test results:

Alkaline phosphatase = 820 U/L (50-120 U/L) (SI: 13.7 µkat/L [0.74-2.00 µkat/L])
Total bilirubin = 1.1 mg/dL (0.3-1.2 mg/dL) (SI: 18.1 µmol/L [5.1-20.5 µmol/L])
Total cholesterol = 487 mg/dL (<200 mg/dL [optimal]) (SI: 12.61 mmol/L [<5.18 mmol/L])
Triglycerides = 286 mg/dL (<150 mg/dL [optimal]) (SI: 3.23 mmol/L [<1.70 mmol/L])
HDL cholesterol = 38 mg/dL (>60 mg/dL [optimal]) (SI: 0.98 mmol/L [>1.55 mmol/L])
LDL cholesterol = 392 mg/dL (<100 mg/dL [optimal]) (SI: 10.15 mmol/L [<2.59 mmol/L])

Which of the following is the most likely explanation for her lipid profile?

A. Accumulation of lipoprotein (a)
B. Accumulation of lipoprotein X
C. A complication of ursodeoxycholic acid treatment
D. Lecithin-cholesterol acyltransferase (LCAT) deficiency
E. Liver disease causing increased apolipoprotein B production

20 A 30-year-old woman with systemic lupus erythematosus and the following lipid profile is referred for evaluation:

Total cholesterol = 300 mg/dL (<200 mg/dL [optimal]) (SI: 7.77 mmol/L [<5.18 mmol/L])
HDL cholesterol = 30 mg/dL (>60 mg/dL [optimal]) (SI: 0.78 mmol/L [>1.55 mmol/L])
Triglycerides = 1000 mg/dL (<150 mg/dL [optimal]) (SI: 11.30 mmol/L [<1.70 mmol/L])

LDL cholesterol cannot be estimated. Her current medications include prednisone, 20 mg daily; hydrochlorothiazide; lisinopril; metoprolol; and infliximab.

There is concern that medications could be contributing to her dyslipidemia. Which of the following adjustments should be recommended?

A. Discontinue lisinopril
B. Switch hydrochlorothiazide to chlorthalidone
C. Switch infliximab to apremilast
D. Switch metoprolol to amlodipine
E. Switch prednisone to dexamethasone

21 A 35-year-old Japanese-American woman with the following lipid panel is referred for evaluation:

Total cholesterol = 245 mg/dL (<200 mg/dL [optimal]) (SI: 6.35 mmol/L [<5.18 mmol/L])
LDL cholesterol = 110 mg/dL (<100 mg/dL [optimal]) (SI: 2.85 mmol/L [<2.59 mmol/L])
HDL cholesterol = 120 mg/dL (>60 mg/dL [optimal]) (SI: 3.11 mmol/L [>1.55 mmol/L])
Triglycerides = 75 mg/dL (<150 mg/dL [optimal]) (SI: 0.85 mmol/L [<1.70 mmol/L])

Which of the following is the most likely cause of this lipid profile?

A. ABCA1 deficiency
B. Cholesterol ester transfer protein (CETP) deficiency
C. Hepatic lipase deficiency
D. Lecithin cholesterol acyltransferase (LCAT) deficiency
E. Scavenger receptor B1 (SR-B1) deficiency

22 A 22-year-old college student comes to the student health clinic because of an upper respiratory infection. The treating physician notices that she has gained 5 lb (2.3 kg) over the last year. The clinician asks about the student's usual sleep habits, and she reports that during the week she only gets about 4 hours of sleep each night.

Which of the following statements about the adaptive responses to shortened sleep time best describes the factors that promote weight gain in this student?

A. A marked reduction in total daily energy expenditure and an increase in leptin levels
B. A marked reduction in total daily energy expenditure and no change in leptin or ghrelin levels
C. An increase in cortisol levels and insulin resistance and no change in ghrelin, leptin, or energy expenditure
D. A reduction in energy expended from physical activity and an increase in ghrelin
E. No change in total daily energy expenditure and a decrease in leptin

23 A 38-year-old man with an 8-year history of coronary artery disease and multiple hospitalizations for coronary artery stent placements is referred for evaluation. The patient's family has a strong history of heart disease: his father and 2 paternal uncles died before age 50 years. The patient has been taking atorvastatin, 80 mg daily, for the last 5 years.

Laboratory test results:

Total cholesterol = 210 mg/dL (<200 mg/dL [optimal]) (SI: 5.44 mmol/L [<5.18 mmol/L])
LDL cholesterol = 150 mg/dL (<100 mg/dL [optimal]) (SI: 3.89 mmol/L [<2.59 mmol/L])
HDL cholesterol = 40 mg/dL (>60 mg/dL [optimal]) (SI: 1.04 mmol/L [>1.55 mmol/L])
Triglycerides = 100 mg/dL (<150 mg/dL [optimal]) (SI: 1.13 mmol/L [<1.70 mmol/L])

On physical examination, you should look for which of the following findings?

A. Arthropathy
B. Corneal arcus
C. Eruptive xanthomas
D. Lipemia retinalis
E. Palmar xanthomas

24 A 70-year-old woman is referred for lipid management. She has moderately well-controlled type 2 diabetes mellitus with a hemoglobin A_{1c} level of 7.8% (62 mmol/mol). She has a history of several episodes of pancreatitis, as well as a myocardial infarction at age 68 years. After her heart attack, she started atorvastatin, 40 mg daily, which brought her LDL-cholesterol concentration down from 158 mg/dL (4.09 mmol/L) to 88 mg/dL (2.28 mmol/L), but her fasting triglycerides are persistently elevated at 760 mg/dL (8.59 mmol/L). She had been prescribed gemfibrozil but has not yet started it.

Which of the following is the best next step in managing this patient's cholesterol?

A. Continue atorvastatin and add fenofibrate
B. Continue atorvastatin and add gemfibrozil
C. Continue atorvastatin and add niacin
D. Increase atorvastatin to the maximum dosage
E. Stop atorvastatin and start fenofibrate

25 A 31-year-old man with type 2 diabetes mellitus treated with metformin, pioglitazone, atorvastatin, and fenofibrate is referred for the following lipid panel:

HDL cholesterol = 5 mg/dL (>60 mg/dL [optimal]) (SI: 0.13 mmol/L [>1.55 mmol/L])
LDL cholesterol = 120 mg/dL (<100 mg/dL [optimal]) (SI: 3.11 mmol/L [<2.59 mmol/L])
Triglycerides = 300 mg/dL (<150 mg/dL [optimal]) (SI: 3.39 mmol/L [<1.70 mmol/L])

On a previous lipid profile 5 years ago, his HDL-cholesterol concentration was 25 mg/dL (0.65 mmol/L). His BMI is 37 kg/m^2, and his hemoglobin A_{1c} value is 6.3% (45 mmol/mol).

This marked reduction in HDL cholesterol is most likely due to which of the following?

A. Acquired lecithin-cholesterol acyltransferase deficiency
B. Erroneous apolipoprotein B precipitation
C. Fenofibrate therapy
D. Metformin inhibition of ABCA1
E. Statin-induced hypoalphalipoproteinemia

26 A 58-year-old woman has the physical finding shown in the photograph. She has been in good health and has no personal or family history of vascular disease. She is unaware of having a dyslipidemia and is sure that her cholesterol was checked when she was younger. After menopause, she gained 20 lb (9.1 kg), and during the past year she has attempted to reduce her weight with a high-fat, low-carbohydrate diet. On this diet, her BMI has decreased from 35 to 27 kg/m^2. Her total cholesterol concentration has increased to greater than 600 mg/dL (>15.54 mmol/L) with an equal increase in triglycerides. Thyroid function is normal.

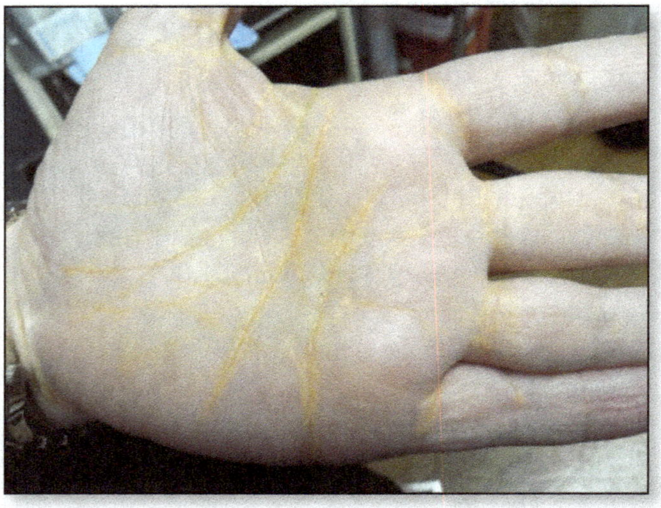

To make the definitive diagnosis of this patient's disorder, which of the following tests should be ordered?

A. Apolipoprotein AI radioimmunoassay
B. Apolipoprotein E genotyping
C. Assessment of LDL particle size
D. Lipoprotein(a) gene analysis

Pituitary Board Review

John D. Carmichael, MD

1 A 32-year-old woman has a history of panhypopituitarism secondary to craniopharyngioma resection 2 years ago followed by fractionated stereotactic radiation. She has been treated with desmopressin spray twice daily; hydrocortisone, 15 mg daily in divided doses; levothyroxine, 125 mcg daily; an estrogen- and progesterone-containing oral contraceptive; and GH, 0.4 mg daily. She is here for routine follow-up and reports a new symptom of fatigue. She is otherwise asymptomatic. Her primary care physician recently ordered routine bloodwork at her annual physical appointment. Laboratory test results were unremarkable except for undetectable TSH with a normal free T_4 level. Her levothyroxine dosage was decreased to 25 mcg daily, and she was asked to make an appointment with endocrinology for further management.

Which of the following is the best next step in this patient's management?

A. Change the hormone replacement regimen to an estrogen transdermal patch with intermittent oral progesterone
B. Discontinue levothyroxine and initiate methimazole, 10 mg daily
C. Measure serum T_3
D. Perform ^{123}I radioactive iodine uptake and scan
E. Restart levothyroxine, 125 mcg daily

2 A 35-year-old woman presents to her primary care office with an 8-month history of amenorrhea. She has no notable medical history. She had 1 pregnancy followed by an uncomplicated spontaneous vaginal delivery 1 year ago. Breastfeeding stopped 9 months ago. She reports having 1 menstrual period after delivery but none since.

On physical examination, her weight is 136.5 lb (62 kg), blood pressure is 122/74 mm Hg, and pulse rate is 62 beats/min. Examination findings are notable for full visual fields to confrontation, thyromegaly (gland is twice normal size with no dominant nodules), and bilateral galactorrhea.

A urine pregnancy test is negative, and her prolactin concentration is 82 ng/mL (3.6 nmol/L). Pituitary MRI with and without gadolinium demonstrates a 12 × 15 × 8-mm seller mass with homogeneous enhancement and suprasellar extension, but no optic chiasm compression or evidence of cavernous sinus invasion. The patient is referred to endocrinology for evaluation and management of the pituitary mass.

Laboratory test results:

IGF-1 = 182 ng/mL (113-297 ng/mL) (SI: 23.8 nmol/L [14.8-38.9 nmol/L])
TSH = 282 mIU/L (0.5-5.0 mIU/L)
Free T_4 = 0.2 ng/dL (0.8-1.8 ng/dL) (SI: 2.6 pmol/L [10.30-23.17 pmol/L])
Prolactin (with serial dilutions) = 98 ng/mL (4-30 ng/mL) (SI: 4.3 nmol/L [0.17-1.30 nmol/L])
LH = 0.1 mIU/mL (1.0-18.0 mIU/mL) (SI: 0.1 IU/L [1.0-18.0 IU/L])
FSH = 0.2 mIU/mL (2.0-12.0 mIU/mL) (SI: 0.2 IU/L [2.0-12.0 IU/L])
Cortisol (8 AM) = 16.2 µg/dL (5-25 µg/dL) (SI: 466.9 nmol/L [137.9-689.7 nmol/L])
Estradiol = 8 pg/mL (10-180 pg/mL [follicular/luteal]; <10 pg/mL [postmenopausal]) (SI: 29.4 pmol/L [36.7-660.8 pmol/L (follicular/luteal); <36.7 pmol/L (postmenopausal)])

Which of the following is the best next step in this patient's treatment?

A. Initiate cabergoline, 0.5 mg tablet twice weekly
B. Initiate levothyroxine, 100 mcg daily
C. Measure α-subunit
D. Perform ^{123}I radioactive iodine uptake and scan
E. Refer to neurosurgery for transsphenoidal surgery of the pituitary mass

3 A 52-year-old man is referred for evaluation and management of a pituitary tumor found on MRI after a car accident. The mass is 11 mm in greatest diameter, solid, and hypoenhancing. MRI shows suprasellar extension without contact with the optic chiasm. Formal visual fields performed by an ophthalmologist confirm no visual deficits. His initial hormonal evaluation after the accident did not demonstrate any pituitary deficiencies, and his prolactin concentration was normal. The patient is counseled to undergo imaging again in 6 months and have screening to monitor for any new hormone deficiencies. He is told to contact the clinic if new neurologic symptoms develop. Six months later, pituitary MRI demonstrates growth of 4 mm (greatest diameter is 15 mm). The mass is solid and hypoenhancing with no signs of hemorrhage. However, there is new abutment with the optic chiasm. Visual field testing is normal.

Laboratory test results:

Prolactin = 42 ng/mL (4-23 ng/mL) (SI: 1.83 nmol/L [0.17-1.00 nmol/L])
Total testosterone = 125 ng/dL (300-900 ng/dL) (SI: 4.3 nmol/L [10.4-31.2 nmol/L])
LH = 0.2 mIU/mL (1.0-9.0 mIU/mL) (SI: 0.2 IU/L [1.0-9.0 IU/L])
FSH = 0.3 mIU/mL (1.0-13.0 mIU/mL) (SI: 0.3 IU/L [1.0-13.0 IU/L])

He reports his libido has decreased over the last year, but he attributes this to aging and work-related stress. His only interim medical history is a 2-mm prostate lesion identified after a screening PSA measurement was found to be mildly elevated. He is being followed by urology with observation.

Which of the following is the best next step in this patient's management?

A. Initiate cabergoline, 0.5 mg twice weekly
B. Initiate testosterone replacement, with close surveillance of PSA
C. Recommend prostate surgery to his urologist to allow safe testosterone treatment
D. Refer to neurosurgery for transsphenoidal surgery
E. Refer to radiation oncology for single-dose stereotactic radiosurgery

4 A 22-year-old man is transitioning from his pediatric endocrinology office to adult endocrinology. He has a history of delayed puberty and has been treated with testosterone for the past 4 years. He reports that pubertal changes started at age 14 years but further development stopped by age 15. He describes an inability to smell. Initial workup at age 15 years revealed the following laboratory test results:

Serum total testosterone = 55 ng/dL (300-900 ng/dL) (SI: 1.9 nmol/L [10.4-31.2 nmol/L])
Serum LH = 2.2 mIU/mL (1.0-9.0 mIU/mL) (SI: 2.2 IU/L [1.0-9.0 IU/L])
FSH = 4.3 mIU/mL (1.0-13.0 mIU/mL) (SI: 4.3 IU/L [1.0-13.0 IU/L])

Low testosterone was confirmed on multiple occasions before starting testosterone therapy.

Physical examination findings are notable for a eunuchoid habitus with arm span longer than height. His height is 70.1 in (178 cm), and weight is 175.0 lb (79.4 kg) (BMI = 25 kg/m^2). He has no facial or body hair. Body habitus is prepubertal, with little pubertal muscle development. On genital examination, he has normal pubic hair, no hypospadias, and bilateral descended testes (approximately 4 mL bilaterally). The patient is currently interested in fertility.

Laboratory test results (while taking topical testosterone gel):

Prolactin = 12.5 ng/mL (4-23 ng/mL) (SI: 0.54 nmol/L [0.17-1.00 nmol/L])
Total testosterone = 463 ng/dL (SI: 16.1 nmol/L)
FSH = <0.1 mIU/mL (SI: <0.1 IU/L)

LH = <0.1 mIU/mL (SI: <0.1 IU/L)
IGF-1 = 217 ng/mL (116-341 ng/mL)
(SI: 28.4 nmol/L [15.2-44.7 nmol/L])

Semen analysis demonstrates azoospermia.

Which of the following is the best next step for fertility induction in this patient?

A. Continue topical testosterone and add anastrozole, 1 mg orally daily
B. Refer to urology for testicular sperm extraction
C. Stop topical testosterone and begin clomiphene citrate, 25 orally mg daily
D. Stop topical testosterone and begin hCG, 2000 IU subcutaneous injection 3 times weekly
E. Stop topical testosterone and begin testosterone enanthate, 100 mg intramuscular injection weekly

5 A 52-year-old man presents for evaluation of fatigue. He was previously in good health until a year ago when he injured his back and was placed on a 6-week course of corticosteroids and opioid pain medications. He has not taken any steroids or pain medications since. He reports that his testosterone was measured around the time of his injury and was found to be low (110 ng/dL [3.8 nmol/L]). He is concerned this is still a problem. He reports weight gain, and medical records corroborate weight gain of 35 lb (15.9 kg) over the past 2 years. His BMI has increased from 25 to 30 over the same timeframe. He stopped exercising 2 years ago after the birth of his son and was unable to restart after his back injury. His libido is not the same as it was when he was younger, but it is still present and he can attain and maintain erections during intercourse. He uses continuous positive airway pressure for a recent diagnosis of obstructive sleep apnea.

On physical examination, his blood pressure is 135/85 mm Hg and pulse rate is 88 beats/min. His weight is 209.5 lb (95 kg) (BMI = 30 kg/m^2). There is no facial plethora, striae, or bruising. He has normal findings on genital examination, with testicular size of 20 mL bilaterally with normal consistency.

Laboratory test results:

Complete blood cell count, normal
Glucose = 109 mg/dL (70-99 mg/dL)
(SI: 6.0 mmol/L [3.9-5.5 mmol/L])
AST = 58 U/L (20-48 U/L) (SI: 0.97 µkat/L [0.33-0.80 µkat/L])
ALT = 64 U/L (10-40 U/L) (SI: 1.07 µkat/L [0.17-0.67 µkat/L])
Alkaline phosphatase, normal
Hemoglobin A_{1c} = 6.3% (4.0%-5.6%)
(45.4 mmol/mol [20-38 mmol/mol])
Total cholesterol = 230 mg/dL
(<200 mg/dL [optimal])
(SI: 5.96 mmol/L [<5.18 mmol/L])
Triglycerides = 310 mg/dL (<150 mg/dL [optimal])
(SI: 3.50 mmol/L [<1.70 mmol/L])
HDL cholesterol = 32 mg/dL
(>60 mg/dL [optimal])
(SI: 0.83 mmol/L [>1.55 mmol/L])
LDL cholesterol = 168 mg/dL
(<100 mg/dL [optimal])
(SI: 4.35 mmol/L [<2.59 mmol/L])
Total testosterone = 238 ng/dL (300-900 ng/dL)
(SI: 8.3 nmol/L [10.4-31.2 nmol/L])
Prolactin = 12 ng/mL (4-23 ng/mL)
(SI: 0.52 nmol/L [0.17-1.00 nmol/L])
TSH = 1.78 mIU/L (0.5-5.0 mIU/L)
Free T_4 = 1.1 ng/dL (0.8-1.8 ng/dL)
(SI: 14.1 pmol/L [10.30-23.17 pmol/L])
LH = 8.1 mIU/mL (1.0-9.0 mIU/mL) (SI: 8.1 IU/L [1.0-9.0 IU/L])
FSH = 5.2 mIU/mL (1.0-13.0 mIU/mL)
(SI: 5.2 IU/L [1.0-13.0 IU/L])

Free and total testosterone are retested on a subsequent morning at 8 AM (equilibrium dialysis and liquid chromatography/mass spectrometry methods):

Total testosterone = 225 ng/dL (300-900 ng/dL)
(SI: 7.8 nmol/L [10.4-31.2 nmol/L])
Free testosterone = 12.0 ng/dL (9.0-30.0 ng/dL)
(SI: 0.42 nmol/L [0.31-1.04 nmol/L])
SHBG = 1.1 µg/mL (1.1-6.7 µg/mL) (SI: 10 nmol/L [10-60 nmol/L])

Which of the following is the best next step in this patient's initial management?

A. Perform pituitary MRI
B. Recommend exercise, calorie counting, and nutrition referral
C. Start clomiphene, 25 mg daily
D. Start hCG, 2000 IU 3 times weekly
E. Start topical testosterone gel 1.62%, 40.5 mg daily

6 A 32-year-old woman presents with a history of abrupt weight gain of 22 lb (10 kg) over 12 months. She reports new onset of facial plethora, rounding of the face and shoulders, easy bruising, and prominent stretch marks. She has had difficulty climbing stairs over the past month. Prior to 6 months ago, she was a yoga instructor at her local gym, but she had to stop due to weakness in her upper arms and an inability to hold the positions. Menstrual periods were always regular until 8 months ago when they stopped. Pregnancy testing is negative. She is currently not taking any medications or supplements.

On physical examination, her blood pressure is 138/87 mm Hg. Her height is 61.8 in (157 cm), and weight is 141 lb (64 kg) (BMI = 26 kg/m^2). She has a rounded, plethoric face and dorsocervical dysplasia. There are signs of recent and older bruises on her forearms and legs. The skin is thin on the dorsum of her hands. Her weight is centrally located with 1-cm violaceous striae noted on the lower abdomen. She is unable to rise from a squatting position without using her arms.

Results from screening for hypercortisolemia:

Serum cortisol (after 1-mg overnight dexamethasone-suppression test) = 15.7 μg/dL (<1.8 μg/dL) (SI: 433.1 nmol/L [<50 nmol/L])
Urinary free cortisol (2 samples) = 255 μg/24 h (SI: 704 nmol/d) and 301 μg/24 h (SI: 831 nmol/d) (4-50 μg/24 h [SI: 11-138 nmol/d])
Salivary cortisol (2 samples, obtained at bedtime) = 0.28 μg/dL (SI: 7.7 nmol/L) and 0.34 μg/dL (SI: 9.4 nmol/L) (<0.09 μg/dL [SI: <2.5 nmol/L])

Which of the following is the best next step in this patient's diagnosis?

A. CT of the abdomen with adrenal protocol
B. Inferior petrosal sinus sampling at an expert center
C. Measurement of morning plasma ACTH
D. Measurement of morning serum cortisol after 8-mg overnight dexamethasone administration
E. MRI of the pituitary with and without contrast

7 A 33-year-old woman is referred for suspected Cushing syndrome. She was seen by her primary care physician because she was concerned about a 5-year history of weight gain. She reports 2 pregnancies, one at age 24 and another at age 27. She was able to lose weight after her first pregnancy but not after the second. She has subsequently gained 15 lb (6.8 kg) over 5 years. She was diagnosed with postpartum depression and treated with antidepressant therapy after her second delivery. This medication was discontinued 2 years ago, as it was thought to be contributing to her weight gain. She is currently taking no medications.

Results of initial screening by her primary care physician:

Cortisol (8 AM) after 1-mg overnight dexamethasone-suppression test = 5.3 μg/dL (<1.8 μg/dL) (SI: 146.2 nmol/L [<50 nmol/L])
Urinary free cortisol (2 samples) = 52 μg/24 h (SI: 143.5 nmol/d) and 80 μg/24 h (SI: 220.8 nmol/d) (4-50 μg/24 h) (SI: [11-138 nmol/d])
Salivary cortisol (2 samples) = 0.08 μg/dL (SI: 2.2 nmol/L) and 0.13 μg/dL (SI: 3.6 nmol/L) (<0.09 μg/dL [SI: <2.5 nmol/L])
ACTH (8 AM) = 56 pg/mL (10-60 pg/mL) (SI: 12.3 pmol/L [2.2-13.2 pmol/L])

Finding on pituitary MRI are normal.

On physical examination, her blood pressure is 135/84 mm Hg and pulse rate is 88 beats/min. Her height is 64 in (162.6 cm), and weight is 162 lb (73.5 kg) (BMI = 27.8 kg/m^2). Her face is nonplethoric but shows facial rounding compared with prepregnancy photos. There is no supraclavicular fullness or dorsal cervical dysplasia. She has mild central adiposity with pale, white striae approximately 1 cm wide on her lower abdomen. There is no bruising on the extremities, and strength is 5/5 throughout.

Which of the following is the best next step in this patient's management?

A. Bilateral inferior petrosal sinus sampling
B. Chest CT with and without contrast
C. Desmopressin-stimulation test
D. ^{68}Ga-DOTATATE scan
E. 8-mg overnight dexamethasone-suppression test

8 An 18-year-old girl develops severe headaches. Head MRI shows a 2.8 × 2.8 × 2.2-cm cystic sellar and suprasellar mass with calcifications (*see image*). In retrospect, she has been tired, and her menses, which began at age 12 years, stopped 1 year ago.

On physical examination, her vision is normal, and findings are only notable for bilateral galactorrhea.

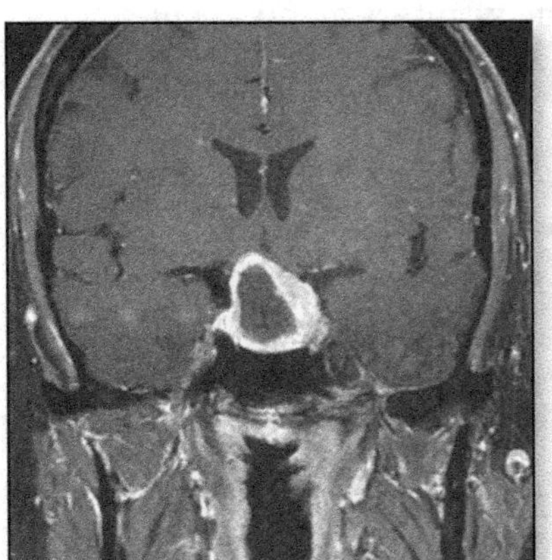

Laboratory test results:

Free T_4 = 0.9 ng/dL (0.8-1.8 ng/dL)
(SI: 11.6 pmol/L [10.30-23.17 pmol/L])
Cortisol (8 AM) = 7.1 μg/dL (5-25 μg/dL)
(SI: 195.9 nmol/L [137.9-689.7 nmol/L])
Estradiol = 22 pg/mL (27-123 pg/mL)
(SI: 81 pmol/L [99-452 pmol/L])
Prolactin = 355 ng/mL (4-30 ng/mL)
(SI: 15.4 nmol/L [0.17-1.30 nmol/L])
IGF-1 = 122 ng/mL (162-541 ng/mL)
(SI: 16.0 nmol/L [21.2-70.9 nmol/L])

On the basis of the presented information, which of the following treatments should be recommended?

A. Conventional fractionated irradiation
B. Dopamine agonist
C. Stereotactic radiosurgery
D. Transcranial surgery
E. Transsphenoidal surgery

9 A 48-year-old man is referred after head MRI performed for evaluation of headache showed a 0.9-cm right-sided pituitary adenoma without parasellar extension (*see image*). He has been feeling well. He has no vision symptoms.

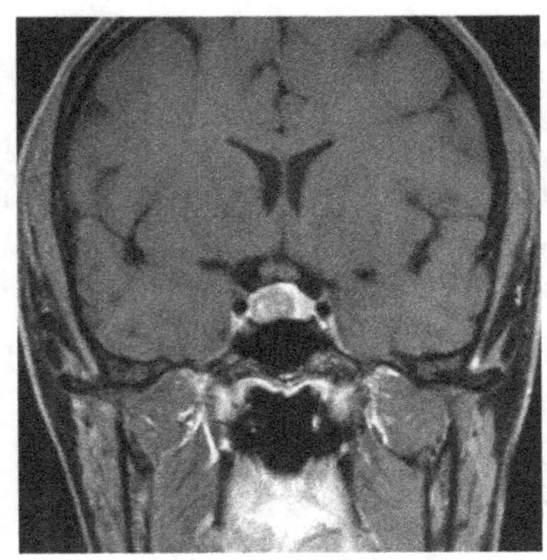

Courtesy of William Young.

On physical examination, his blood pressure is 136/70 mm Hg and pulse rate is 74 beats/min. His skin has normal texture, and his reflexes are normal. He saw a local neurosurgeon who recommended surgery.

Laboratory test results (8 AM):

Testosterone = 325 ng/dL (300-900 ng/dL)
(SI: 11.3 nmol/L [10.4-31.2 nmol/L])
LH = 2.3 mIU/mL (1.0-9.0 mIU/L) (SI: 2.3 IU/L [1.0-9.0 IU/L])
FSH = 1.4 mIU/mL (1.0-13.0 mIU/L) (SI: 1.4 IU/L [1.0-13.0 IU/L])
Cortisol (8 AM) = 15.7 μg/dL (5-25 μg/dL)
(SI: 433.1 nmol/L [137-39-689.7 nmol/L])
Prolactin = 5.7 ng/mL (4-23 ng/mL)
(SI: 0.25 nmol/L [0.17-1.00 nmol/L])
Free T_4 = 1.2 ng/dL (0.8-1.8 ng/dL)
(SI: 15.4 pmol/L [10.3-23.2 pmol/L])
Serum sodium = 143 mEq/L (136-142 mEq/L)
(SI: 143 mmol/L [136-142 mmol/L])

Which of the following is the best next step in this patient's management?

A. Another MRI in 12 months
B. Radiotherapy
C. Transsphenoidal surgery
D. Visual field testing

10 A 53-year-old woman has a medical history of stage 2 breast cancer diagnosed 4 years ago, status post mastectomy, local radiation therapy, and adjuvant chemotherapy. She recently slipped and struck her head, without loss of consciousness. However, given persistent headaches, she underwent head CT, which revealed a 1.5-cm sellar mass with suprasellar extension. In retrospect, she noted abrupt onset of frequent urination and increased thirst in the previous 3 weeks. MRI is performed 4 weeks later and shows that the mass is now 2 cm.

On physical examination, she appears tired. Her blood pressure is 98/66 mm Hg, pulse rate is 92 beats/min, and BMI is 21.1 kg/m^2.

Laboratory test results:

Serum sodium = 152 mEq/L (136-142 mEq/L) (SI: 152 mmol/L [136-142 mmol/L])
Prolactin = 122 ng/mL (4-30 ng/mL) (SI: 5.30 nmol/L [0.17-1.30 nmol/L])
FSH = 15.0 mIU/mL (>30.0 mIU/mL [postmenopausal]) (SI: 15.0 IU/L [>30.0 IU/L])
LH = 12.0 mIU/mL (>30.0 mIU/mL [postmenopausal]) (SI: 12.0 IU/L [>30.0 IU/L])
Plasma glucose = 89 mg/dL (70-99 mg/dL) (SI: 4.9 mmol/L [3.9-5.5 mmol/L])

Chest CT shows no evidence of lesion or adenopathy.

Which of the following is this patient's most likely diagnosis?

A. Clinically nonfunctioning pituitary adenoma
B. Craniopharyngioma
C. Metastasis
D. Neurosarcoidosis
E. Prolactinoma

11 A 51-year-old man presents with new-onset atrial fibrillation and a 10-lb (4.5-kg) weight loss. In retrospect, he has noticed some fatigue, a mild tremor, and heat intolerance for several months. His sister has hypothyroidism.

On physical examination, his blood pressure is 139/67 mm Hg, pulse rate is 92 beats/min (irregular), and BMI is 24.1 kg/m^2. He has no proptosis but does have slight lid-lag. His thyroid gland is about 2-fold diffusely enlarged and is soft. He has brisk reflexes and a fine tremor of his outstretched hands.

Laboratory test results:

Free T_4 = 4.5 ng/dL (0.8-1.8 ng/dL) (SI: 57.9 pmol/L [10.30-23.17 pmol/L])
Total T_3 = 482 ng/dL (70-200 ng/dL) (SI: 7.4 nmol/L [1.08-3.08 nmol/L])
TSH = 9.47 mIU/L (0.5-5.0 mIU/L)
Thyroid-stimulating immunoglobulin index = 1.4 (<1.3)

Results from repeated tests are similar. Findings on MRI of the pituitary gland are normal.

Which of the following tests would be the most helpful in determining the etiology of his hyperthyroidism?

A. Measurement of β-subunit
B. Measurement of HAMA (human anti-mouse antibodies)
C. Measurement of thyrotropin-binding inhibitory immunoglobulin (TBII)
D. Petrosal sinus sampling for TSH measurements
E. T_3-suppression test

12 A 43-year-old woman with acromegaly has a GH concentration of 11.7 ng/mL (11.7 μg/L) and an IGF-1 concentration of 890 ng/mL (116.6 nmol/L) after surgery. Octreotide LAR is initiated with a dosage increase to 30 mg intramuscular monthly. On this dosage, her IGF-1 concentration is 625 ng/mL (81.9 nmol/L). She has persistent arthralgias and sweating and modest hyperglycemia with a hemoglobin A_{1c} value of 7.3% (56 mmol/mol). Brain MRI reveals 0.5-cm residual left cavernous sinus disease.

Which of the following options would be most effective in controlling her acromegaly within the next 6 months?

A. Add pegvisomant, 40 mg subcutaneously weekly
B. Change octreotide LAR dosing to every 21 days
C. Perform radiation therapy
D. Stop octreotide LAR and switch to cabergoline
E. Switch to pasireotide LAR, 40 mg monthly

13 A 46-year-old man presents with loss of libido and erectile dysfunction. His primary care physician documented his testosterone concentration to be 180 ng/dL (6.2 nmol/L) and referred him for further evaluation.

Laboratory test results (sample drawn at 8 AM):

Repeated testosterone = 171 ng/dL (300-900 ng/dL) (SI: 5.9 nmol/L [10.4-31.2 nmol/L])
LH = 0.9 mIU/mL (1.0-9.0 mIU/L) (SI: 0.9 IU/L [1.0-9.0 IU/L])
FSH = 1.1 mIU/mL (1.0-13.0 mIU/L) (SI: 1.1 IU/L [1.0-13.0 IU/L])
Prolactin = 2513 ng/mL (4-23 ng/mL) (SI: 109.3 nmol/L [0.17-1.00 nmol/L])
TSH, normal
Cortisol, normal

MRI shows a 1.7-cm adenoma with substantial extension into the left cavernous sinus.

At a cabergoline dosage of 1.0 mg twice weekly, his prolactin level normalizes, his tumor greatly reduces in size, his testosterone level increases to 602 ng/dL (20.9 nmol/L), and his erectile function returns. However, his wife complains that he has recently become obsessed with sexuality, to the point that it is hindering their relationship.

Which of the following is the most likely explanation for his current behavior?

A. An adverse effect of cabergoline
B. Behavior change unrelated to his tumor or treatment
C. Hypothalamic damage from the tumor
D. The normalized testosterone level

14 Following transsphenoidal surgery, a 56-year-old woman with acromegaly has residual tumor in the cavernous sinus. Her postoperative GH concentration is 9.0 ng/mL (9.0 µg/L), and her IGF-1 concentration 12 weeks after surgery is 690 ng/mL (90.4 nmol/L). She has bothersome headaches. She has diet-controlled diabetes mellitus. Her physical examination reveals coarse facial features.

Which of the following treatment options is the best recommendation now?

A. Another transsphenoidal surgery
B. Cabergoline
C. Lanreotide depot monthly
D. Pegvisomant weekly

15 A 19-year-old man presents with delay in puberty and frontal headaches. In retrospect, he has had poor energy, frequent urination, increased thirst, and a 46-lb (20.9-kg) weight gain over the past 2 years. Testing reveals a prolactin concentration of 42.7 ng/mL (1.9 nmol/L) (similar on dilution), panhypopituitarism, and arginine vasopressin deficiency. He has a 2.3-cm cystic sellar mass with suprasellar extension, abutting the optic chiasm. An ophthalmologist identifies bilateral homonymous hemianopsia.

Which of the following is this patient's most likely diagnosis?

A. Craniopharyngioma
B. Gonadotroph adenoma
C. Langerhans cell histiocytosis
D. Prolactinoma
E. Silent corticotroph adenoma

16 Following transsphenoidal surgery, a 45-year-old woman with acromegaly has had persistently elevated concentrations of GH (5.3 ng/mL [5.3 µg/L]) and IGF-1 (456 ng/mL [59.7 nmol/L]). While on lanreotide depot, 90 mg monthly, her GH level decreases to 0.5 ng/mL (0.5 µg/L) and her IGF-1 level is in the reference range. With reduction of her dosage to 60 mg monthly, her GH concentration remains less than

1.0 ng/mL (<1.0 μg/L) and her IGF-1 level is normal for more than 1 year. Although there has been some shrinkage, residual tumor is still visible on MRI.

Which of the following is the best next management step?

A. Add cabergoline, 0.5 mg twice weekly
B. Continue current therapy
C. Increase lanreotide dosage to 120 mg and extend the time between lanreotide depot doses to every 6 weeks
D. Recommend stereotactic radiotherapy
E. Switch to pegvisomant

17 A 52-year-old woman has had hypopituitarism for 10 years after resection of a nonfunctioning pituitary adenoma. She has been treated with levothyroxine, hydrocortisone, a low-dosage oral contraceptive pill, and daily GH injections. Because her sister recently developed breast cancer, the patient has decided to stop her oral contraceptive. During the next month, she notices progressive joint aches and sweating.

Which of the following is the best next step to relieve these new symptoms?

A. Decrease the GH dosage
B. Decrease the hydrocortisone dosage
C. Increase the GH dosage
D. Increase the hydrocortisone dosage
E. Increase the levothyroxine dosage

18 A 75-year-old man is referred because a pituitary incidentaloma was identified on CT performed after he fell on ice and struck his head. Subsequent MRI confirmed a 1.3-cm, T1-hypoenhancing mass that appeared to be a pituitary adenoma, with no suprasellar extension. He states that he has been feeling well, but generally has been slowing down. He attributes this to aging. He has no headaches or vision symptoms. He had a myocardial infarction 10 years ago and subsequent 3-vessel coronary bypass surgery. He has hypertension. His only medications are a statin, a daily baby aspirin, and lisinopril.

On physical examination, his is blood pressure is 136/70 mm Hg and pulse rate is 74 beats/min. His skin has normal texture, and his reflexes are normal. Testes are 15 mL bilaterally.

Laboratory test results (sample drawn at 8 AM):

LH = 2.3 mIU/mL (1.0-9.0 mIU/L) (SI: 2.3 IU/L [1.0-9.0 IU/L])
FSH = 1.4 mIU/mL (1.0-13.0 mIU/L) (SI: 1.4 IU/L [1.0-13.0 IU/L])
Cortisol = 17 μg/dL (5-25 μg/dL) (SI: 469.0 nmol/L [137.9-689.7 nmol/L])
Testosterone = 195 ng/dL (300-900 ng/dL) (SI: 6.8 nmol/L [10.4-31.2 nmol/L])
Free T_4 = 1.1 ng/dL (0.8-1.8 ng/dL) (SI: 14.2 pmol/L [10.30-23.17 pmol/L])
Prolactin = 92 ng/mL (4-23 ng/mL) (SI: 4.00 nmol/L [0.17-1.00 nmol/L])
Creatinine = 1.5 mg/dL (0.7-1.3 mg/dL) (SI: 132.6 μmol/L [61.9-114.9 μmol/L])
IGF-1 = 135 ng/dL (98-261 ng/mL) (SI: 17.7 nmol/L [12.8-34.2 nmol/L])

Which of the following is the best next step in this patient's management?

A. Perform visual field testing
B. Refer to an experienced pituitary surgeon
C. Refer for stereotactic radiosurgery
D. Repeat MRI in 6 months
E. Start dopamine agonist therapy and repeat MRI in 6 months

19 A 34-year-old woman has been diagnosed with a 2.5-cm clinically nonfunctioning pituitary macroadenoma that has caused chiasmal compression. Her preoperative evaluation reveals no evidence of acromegaly, Cushing disease, or salt and water imbalance. She undergoes transsphenoidal surgery, which is uneventful. Twenty hours after surgery, she develops marked increase in thirst and polyuria.

Laboratory test results:

Serum sodium = 152 mEq/L (136-142 mEq/L) (SI: 152 mmol/L [136-142 mmol/L])

Urine osmolality = 110 mOsm/kg (150-1150 mOsm/kg) (SI: 110 mmol/kg [150-1150 mmol/kg])

Which of the following treatment options should be initiated?

A. 1 L fluid restriction
B. DDAVP, 0.1 mg orally as needed for polyuria and hypernatremia
C. DDAVP, 10 mcg intranasally nightly
D. DDAVP, scheduled dosing, 0.2 mg orally twice daily
E. Tolvaptan, 15 mg orally once daily

20 A 19-year-old man is evaluated because of headaches, decreased libido, and progressive fatigue and is found to have what appears to be an 11-mm Rathke cleft cyst on MRI. He recalls having some problems with increased urinary frequency and thirst several years ago, but he no longer has these symptoms.

On physical examination, he has a sallow complexion, a normal-sized phallus and testes, and a sparse beard.

Laboratory test results (8 AM):

Serum sodium = 144 mEq/L (136-142 mEq/L) (SI: 144 mmol/L [136-142 mmol/L])
Urine specific gravity = 1.004
Serum cortisol (8 AM) = 7.0 µg/dL (5-25 µg/dL) (SI: 193.1 nmol/L [137-39-689.7 nmol/L])
Free T_4 = 0.5 ng/dL (0.8-1.8 ng/dL) (SI: 6.44 pmol/L [10.3-23.2 pmol/L])
TSH = 1.4 mIU/L (0.5-5.0 mIU/L)
Testosterone = 293 ng/dL (300-900 ng/dL) (SI: 10.2 nmol/L [10.4-31.2 nmol/L])

Which of the following might be expected with initiation of hydrocortisone and levothyroxine in this patient?

A. Increase in polyuria and polydipsia
B. Orthostatic hypotension
C. Rapid development of hyponatremia
D. Worsening headache

21 A 33-year-old woman is referred because head CT performed in the emergency department after an automobile crash showed an empty sella. She has generally been well, but she has had problems with headaches for years. Her examination findings are normal except for obesity.

Which of the following is the most likely cause of her empty sella?

A. Burnt-out hypothalamic/pituitary sarcoidosis
B. Langerhans cell histiocytosis
C. Pseudotumor cerebri (benign, idiopathic, intracranial hypertension)
D. Trauma-induced pituitary infarction

22 A 33-year-old woman has developed Cushing syndrome during her 16th week of pregnancy. She has hypertension, diabetes mellitus, hirsutism, and wide, purple striae on her abdomen.

Laboratory test results:

Serum cortisol (8 AM) = 37 µg/dL (5-25 µg/dL) (SI: 1020.8 nmol/L [137.9-689.7 nmol/L])
ACTH = 129 pg/mL (10-60 pg/mL) (SI: 28.4 pmol/L [2.2-13.2 pmol/L])
Urinary free cortisol = 475 µg/24 h (4-50 µg/24 h) (SI: 1311 nmol/d [11-138 nmol/d])

MRI shows a 6-mm pituitary adenoma.

Which of the following treatment options is the most appropriate to control her Cushing disease?

A. Cabergoline
B. Mifepristone
C. Pasireotide
D. Transsphenoidal surgery after delivery
E. Transsphenoidal surgery now

Thyroid Board Review

Jacqueline Jonklaas, MD, PhD, MPH

1 An 18-year-old man is referred for symptomatic, new-onset hypothyroidism. One year ago, he had normal thyroid function with a TSH value of 2.7 mIU/L and a free T_4 value of 1.37 ng/dL (17.63 pmol/L).

Current thyroid test results:

TSH = 58.7 mIU/L (0.5-5.0 mIU/L)
Free T_4 = 0.34 ng/dL (0.8-1.8 ng/dL)
(SI: 4.38 pmol/L [10.30-23.17 pmol/L])
TPO antibodies, negative

The patient describes extreme fatigue, constipation, cold sensitivity, and difficulty concentrating. On physical examination, he appears tired. His vital signs are normal, and his skin is cool and dry.

The patient's medical history is notable for metastatic neuroblastoma, which had progressed despite multiple therapies. Most recently, the patient had enrolled in a clinical trial of radioactive ^{131}I MIBG, and he has thus far had a good response to this therapy.

Which of the following is the most likely explanation for the development of hypothyroidism in this patient?

A. Failure to escape from the Wolff-Chaikoff effect
B. Free radiolabeled iodine reaching the thyroid gland
C. Metastatic neuroblastoma to the thyroid gland
D. Pathogenic variant in the gene encoding the sodium-iodide transporter
E. TPO antibody negative–Hashimoto thyroiditis

2 A 74-year-old man feels weak and has a racing heart, anxiety, and weight loss shortly after having a COVID vaccination. Later, his racing heart worsens and he is found to have new-onset atrial fibrillation. He is treated with a β-adrenergic blocker and anticoagulation. Subsequently, he reverts to normal sinus rhythm. His anxiety and weight loss continue, and an evaluation by his primary care physician is unrevealing. Several weeks later, the patient is found to have recurrent atrial fibrillation. Thyroid function is assessed, and the patient is determined to have hyperthyroidism. His thyroid gland is normal-sized, has irregular

	Timeline				
Results	Time of diagnosis of hyperthyroidism	1-3 Months later	4 Months later	5 Months later	6 Months later
TSH	0.05 mIU/L	0.0-0.02 mIU/L	0.01 mIU/L	0.02 mIU/L	0.01 mIU/L
Free T_4	3.5 ng/dL (SI: 45.0 pmol/L)	3-1-3.3 ng/dL (SI: 39.9-42.5 pmol/L)	2.9 ng/dL (SI: 37.3 pmol/L)	2.9 ng/dL (SI: 37.3 pmol/L)	3.0 ng/dL (SI: 38.6 pmol/L)
Total T_3	325 ng/dL (SI: 5.00 nmol/L)	250-295 ng/dL (SI: 3.85-4.54 nmol/L)	220 ng/dL (SI: 3.39 nmol/L)	230 ng/dL (SI: 3.54 nmol/L)	230 ng/dL (SI: 3.54 nmol/L)
TSI	Negative	...	...	...	...
TRAb	Negative	...	...	...	...
Thyroglobulin	60 ng/mL (SI: 60 μg/L)	...	...	...	...
^{123}I Radioactive iodine and scan	<2%	...	...	...	...
Therapy	None	Prednisone	Prednisone and methimazole	Prednisone and methimazole	Prednisone

texture, and is nontender. A thyroid scan and uptake is performed, and uptake is less than 2% at 24 hours. The patient states he has not received amiodarone or intravenous contrast. The patient is started on prednisone for a diagnosis of thyroiditis. Over a 3-month period, there is no decline in his free T_4 levels. Methimazole is added, resulting in a marginal decrease in free T_4 levels. Methimazole is discontinued, and prednisone is maintained (*see table on preceding page*).

A single additional evaluation is then performed, which provides information about why the patient's hyperthyroidism had not responded to the therapies that were used.

Which of the following is the most likely evaluation that was performed?

A. COVID antibody titer
B. COVID PCR test
C. Serum hCG level
D. Spot urine iodine
E. Whole-body iodine scan

3 A 23-year-old woman presents to establish care. She had a thyroidectomy and is taking levothyroxine for postsurgical hypothyroidism. She says she was noted to have had a goiter as a child, but her thyroid function was normal. Five years ago, 2 thyroid nodules (4 cm and 2 cm) were detected. She explains that it could not be determined whether they were cancerous, and she underwent thyroidectomy. Pathology showed several colloid-filled cysts and multiple macroscopic and adenomatoid nodules. There was no evidence of autoimmune thyroiditis. The patient is hearing impaired and has bilateral cochlear implants, but she is otherwise healthy.

Her younger brother is being monitored for an enlarged thyroid in the setting of normal thyroid function and has a unilateral cochlear implant. Additional questions about family history reveal other family members with hearing impairment at a young age and goiters.

Current thyroid test results:

TSH = 0.56 mIU/L (0.5-5.0 mIU/L)
Free T_4 = 1.3 ng/dL (0.8-1.8 ng/dL)
(SI: 16.73 pmol/L [10.30-23.17 pmol/L])
Total T_3 = 90 ng/dL (70-200 ng/dL)
(SI: 1.39 nmol/L [1.08-3.08 nmol/L])

Which of the following is likely to be present in this patient and the family members described?

A. Autosomal dominant transmission of the condition
B. Normal results on perchlorate discharge test
C. Pathogenic variant in the gene encoding the chloride-iodide cotransporter in the thyroid, inner ear, and kidney
D. Positive thyroid autoantibodies
E. Unremarkable MRI of the auditory canals

4 A 20-year-old man presents after transferring care from his pediatric endocrinologist for management of papillary thyroid cancer. He appears to have had an excellent response to his therapy and currently has undetectable thyroglobulin. Neck ultrasonography does not show abnormal cervical lymph nodes.

His medical records document a total thyroidectomy and cervical node dissection 3 years ago. He was then treated with 125 mCi of ^{131}I radioiodine following a recombinant human TSH-stimulated diagnostic iodine scan that showed thyroid bed uptake and a stimulated thyroglobulin concentration of 2 ng/mL. A posttherapy whole-body scan showed mediastinal uptake in a pyramidal pattern that was interpreted as being consistent with metastatic disease to mediastinal lymph nodes (*see images*).

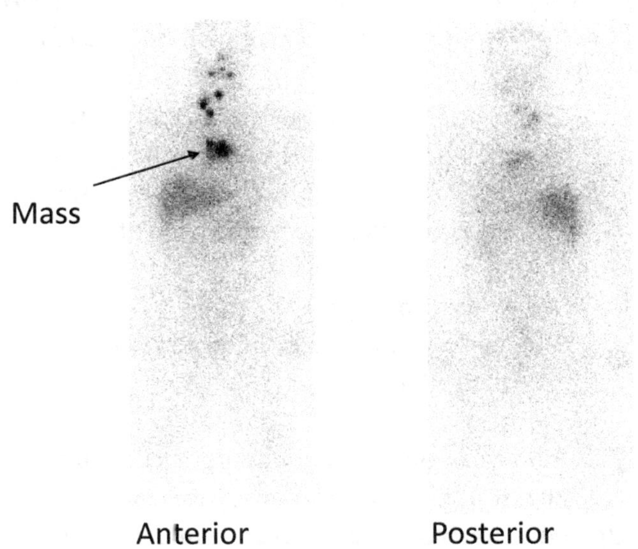

CT showed an anterior mediastinal mass. The patient then underwent a video-assisted thorascopic surgery to resect the mass.

Which of the following was the most likely finding on pathologic examination of this patient's resected mediastinal mass 3 years ago?

A. Ectopic thyroid tissue
B. Metastatic papillary thyroid cancer in the thymus
C. Normal mediastinal lymph nodes
D. Parathyroid tissue
E. Thymic tissue

5 A 67-year-old woman is found to have a thyroid nodule on thyroid ultrasonography after a left-sided thyroid nodule was incidentally identified following chest CT performed during assessment of her breast cancer. The nodule is 0.8 × 0.9 × 0.6 cm and is considered suspicious. FNA biopsy of the nodule is initially not advised based on its small size, although it is subsequently performed as part of the patient's breast cancer staging to rule out metastatic breast cancer to the thyroid. The nodule cytology suggests papillary thyroid cancer. The patient's complete evaluation determines that her breast cancer has not metastasized. The patient expresses an interest in having her thyroid cancer followed without current treatment using an "active surveillance" protocol being conducted locally.

If present, which of the following features would support the patient's decision to opt for active surveillance of her papillary thyroid cancer?

A. Apparent extrathyroidal extension of the thyroid nodule as imaged by ultrasonography
B. Evidence of coexistent hyperparathyroidism with a serum calcium concentration of 11 mg/dL (2.75 mmol/L)
C. New-onset hoarseness
D. Presence of palpable cervical lymph nodes
E. The patient's older age

6 A 56-year-old woman undergoes thyroid ultrasonography after her gynecologist palpated a thyroid nodule. Several small nodules of similar appearance and size are seen throughout both lobes of the thyroid gland. A representative left-sided nodule is shown (*see image*). The radiology report describes the nodules using the American College of Radiology (ACR) Thyroid Imaging Reporting and Data System (TI-RADS) risk stratification system.

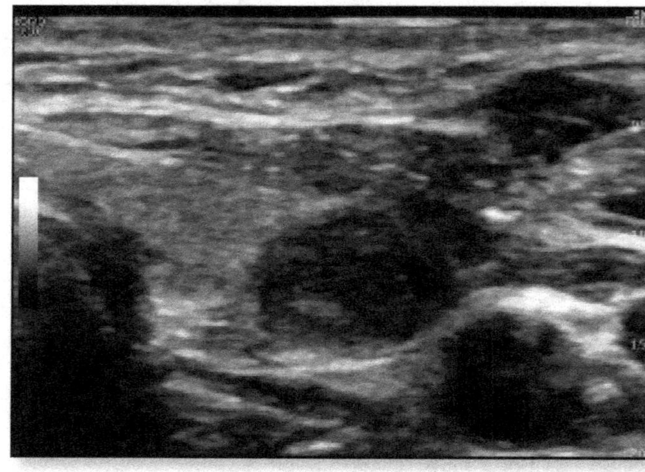

Which of the following options likely best matches the radiologist's description of the left-sided nodule depicted in the image?

Answer	Composition	Echogenicity	Margin	Echogenic foci
A.	Mixed cystic and solid	Isoechoic	Smooth	None
B.	Spongiform	Not applicable	Not applicable	Not applicable
C.	Mixed cystic and solid	Hypoechoic	Extra-thyroidal extension	None
D.	Almost completely solid	Isoechoic	Ill-defined	Peripheral calcifi-cations
E.	Almost completely solid	Hypoechoic	Ill-defined	Punctate echogenic foci

7 A 41-year-old woman presents to an obstetrician after a positive home pregnancy test. She is confirmed to be at 8 weeks' gestation. She was diagnosed with Graves disease at age 14 years and was treated with radioactive iodine ablation followed by levothyroxine replacement therapy. She is now being prescribed 125 mcg of levothyroxine daily, although her weight-based dose before pregnancy was 112 mcg daily. She has a history of nonadherence to her treatment regimen and discontinued levothyroxine completely on prior occasions, citing anxiety, depression, and palpitations as the reasons for the discontinuation. Prior cardiac evaluations have not revealed any underlying pathology. The patient has not tolerated medications for anxiety and depression.

Medical records from 4 years ago show a TSH concentration of 119 mIU/L and a free T_4 concentration of 0.52 ng/dL (6.69 pmol/L) when the patient had stopped taking her levothyroxine and a TSH concentration of 4.5 mIU/L when adherence with 125 mcg of levothyroxine was reestablished.

Current laboratory test results:

TSH = 257 mIU/L (0.5-5.0 mIU/L)
Free T_4 = 0.35 ng/dL (0.8-1.8 ng/dL)
(SI: 4.50 pmol/L [10.30-23.17 pmol/L])

The patient states that she has not been taking her levothyroxine (for an unspecified length of time) because of anxiety and palpitations.

Assuming close monitoring to titrate and adjust her dosage, which of the following is the best approach to restarting this patient's thyroid hormone?

A. 50% of her prior dose of 125 mcg levothyroxine daily
B. 112 mcg levothyroxine daily
C. 125 mcg levothyroxine daily
D. 125 mcg levothyroxine and 5 mcg liothyronine daily
E. At least 150 mcg daily

8 A 71-year-old woman requires an extended stay in the intensive care unit following resection of a meningioma. The meningioma was in close proximity to the hypothalamus and pituitary gland, and the patient had been experiencing worsening visual field defects. Prior to her admission to the neurosurgery service, she had been documented to have a normal pituitary axis (normal thyroid and adrenal axes, and an appropriately elevated FSH and LH for her menopausal state). The patient's postoperative course has been complicated by meningitis, cerebral edema, and new-onset seizure activity. A few weeks postoperatively, the patient had normal concentrations of serum TSH and free T_4. She remains hospitalized for treatment of various complications. Thyroid function tests were performed approximately 6 weeks later after the patient's steroid regimen had been tapered to physiologic hydrocortisone from high-dosage dexamethasone given for cerebral edema. The patient was also receiving parenteral nutrition, but she has been weaned off pressors and dopamine. Additional thyroid function tests obtained 11 weeks postoperatively triggered an endocrine consultation.

Serial thyroid function test results are shown in the Table.

The endocrinology consult team is specifically requested to give an opinion as to whether the patient has thyroid abnormalities due to nonthyroidal illness syndrome or whether she has central hypothyroidism.

Analyte	3 weeks postoperatively	9 weeks postoperatively	11 weeks postoperatively	Reference range
TSH	0.7 mIU/L	0.1 mIU/L	0.05 mIU/L	0.5-5.0 mIU/L
Free T_4	0.85 ng/dL (SI: 10.94 pmol/L)	0.30 ng/dL (SI: 3.86 pmol/L)	0.23 ng/dL (SI: 2.96 pmol/L)	0.8-1.8 ng/dL (SI: 10.30-23.17 pmol/L)
Total T_3	71 ng/dL (SI: 1.09 nmol/L)	22 ng/dL (SI: 0.34 nmol/L)	11 ng/dL (SI: 0.17 nmol/L)	70-200 ng/dL (SI: 1.08-3.08 nmol/L)
Total T_4	6.0 μg/dL (SI: 77.22 nmol/L)	1.8 μg/dL (SI: 23.17 nmol/L)	0.8 μg/dL (SI: 10.30 nmol/L)	5.5-12.5 μg/dL (SI: 70.79-160.88 nmol/L)

In addition to the low TSH, which of the following test results or combination of test results would be helpful in pointing to a diagnosis of nonthyroidal illness syndrome, rather than central hypothyroidism?

A. Elevated FSH
B. Low free T_3 and high FSH
C. Low free T_3 and high reverse T_3
D. Low free T_3 and negative TPO antibody titer
E. Low free T_3 and positive TPO antibody titer

9 A 38-year-old woman is referred for a diagnosis of Hashimoto thyroiditis. She brings with her laboratory results documenting a TSH concentration of 7.1 mIU/L and an elevated TPO antibody titer. Thyroid ultrasonography shows heterogeneous thyroid parenchyma consistent with Hashimoto thyroiditis and multiple nodules, including a 1.7-cm, solid, hypoechoic nodule with irregular margins within the left lobe. She was recently diagnosed with breast cancer for which she underwent treatment and subsequently appears to be in remission. Her history is also notable for oral papillomatosis affecting her tongue, acral keratoses, and lipomas. Her family history is notable for a younger sister who is undergoing an evaluation for headache and vertigo, a father with colon cancer, and a mother with uterine cancer.

Physical examination findings are notable for cutaneous lesions and a diffusely enlarged, irregularly textured thyroid gland with left-sided fullness and firmness.

The patient's 1.7-cm thyroid nodule is biopsied, and the cytologic findings suggest papillary thyroid cancer.

Which of the following is the most significant underlying risk factor for thyroid cancer in this patient?

A. Familial adenomatous polyposis
B. Hashimoto thyroiditis
C. *PTEN* hamartoma tumor syndrome
D. Serum TSH above the normal range
E. Werner syndrome

10 A 39-year-old woman presents to discuss whether her Hashimoto disease has resolved. She was first seen by an endocrinologist at age 28 years. At that time, she had a TSH concentration of 11.0 mIU/L and an elevated TPO titer of 816 IU/L. She was reluctant to start levothyroxine, but she was strongly advised to do so because she was planning a pregnancy. She began treatment with levothyroxine and maintained this therapy during her 3 ensuing pregnancies with maintenance of a normal TSH concentration throughout and with uncomplicated pregnancies and no adverse fetal outcomes. However, she frequently noted palpitations associated with levothyroxine therapy.

She is not planning additional pregnancies and wishes to pursue a more natural and holistic approach to her health. Over a 6-month period, she self-tapered herself off levothyroxine (137 mcg daily) and is not currently taking any prescribed medications. She feels well, has improved energy, and has no symptoms of either hypothyroidism or hyperthyroidism.

On physical examination, she has normal vital signs, no palpable thyroid tissue, and a subtle tremor of her outstretched hands.

Thyroid ultrasonography identifies an atrophic appearance to her thyroid gland bilaterally.

Thyroid function test results:

TSH = <0.001 mIU/L (0.5-5.0 mIU/L)
Free T_4 = 2.2 ng/dL (0.8-1.8 ng/dL)
(SI: 28.3 pmol/L [10.30-23.17 pmol/L])

In addition to requesting that the patient bring her over-the-counter medications and supplements for review, which of the following should be measured to confirm her diagnosis?

A. Current TPO antibody titer
B. Random urinary iodine
C. Serum selenium
D. Serum T_3
E. Thyroid-stimulating immunoglobulin

11 An 86-year-old man is referred for an elevated serum TSH value. The patient has been in good health, with no history of thyroid dysfunction. He generally feels well.

On physical examination, his pulse rate is 72 beats/min and he has no goiter.

Laboratory test results:

Serum TSH = 6.2 mIU/L (0.5-5.0 mIU/L)
Free T_4 = 1.1 ng/dL (0.8-1.8 ng/dL)
(SI: 14.2 pmol/L [10.30-23.17 pmol/L])

These results are stable on repeated testing, and TPO antibodies are not detected.

Which of the following is the best way to counsel this patient?

A. A TSH value in this range is associated with decreased systemic vascular resistance
B. He has apathetic hypothyroidism
C. He should be started on a statin
D. His TSH value is normal for octogenarians
E. Levothyroxine treatment will improve his quality of life

12 A 22-year-old man presents with nervousness, palpitations, itchy eyes, and weight loss of 20 lb (9.1 kg) over the last 3 months.

On physical examination, his pulse rate is 110 beats/min. He has moderate proptosis, a diffuse goiter with bruit, and moderate tremor.

His serum free T_4 and T_3 levels are moderately elevated, and baseline liver function and complete blood cell count are normal.

Methimazole, 30 mg daily, and atenolol are started and his symptoms improve, but he develops hepatic transaminase enzyme elevations (5 times the upper normal limit). Methimazole is stopped. Radioiodine therapy is recommended, but the patient declines this treatment. Atenolol is changed to propranolol. One week later, his thyroid hormone levels have doubled and his liver enzyme levels continue to rise.

Which of the following is the best approach now?

A. Give supersaturated potassium iodide (SSKI) for 3 to 4 weeks and refer for thyroidectomy
B. Maximize β-adrenergic blockade and refer for thyroidectomy
C. Resume methimazole at a 50% lower dosage
D. Start hydrocortisone, start SSKI, and optimize β-adrenergic blockade before surgery
E. Start propylthiouracil and closely follow liver function

13 A 39-year-old woman with postsurgical hypothyroidism and type 2 diabetes mellitus is referred for a progressively increasing levothyroxine dosage requirement over the past 12 months. Other medications include metformin, lisinopril, and aspirin. She acknowledges some recent weight gain, but she reports strict adherence to her therapeutic regimen and takes no over-the-counter preparations.

On physical examination, her blood pressure is 140/88 mm Hg. She has no palpable tissue in the thyroid bed, normal deep-tendon reflexes, and moderate lower-extremity edema.

Laboratory test results:

Serum TSH = 8.7 mIU/L (0.5-5.0 mIU/L)
Free T_4 = 1.0 ng/dL (0.8-1.8 ng/dL)
(SI: 12.87 pmol/L [10.30-23.17 pmol/L])
Total cholesterol = 305 mg/dL (<200 mg/dL [optimal]) (SI: 7.90 mmol/L [<5.18 mmol/L])
Triglycerides = 880 mg/dL (<150 mg/dL [optimal]) (SI: 9.94 mmol/L [<1.70 mmol/L])
25-Hydroxyvitamin D = 20 ng/mL (30-80 ng/mL [optimal]) (SI: 49.9 nmol/L [74.9-199.7 nmol/L])
Serum albumin = 2.6 g/dL (3.5-5.0 g/dL) (SI: 26 g/L [35-50 g/L])
Hemoglobin A_{1c} = 7.1% (4.0%-5.6%) (54 mmol/mol [20-38 mmol/mol])
Urinalysis, positive for protein (2.2 g/g creat)

Which of the following is the most likely cause of this patient's increasing levothyroxine dosage requirement?

A. Celiac disease
B. Euthyroid sick syndrome
C. Medication nonadherence
D. Metformin therapy
E. Nephrotic syndrome

14 A 27-year-old man was diagnosed with Graves hyperthyroidism 2 months ago, and methimazole, 40 mg daily, was prescribed. He takes his medication regularly. He has developed a sore throat and fever and now presents to the emergency department.

On physical examination, his temperature is 101.8°F (38.8°C), pulse rate is 90 beats/min, pharynx is without exudate, and there is no cervical adenopathy.

Laboratory test results (2 weeks ago):

Free T_4 = 2.1 ng/dL (0.8-1.8 ng/dL) (SI: 27.03 pmol/L [10.30-23.17 pmol/L])
TSH = 0.01 mIU/L (0.5-5.0 mIU/L)
Liver-associated enzymes, normal
Complete blood cell count with differential, normal

Which of the following is the best next step in this patient's management?

A. Admit to the hospital for impending thyroid storm
B. Increase the methimazole dosage
C. Obtain throat culture and start amoxicillin
D. Repeat complete blood cell count with differential
E. Switch methimazole to propylthiouracil

15 A 46-year-old woman with longstanding hypothyroidism is referred because of very high levothyroxine dosage requirements. Previously, she had maintained normal TSH values while taking levothyroxine, 112 mcg daily. However, over the past 2 years, the patient's levothyroxine dosage has been as high as 600 mcg daily without good biochemical control of her hypothyroidism. She reports strict adherence to her treatment regimen.

On physical examination, there is no goiter, but a large abdominal mass is noted that extends into the pelvis.

Laboratory test results:

Serum TSH = 178 mIU/L (0.5-5.0 mIU/L)
Free T_4 = 0.4 ng/dL (0.8-1.8 ng/dL) (SI: 5.1 pmol/L [10.30-23.17 pmol/L])
Free T_3 = 0.26 pg/mL (2.3-4.2 pg/mL) (SI: 0.4 pmol/L [3.53-6.45 pmol/L])
Reverse T_3 = 413 ng/dL (10-24 ng/dL) (SI: 6.4 nmol/L [0.15-0.37 nmol/L])

The tumor is most likely to contain excessive amounts of which of the following?

A. Monocarboxylase transporter 8
B. Pendrin
C. Sodium-iodide transporter
D. TPO
E. Type 3 deiodinase

16 A 63-year-old man with stage 4 medullary thyroid cancer is referred for consideration of further therapy. Medullary thyroid cancer was diagnosed 8 years earlier and was believed to be sporadic. He has had a persistent postoperative elevation of serum calcitonin. Distant metastases to the lungs bilaterally and ribs were detected 1 year ago, with disease progression over the past 6 months. Testing for germline and somatic *RET* pathogenic variants is negative.

Physical examination reveals a well-healed thyroidectomy scar, and findings are otherwise unremarkable.

Laboratory test results:

Serum calcitonin = 14,000 pg/mL (<10 pg/mL) (SI: 4088 pmol/L [<2.9 pmol/L])
Carcinoembryonic antigen = 72 ng/mL (<2.5 ng/mL) (SI: 72 μg/L [<2.5 μg/L])

Which of the following is the most appropriate next step in this patient's management?

A. Chemotherapy with doxorubicin and cisplatin
B. Octreotide therapy
C. Radioactive iodine treatment
D. Radiotherapy to the lung and rib lesions
E. Vandetanib therapy

17 A 37-year-old man is found to have a left thyroid nodule. Thyroid ultrasonography shows a 4.6-cm hypoechoic nodule without calcification or hypervascularity, with no suspicious lymph nodes. The patient undergoes FNA biopsy of the nodule with cytologic findings of follicular neoplasm (Bethesda class IV). Repeated FNA biopsy with molecular analysis reveals a *RET/PTC* rearrangement.

Which of the following is the most appropriate next step in this patient's management?

A. Referral for lobectomy
B. Referral for total thyroidectomy
C. Referral for total thyroidectomy with bilateral neck dissection
D. Repeated FNA biopsy in 6 months
E. Repeated thyroid ultrasonography in 6 months

18 A 42-year-old woman presents for a routine physical examination. There is a family history of Hashimoto thyroiditis in her mother. The patient reports anxiety and recent hair loss, but has no other symptoms.

On physical examination, her pulse rate is 76 beats/min. She has no exophthalmos, lid lag, or stare. Her thyroid gland is 20 g in size without nodules, and there is no tremor of her outstretched hands.

She is not taking any prescription medications. She reports taking a multivitamin; biotin, 4500 mcg daily; and a selenium supplement, 300 mcg daily. She started the biotin to treat hair loss. Her serum TSH level is documented to be less than 0.01 mIU/L.

Results of repeated laboratory testing 3 days later:

TSH = <0.01 mIU/L (0.5-5.0 mIU/L)
Free T_4 = 3.2 ng/dL (0.8-1.8 ng/dL)
(SI: 41.2 pmol/L [10.30-23.17 pmol/L])
Total T_3 = 374 ng/dL (70-200 ng/dL)
(SI: 5.8 nmol/L [1.08-3.08 nmol/L])

Which of the following is the best next step for establishing this patient's diagnosis?

A. Initiation of methimazole
B. Inquire about other hair loss products
C. Measurement of serum thyroid-stimulating immunoglobulin
D. Radioactive iodine uptake and scan
E. Repeated blood tests after stopping biotin for 7 days

19 A 23-year-old man is seen for follow-up of hypothyroidism. He has been treated with levothyroxine, 150 mcg daily, since age 15 years. His dosage has been stable for several years, and his most recent TSH value 10 months ago was 1.34 mIU/L. He reports strict adherence to his levothyroxine regimen. He notes that since his last visit he has entered body-building competitions and has started using a regimen of anabolic steroids and aromatase inhibitors that he obtains over the internet.

Which of the following patterns is most likely in this patient?

Answer	TSH	Total T_4	Total T_3	Free T_4
A.	10.0 mIU/L	15.0 µg/dL (193.1 nmol/L)	280 ng/dL (4.3 nmol/L)	0.7 ng/dL (9.0 pmol/L)
B.	1.2 mIU/L	15.0 µg/dL (193.1 nmol/L)	280 ng/dL (4.3 nmol/L)	1.4 ng/dL (18.0 pmol/L)
C.	1.2 mIU/L	10.0 µg/dL (128.7 nmol/L)	150 ng/dL (2.3 nmol/L)	1.4 ng/dL (18.0 pmol/L)
D.	1.2 mIU/L	5.0 µg/dL (64.4 nmol/L)	70 ng/dL (1.1 nmol/L)	1.4 ng/dL (18.0 pmol/L)
E.	0.01 mIU/L	5.0 µg/dL (64.4 nmol/L)	70 ng/dL (1.1 nmol/L)	2.8 ng/dL (36.0 pmol/L)

Reference ranges: TSH, 0.5-5.0 mIU/L; total T_4, 5.5-12.5 µg/dL (94.02-213.68 nmol/L); total T_3, 70-200 ng/dL (1.08-3.08 nmol/L); free T_4, 0.8-1.8 ng/dL (10.30-23.17 pmol/L)

20 A 75-year-old woman is admitted to the medical intensive care unit with progressive obtundation and is found to be in myxedema coma. She is treated with intravenous levothyroxine therapy, stress-dose hydrocortisone, and empiric antibiotics while awaiting blood culture results. After 48 hours, the patient has gradually improved sensorium but develops progressive hypotension with narrowing of the pulse pressure and diminished heart sounds. Electrocardiography shows low voltage in all leads.

Laboratory test results:

- Free T_4 = 1.0 ng/dL (0.8-1.8 ng/dL) (SI: 12.9 pmol/L [10.30-23.17 pmol/L])
- TSH = 12.8 mIU/L (0.5-5.0 mIU/L)
- Serum cortisol = 2.8 μg/dL (5-25 μg/dL) (SI: 77.3 nmol/L [137.9-689.7 nmol/L])
- Creatine kinase = 280 U/L (50-200 U/L) (SI: 4.7 μkat/L [0.84-3.34 μkat/L]) with 12% MB fraction but normal troponin levels

Which of the following is the most likely cause of this patient's change in clinical status?

A. Adrenal insufficiency
B. Cardiac ischemia
C. Cardiac tamponade
D. Cardiomyopathy
E. Inadequate thyroid hormone replacement

21 A 26-year-old woman presents for evaluation. She is currently 15 weeks' pregnant with her first child. At an initial antenatal visit at 11 weeks' gestation, her serum TSH concentration was 0.03 mIU/L.

Laboratory test results at a follow-up obstetric visit 2 days ago:

- Serum TSH = 0.11 mIU/L (0.5-5.0 mIU/L)
- Free T_4 index = 3.6 (1-4)
- Total T_4 = 15.5 μg/dL (5.5-12.5 μg/dL) (SI: 199.5 nmol/L [94.02-213.68 nmol/L])
- Total T_3 = 280 ng/dL (70-200 ng/dL) (SI: 4.31 nmol/L [1.08-3.08 nmol/L])
- Thyroid-stimulating immunoglobulin = 140% (reference range ≤120% of basal activity)

She reports mild fatigue but otherwise feels well. She had some morning sickness earlier in her pregnancy, but this has resolved in the last 3 weeks.

On physical examination, her pulse rate is 92 beats/min. On palpation, her thyroid gland is nontender and 20 g in size without nodules. She has no proptosis.

Which of the following is the best option?

A. Plan thyroidectomy in the second trimester
B. Repeat thyroid function tests in 4 to 6 weeks
C. Start atenolol
D. Start methimazole, 5 mg daily
E. Start propylthiouracil, 50 mg 3 times daily

22 A 25-year-old woman with a history of suboptimally controlled thyrotoxicosis becomes pregnant. She is currently treated with methimazole.

If the patient continues her current treatment regimen, her fetus would be at increased risk of developing which of the following?

A. Biliary atresia
B. Cleft palate
C. Omphalocele
D. Placenta previa
E. Spina bífida

23 An 83-year-old man with refractory atrial fibrillation is prescribed amiodarone. Three months later, he reports increasing palpitations and diaphoresis.

On physical examination, his pulse rate is 90 beats/min and regular, his thyroid gland is of normal size and is nontender, and he has a fine tremor.

Which of the following would be the most specific indicator of thyrotoxicosis in this patient?

A. Clinical signs and symptoms
B. Elevated free T_4 level
C. Elevated total T_4 level
D. Low radioactive iodine uptake
E. Suppressed serum TSH level

24 An 18-year-old woman presents with pain in the left neck radiating to the left ear. After an initial ultrasound examination, she is informed that she has a hypoechoic thyroid nodule. While awaiting the recommended FNA biopsy, she develops dysphagia and fever (temperature up to 101.1°F [38.4°C]). She has a firm, tender, enlarged left thyroid lobe that is not fluctuant.

Her white blood cell count is 15,200/µL (15.2×10^9/L), and serum TSH concentration is 0.9 mIU/L.

Thyroid ultrasonography now shows an ill-defined abnormality with cystic changes in the left lobe, aspiration of which confirms infection with streptococcus pyogenes. The patient relates 2 similar episodes, 3 and 5 years earlier, that were treated with intravenous antibiotic therapy.

Which of the following is the most likely source of this patient's recurrent episodes?

A. Chronic sinusitis
B. Intravenous drug abuse
C. Pyriform sinus fistula
D. Recurrent dental abscess
E. Thyroglossal duct cyst

25 A 54-year-old woman presents with a left lateral neck mass, determined via FNA biopsy to be papillary thyroid cancer metastatic to a level III lymph node. She undergoes total thyroidectomy with central and left lateral neck dissection, with removal of a 1.0-cm tall-cell variant of papillary thyroid cancer and involved lymph nodes in both left central and left lateral compartments. Postoperatively, she receives 150 mCi ^{131}I, and a posttreatment scan reveals thyroid bed uptake and numerous pulmonary metastases.

Which of the following corresponds to the correct AJCC-8 staging (American Joint Committee on Cancer Staging System, 8th edition) for this patient's thyroid cancer?

A. Stage II
B. Stage III
C. Stage IVA
D. Stage IVB
E. Stage IVC

26 A 21-year-old man with attention deficit disorder is referred for palpitations and abnormal thyroid function test results. He has no compressive symptoms.

On physical examination, his pulse rate is 96 beats/min and regular. He has a diffuse goiter, without nodules or bruit. Tremor is absent, and he has normal deep tendon reflexes.

Laboratory test results:

Free T_4 = 2.7 ng/dL (0.8-1.8 ng/dL) (SI: 34.8 pmol/L [10.30-23.17 pmol/L])
TSH = 4.3 mIU/L (0.5-5.0 mIU/L)
Radioactive iodine uptake = 35% at 24 hours (15%-30% at 24 hours)
α-Subunit of pituitary glycoprotein hormones = 0.3 ng/mL (<1.2 ng/mL) (SI: 0.3 µg/L [<1.2 µg/L])
SHBG = 3.0 µg/mL (1.1-6.7 µg/mL) (SI: 26.7 nmol/L [10-60 nmol/L])

MRI shows a normal-appearing pituitary gland. Results from a test for heterophile antibodies are negative.

Which of the following is the most appropriate next step in this patient's management?

A. No intervention at this time
B. Refer for thyroidectomy
C. Start methimazole
D. Start propranolol
E. Treat with radioiodine

27 A 32-year-old man with widely invasive follicular thyroid cancer undergoes total thyroidectomy followed by radioiodine remnant ablation using 150 mCi ^{131}I. He subsequently develops lung metastases and is treated with an additional 200 mCi ^{131}I, with an objective decrease in the size of the lung metastases and reduction in serum thyroglobulin levels.

Which of the following is the most likely adverse effect from this patient's radioiodine therapy?

A. Azoospermia
B. Hypoparathyroidism
C. Increased risk of dental caries
D. Leukemia
E. Permanent loss of taste

28 A 42-year-old man is seen for follow-up of a right-sided thyroid nodule. His nodule was first assessed 8 years ago, after being noted incidentally on a chest CT. He has no family history of thyroid cancer and no personal history of head or neck radiation exposure. Findings on FNA biopsy performed at another institution 8 years ago were interpreted as Bethesda II (benign). The nodule was biopsied a second time 3 years ago for growth in maximal dimension from 1.9 to 3.1 cm. The second biopsy findings were again interpreted as benign. On ultrasonography now, the nodule measures 2.8 cm × 2.4 cm × 3.8 cm (*see image*). There is no cervical lymphadenopathy. He has no compressive symptoms. His serum TSH concentration is 2.01 mIU/L (0.5-5.0 mIU/L).

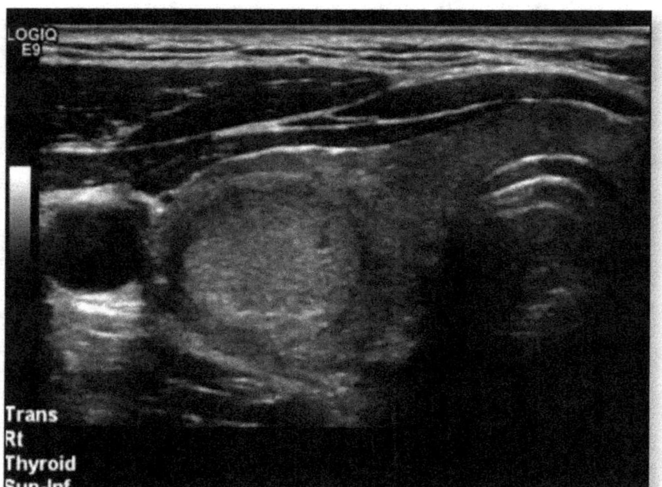

Reprinted from Bahn RS & Castro MR. *J Clin Endocrinol Metab*, 2011; 96(5):1202-1212. © The Endocrine Society.

Which of the following is the most appropriate next step in the management of this nodule?

A. Another ultrasound-guided FNA biopsy
B. Continued monitoring for compressive symptoms
C. Core biopsy
D. Thyroid lobectomy
E. Ultrasonography again in 6 months

29 A 72-year-old woman has a history of papillary thyroid cancer. Five years ago, she underwent total thyroidectomy for a 4.2-cm papillary cancer with extrathyroidal extension. She was subsequently treated with 100 mCi radioactive iodine. On her initial posttreatment scan, there was uptake only in the thyroid bed. Three years ago, she underwent repeated radioactive iodine treatment with 100 mCi for persistent thyroglobulin elevation, with no uptake on her posttreatment scan and no subsequent change in her serum thyroglobulin levels. She feels well. She is currently taking levothyroxine, 137 mcg daily.

On physical examination, her blood pressure is 128/72 mm Hg and pulse rate is 84 beats/min. There is no palpable thyroid tissue or cervical lymphadenopathy.

Laboratory test results:

TSH = 0.2 mIU/L (0.5-5.0 mIU/L)
Thyroglobulin antibodies = <4.0 IU/mL (≤4.0 IU/mL) (SI: <4.0 kIU/L [≤4.0 kIU/L])
Thyroglobulin = 11 ng/mL (3-42 ng/mL) (SI: 11 μg/L [3-42 μg/L])

Her serum thyroglobulin has been stable for the last 3 years. Neck ultrasonography shows no sign of tumor recurrence. No tumor foci are observed on PET/CT imaging. On a recent DXA, her T-score was −2.7 at the spine and −2.6 at the hip. She has not sustained a fracture.

Which of the following management strategies is most appropriate for this patient?

A. Continue current levothyroxine
B. Increase levothyroxine for goal TSH less than 0.01 mIU/L
C. Perform a diagnostic ^{123}I iodine scan
D. Treat with radioactive iodine
E. Treat with sorafenib

30 A 49-year-old woman has just undergone total thyroidectomy for a 3-cm nodule interpreted as Bethesda VI (malignant) on cytopathology. Surgical pathology showed a right-sided, 3.2-cm, unifocal classic variant of papillary thyroid cancer. Two of 6 resected central compartment lymph nodes were positive for tumor (with tumor foci measuring <0.2 cm in largest dimension). Surgical margins were negative, extrathyroidal extension was absent, vascular and lymphatic invasion was absent, and perineural invasion was not identified. She would like to discuss the next step in her treatment.

Which of the following is the best next step in this patient's management?

A. 30 mCi radioactive iodine
B. 75 mCi radioactive iodine
C. 100 mCi radioactive iodine
D. A second surgery for additional exploration of the central compartment
E. No radioactive iodine

31 A 77-year-old woman with a history of Hashimoto hypothyroidism since age 42 years presents with rapid thyroid enlargement over the course of several weeks. She reports a sensation of discomfort and pressure in her neck. While taking levothyroxine, her serum TSH concentration is 1.34 mIU/L and her TPO antibody level is 462 IU/mL (462 kIU/L). Ultrasonography shows a markedly heterogeneous gland with a 5.4-cm left-sided nodule. FNA biopsy of the nodule is performed (*see image*).

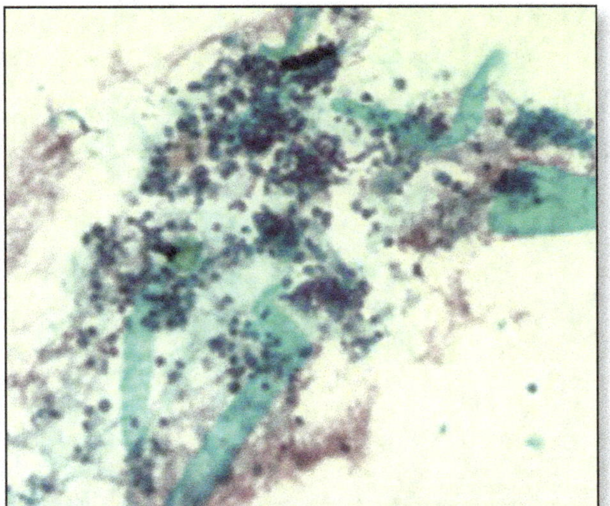

Which of the following is the best next step in this patient's management?

A. ^{123}I scan
B. Repeated FNA biopsy with flow cytometry
C. Repeated FNA biopsy with gene classifier testing
D. Repeated FNA with testing for the pathogenic variants associated with thyroid cancer
E. Total thyroidectomy

32 A 66-year-old man is taking amiodarone for refractory atrial fibrillation. Baseline thyroid function test results are normal, but one year after starting amiodarone he develops thyrotoxicosis.

On physical examination, the patient has a pulse rate of 92 beats/min, no goiter or thyroid tenderness, a normal lung examination, and no edema.

Laboratory test results:

Serum TSH = <0.01 mIU/L (0.5-5.0 mIU/L)
Free T_4 = 4.3 ng/mL (0.8-1.8 ng/mL)
(SI: 55.3 pmol/L [10.3-23.2 pmol/L])
Total T_3 = 215 ng/dL (70-200 ng/dL)
(SI: 3.3 nmol/L [1.1-3.1 nmol/L])
Radioactive iodine uptake, <1%

Thyroid ultrasonography shows some nodularity with mildly increased vascularity of the nodules. Methimazole, 30 mg daily, is initiated, and the patient has repeated thyroid function testing performed 2 weeks later, which shows no improvement. His cardiologist feels strongly that the amiodarone should not be stopped.

Which of the following is the best next step in this patient's management?

A. Add lithium to methimazole
B. Add prednisone to methimazole
C. Refer for immediate thyroidectomy
D. Replace methimazole with perchlorate
E. Replace methimazole with prednisone

33 A 48-year-old woman with a history of thyrotoxicosis due to a 2.2-cm TSH-producing pituitary macroadenoma invading the cavernous sinus undergoes transsphenoidal surgery. Postoperatively, the patient is noted to have persistent hyperthyroidism.

Thyroid function test results:

Free T_4 = 4.7 ng/mL (0.8-1.8 ng/mL)
(SI: 60.5 pmol/L [10.30-23.17 pmol/L])
TSH = 4.8 mIU/L (0.5-5.0 mIU/L)

MRI of the sella turcica at 1 month shows a persistent but decreased pituitary mass.

Which of the following is the most appropriate initial intervention now?

A. Bromocriptine
B. Methimazole
C. Somatostatin analogue
D. Thyroidectomy
E. Triiodothyroacetic acid (TRIAC)

ENDOCRINE BOARD REVIEW

ANSWERS

Adrenal Board Review

Tobias Else, MD

1 ANSWER: E) No further imaging or biochemical workup needed

This patient has symptoms and signs of acute-onset adrenal insufficiency, including nausea, abdominal pain, and fatigue, as well as hypotension. In addition, she has bilateral adrenal masses, which appear well-rounded and circumscribed and are consistent with the diagnosis of bilateral adrenal hemorrhage. Therefore, no further imaging or testing is necessary now (Answer E). Patients undergoing hip replacement receive perisurgical anticoagulation, and this patient received warfarin, which resulted in bilateral adrenal hemorrhage and adrenal insufficiency. The correct therapy is immediate stress-dose hydrocortisone replacement. The differential diagnoses for bilateral adrenal masses with adrenal insufficiency are congenital adrenal hyperplasia (hyperplasia or myelolipomas), infection (eg, tuberculosis, histoplasmosis), adrenal lymphoma (often bilateral adrenal enlargement, somewhat respecting the adrenal shape), granulomatous disease, and bilateral adrenal hemorrhage. The relatively normal DHEA-S concentration is suggestive of very recent onset of primary adrenal insufficiency (longer half-life than cortisol).

Bilateral adrenal metastases are common in patients with cancer and can be the initial finding for a cancer diagnosis. Both, pan-CT (Answer B) and FDG-PET (Answer D) would be reasonable choices to determine the full extent of disease. However, adrenal metastases from solid tumors rarely cause adrenal insufficiency.

Adrenal mass biopsy (Answer A) is reserved for instances when determining the adrenal mass pathology makes a difference in care (eg, patient with lung cancer who has an adrenal nodule).

Regarding this patient's history, there is no concern for bilateral adrenal pheochromocytomas, which also do not cause adrenal insufficiency. Thus, DOTATATE PET (Answer C) is not necessary.

EDUCATIONAL OBJECTIVE

Diagnose and treat patients with adrenal insufficiency in the setting of bilateral adrenal masses.

REFERENCE(S)

Bornstein SR, Allolio B, Arlt W, et al. Diagnosis and treatment of primary adrenal insufficiency: an Endocrine Society clinical practice guideline. *J Clin Endocrinol Metab.* 2016;101(2):364-389. PMID: 26760044

Badawy M, Gaballah AH, Ganeshan D, et al. Adrenal hemorrhage and hemorrhagic masses; diagnostic workup and imaging findings. *Br J Radiol.* 2021;94(1127):20210753. PMID: 34464549

2 ANSWER: D) Recommend no further evaluation now, follow-up with primary care physician

The workup of adrenal masses or nodules aims to answer 2 questions: (1) Is the mass benign or malignant? (2) Is there evidence of any hormone excess? The first question can usually be answered by reviewing imaging. This mass is small, well-circumscribed, homogeneous, and has a density less than 10 Hounsfield units. Therefore, it is a benign adrenal nodule—a lipid-rich adenoma.

FDG-PET (Answer C), which is used for the differential diagnosis of benign and malignant nodules, is not necessary.

Biochemical evaluation for pheochromocytoma (Answer B) is only indicated if the mass has imaging criteria suggestive of pheochromocytoma or if there is clinical suspicion for a catecholamine-secreting tumor. This patient does not have classical spell-like symptoms, hypertension, or imaging consistent with a pheochromocytoma (Hounsfield units >10, commonly >20). She does not have symptoms or signs of overt adrenocortical hormone excess.

Screening for primary aldosteronism (Answer A) would only be necessary if she had hypertension or hypokalemia.

Despite the absence of overt hypercortisolism, screening for mild autonomous cortisol access (1-mg dexamethasone-suppression test) was performed, and the results were normal.

Initial workup of adrenal nodules should attempt to make a final diagnosis and define which patients would benefit from surgery. Only very few patients need to be followed (eg, patients with indeterminate nodules who do not wish to undergo surgery, or those who have small, indeterminate nodules with mainly benign features). This patient has a nonfunctional, benign, lipid-rich adenoma. Such adenomas are present in 1% to 5% of the population and do not need dedicated follow-up (thus, Answer D is correct and Answer E is incorrect).

EDUCATIONAL OBJECTIVE

Interpret diagnostic procedures for incidentally discovered adrenal nodules.

REFERENCE(S)

Fassnacht M, Arlt W, Bancos I, et al. Management of adrenal incidentalomas: European Society of Endocrinology Clinical Practice Guideline in collaboration with the European Network for the Study of Adrenal Tumors. *Eur J Endocrinol.* 2016;175(2):G1-G34. PMID: 27390021

Vaidya A, Hamrahian A, Bancos I, Fleseriu M, Ghayee HK. The evaluation of incidentally discovered adrenal masses. *Endocr Pract.* 2019;25(2):178-192. PMID: 30817193

Yip L, Duh QY, Wachtel H, et al. American Association of Endocrine Surgeons guidelines for adrenalectomy: executive summary. *JAMA Surg.* 2022;157(10):870-877. PMID: 35976622

3 ANSWER: A) CT of the abdomen

This patient has a classic presentation of pheochromocytoma with tachycardia, palpitation, hypertension, headache, pallor, and nausea. Biochemical testing reveals elevated metanephrine and normetanephrine levels. Several imaging modalities can be used to localize a pheochromocytoma or paraganglioma. Typical locations for a functional paraganglioma are abdomen, pelvis, or chest. Head and neck paragangliomas rarely produce catecholamines. This patient has an elevated metanephrine concentration, and this is almost exclusively observed in patients with adrenal pheochromocytoma. Therefore, CT of the abdomen (Answer A) is the correct initial imaging modality.

Whole-body MRI (Answer E) is mainly used for regular screening in carriers of *SDHx* pathogenic variants with a diagnosis of hereditary paraganglioma syndrome, and it is unnecessary in this patient.

Functional scans are largely reserved for defining tumor extent (eg, metastasis). MIBG scan (Answer D) is used in the evaluation of patients with metastatic disease who would benefit from ^{131}I-MIBG therapy. If this patient had only normetanephrine elevation, FDG-PET (Answer C) or DOTATATE-PET (Answer B) could be considered for tumor localization. However, even in that setting, starting with abdominal imaging, which will reveal most tumors, is the more cost-effective method.

EDUCATIONAL OBJECTIVE

Perform cost-effective and rational imaging workup in patients with elevated plasma free metanephrines.

REFERENCE(S)

Neumann HPH, Young WF Jr, Eng C. Pheochromocytoma and paraganglioma. *N Engl J Med.* 2019;381(6):552-565. PMID: 31390501

Lenders JWM, Duh Q-Y, Eisenhofer G, et al; Endocrine Society. Pheochromocytoma and paraganglioma: an Endocrine Society clinical practice guideline. *J Clin Endocrinol Metab.* 2014;99(6):1915-1942. PMID: 24893135

4 ANSWER: A) Continue hydrocortisone orally, 20 mg in the morning and 10 mg in the early afternoon, and measure aldosterone and renin in 2 days

This patient has a classic presentation of immunotherapy-related hypophysitis with secondary adrenal insufficiency. While cosyntropin-stimulation testing is a very good way to assess for primary adrenal insufficiency or longstanding secondary adrenal insufficiency (>3 weeks, time to adrenal atrophy without ACTH stimulus), it is not a good test for recent-onset secondary adrenal insufficiency. The best confirmatory test for secondary adrenal insufficiency is insulin-tolerance testing, but it will not change clinical management in this case. Primary adrenal insufficiency can occur with immunotherapy, but this is rare.

Follow-up testing for hypoaldosteronism once the patient is on a lower dosage of hydrocortisone (Answer A) is reasonable.

Measuring 21-hydroxylase antibodies (Answer B), which are specific for patients with sporadic autoimmune adrenal insufficiency, is unnecessary and would not change management.

With this classic presentation, there is no need for repeated testing (Answer E).

Although affected patients often have headaches and an enlarged pituitary gland, imaging with MRI (Answer D) is not necessary. This imaging could be entertained if the patient had progressive disease and metastasis to the pituitary is suspected or if she developed diabetes insipidus, which is rare in the setting of immunotherapy-associated hypophysitis.

There is no reason to believe that she is regularly exposed to exogenous steroids (Answer C). If she were currently on exogeneous glucocorticoids, she would not have developed an adrenal crisis. If the low cortisol value respresented an asymptomatic laboratory abnormality, any past exposure to glucocorticoids (eg, intraarticular injections, topical steroids) should be explored.

EDUCATIONAL OBJECTIVE

Guide the diagnostic workup of secondary adrenal insufficiency of recent onset.

REFERENCE(S)

Reimondo G, Bovio S, Allasino B, Terzolo M, Angeli A. Secondary hypoadrenalism. *Pituitary.* 2008;11(2):147-154. PMID: 18418713

Bornstein SR, Allolio B, Arlt W, et al. Diagnosis and treatment of primary adrenal insufficiency: an Endocrine Society clinical practice guideline. *J Clin Endocrinol Metab.* 2016;101(2):364-389. PMID: 26760044

5 ANSWER: D) Refer for laparoscopic right adrenalectomy

This patient has a diagnosis of mild autonomous cortisol excess (ie, subclinical Cushing syndrome). Despite the recommendation of surgical removal of the adrenal tumor in all patients with mild autonomous cortisol excess by some expert opinion (American Association of Endocrine Surgeons), the general opinion is that patients for whom adrenalectomy might be beneficial should be very carefully selected. There is a growing body of literature that documents the long-term health consequences of mild autonomous cortisol excess derived from adrenal adenomas. These tumors are typically larger than 2.5 cm in diameter, as in this patient, and although exact minimal criteria for mild autonomous cortisol excess are debated, the 3 main tests (ACTH, DHEA-S, and dexamethasone-suppressed cortisol) are all consistently abnormal in this patient. She was initially clinically observed because she had only osteoporosis and borderline hypertension as possible manifestations of hypercortisolism. However, hypertension has now worsened, and she has developed obesity and diabetes. The DHEA-S concentration has further decreased because of persistent hypercortisolism of adrenal origin (suppression of pituitary ACTH drive). The major morbidity that improves with adrenalectomy is hypertension. However, autonomous cortisol excess from adrenal adenomas is associated with a host of other conditions, such as osteoporosis, glucose intolerance, cardiovascular events, and death, thus justifying the recommendation for surgical right adrenalectomy (Answer D). Retrospective and prospective studies have shown that patients without elevated urinary free cortisol excretion might benefit from surgery.

Delaying medical or surgical therapy until urinary free cortisol is clearly elevated (Answer A) is incorrect. Also, this degree of cortisol excess can cause morbidities.

The patient does not have ACTH-dependent Cushing syndrome and therefore a high-dose dexamethasone-suppression test (Answer B) is not indicated.

There is also no concern for adrenocortical carcinoma, as there is only insidious worsening of symptoms and the mass appears to be benign with a density of less than 10 Hounsfield units. Therefore, imaging for malignant transformation (Answer C) is incorrect.

Surgery as a final therapy is preferred over any medical treatment, including mifepristone or osilodrostat (Answer E), which is indicated for patients with unsuccessful surgery or those who are not surgical candidates. Indeed, this patient needed postsurgical hydrocortisone replacement due to suppression of the contralateral adrenal gland—post hoc evidence for presurgical hypercortisolism.

EDUCATIONAL OBJECTIVE

Identify patients with mild autonomous cortisol excess who might benefit from adrenalectomy.

REFERENCE(S)

Chiodini I, Morelli V, Salcuni AS, et al. Beneficial metabolic effects of prompt surgical treatment in patients with an adrenal incidentaloma causing biochemical hypercortisolism. *J Clin Endocrinol Metab.* 2010;95(6):2736-2745. PMID: 20375210

Di Dalmazi G, Vicennati V, Garelli S, et al. Cardiovascular events and mortality in patients with adrenal incidentalomas that are either non-secreting or associated with intermediate phenotype or subclinical Cushing's syndrome: a 15-year retrospective study. *Lancet Diabet Endocrinol.* 2014;2(5):396-405. PMID: 24795253

Elhassan YS, Alahdab F, Prete A, et al. Natural history of adrenal incidentalomas with and without mild autonomous cortisol excess: a systematic review and meta-analysis. *Ann Intern Med.* 2019;171(2): 107-116. PMID: 31234202

Yip L, Duh Q-Y, Wachtel H, et al. American Association of Endocrine Surgeons guidelines for adrenalectomy: executive summary. *JAMA Surg.* 2022;157(10):870-877. PMID: 35976622

6 ANSWER: C) Cortisol withdrawal syndrome

This patient has classic symptoms of steroid withdrawal syndrome (Answer C) following adrenalectomy for adrenal Cushing syndrome.

She is receiving appropriate hydrocortisone replacement therapy for presumed adrenal insufficiency (15-25 mg daily); therefore, a diagnosis of overt adrenal insufficiency (Answer B) is unlikely. Symptoms of adrenal insufficiency are generally more severe, including nausea and vomiting.

The increased ACTH value is a result of a recovering hypothalamic-pituitary-adrenal axis and not of ectopic ACTH production (Answer E).

After removal of the tumor, the patient likely has persistently low adrenal androgen levels. However, whether deficiency of adrenal androgens causes any clinical symptoms is still an ongoing discussion. A presentation as in this patient would not be explained by simple adrenal androgen deficiency (Answer A), which might affect libido and well-being but not lead to headaches, etc.

Incomplete tumor removal (Answer D) would be evident with persistence of elevated cortisol levels and continued ACTH suppression, which are not present in this patient.

EDUCATIONAL OBJECTIVE

Identify steroid withdrawal as a sequela of treatment of hypercortisolism.

REFERENCE(S)

He X, Findling JW, Auchus RJ. Glucocorticoid withdrawal syndrome following treatment of endogenous Cushing syndrome. *Pituitary.* 2022;25(3):393-403. PMID: 35471718

7 ANSWER: B) Hold ibuprofen and advise against further use

This patient has renal tubular acidosis (RTA) type 4, likely caused by the combination of nonsteroidal anti-inflammatory drugs and mild diabetic nephropathy. RTA type 4 is characterized by hypokalemia, mild metabolic acidosis, and hyporeninemic (or normoreninemic) hypoaldosteronism. Therefore, the best next step is to eliminate the offending agent (naproxen) (Answer B).

Although the patient has mild hypertension and hypokalemia, she lacks any other clear symptoms or signs of adrenal insufficiency. Moreover, hypoaldosteronism would only occur in patients with primary adrenal insufficiency and DHEA-S would be expected to be low and ACTH to be elevated. Therefore, the patient does not need any therapy for adrenal insufficiency—neither stress doses (Answer A) nor regular replacement therapy (Answer C). RTA type 4 is usually a state of low aldosterone production and aldosterone resistance, and therapy with fludrocortisone therapy is not warranted.

Although RTA type 4 is associated with low aldosterone levels, treatment with fludrocortisone (Answer D) is not helpful.

While holding metformin in hospitalized patients with potentially acutely worsened kidney function is good practice, advising against future use (Answer E) is not correct.

EDUCATIONAL OBJECTIVE

Identify renal tubular acidosis type 4 as a state of hyporeninemic hypoaldosteronism.

REFERENCE(S)

Batlle D, Arruda J. Hyperkalemic forms of renal tubular acidosis: clinical and pathophysiological aspects. *Adv Chronic Kidney Dis.* 2018;25(4):321-333. PMID: 30139459

8 ANSWER: D) Glucocorticoid resistance

This patient has elevated cortisol following a 1-mg dexamethasone-suppression test, as well as 2-fold elevated urinary cortisol, yet he does not have any symptoms or signs of Cushing syndrome. Therefore, the most likely diagnosis is glucocorticoid resistance (Answer D), which is caused by pathogenic variants in the glucocorticoid receptor gene (*NR3C1*). Glucocorticoid resistance can be inherited in an autosomal dominant or recessive fashion. Generalized glucocorticoid resistance leads to elevated cortisol and ACTH levels (resistance to feedback) and a diminished glucocorticoid effect in peripheral tissues. Although affected patients lack symptoms or signs of classic hypercortisolism, they develop adrenal hyperplasia and enlargement and apparent mineralocorticoid excess due to elevated deoxycorticosterone and overwhelming of renal 11β-hydroxysteroid dehydrogenase, which leads to mineralocorticoid effects of elevated cortisol. In addition, androgens are often elevated and can lead to menstrual irregularities and hirsutism.

ACTH resistance (Answer A) causes adrenal insufficiency.

While 11β hydroxylase deficiency (Answer E) can present in similar fashion, cortisol is low in that setting.

Ectopic ACTH syndrome (Answer C) and Cushing disease (Answer B) cause both ACTH-dependent Cushing syndrome. However, clinical symptoms and signs of hypercortisolism would be expected.

EDUCATIONAL OBJECTIVE

Identify glucocorticoid resistance due to impaired glucocorticoid receptor function.

REFERENCE(S)

Martins CS, de Castro M. Generalized and tissue specific glucocorticoid resistance. *Mol Cell Endocrinol.* 2021;530:111277. PMID: 33864884

Bouligand J, Delemer B, Hecart AC, et al. Familial glucocorticoid receptor haploinsufficiency by non-sense mediated mRNA decay, adrenal hyperplasia and apparent mineralocorticoid excess. *PLoS One.* 2010;5(10):e13563. PMID: 21042587

9 ANSWER: D) Congenital adrenal hyperplasia

This patient's CT shows massive bilateral adrenal myelolipomas. These lesions are easy to identify on CT because they always have very low Hounsfield units (<10). Myelolipomas are benign neoplasms composed of mature adipose tissue, bone, and hematopoietic tissue. Myelolipomas have been reported in patients with congenital adrenal hyperplasia (CAH) (Answer D) due to deficiency of 21-hydroxylase, 17-hydroxylase, or 11-hydroxylase. Most of these individuals have either untreated or poorly treated CAH. Patients with CAH may actually have no ill effects over many months or years from cessation of steroid therapy until serious illness intervenes.

It is speculated that chronic exposure of the adrenal glands to high ACTH concentrations increases the risk of developing myelolipomas. In 1950, Selye and Stone transformed adrenal tissue in rats into adipose and bone marrow elements by injecting pituitary gland extract in combination with methyltestosterone. Myelolipomas have also been reported in patients with other disorders associated with chronic ACTH hypersecretion, including Cushing disease, Addison disease, and Nelson syndrome.

Although some of the answer choices would explain adrenal insufficiency, there are no known reports of adrenal myelolipomas in patients with histoplasmosis (Answer E) or autoimmune adrenal disease (Answer A).

Adrenal enlargement in patients with metastatic disease (Answer C) or bilateral adrenal hemorrhage (Answer B) has a heterogeneous appearance with an indeterminate attenuation value (>20 Hounsfield units).

Decreased fertility is common in men with CAH and may be related to disordered adrenal metabolism and development and growth of testicular adrenal rest tumors. Since these lesions are quite common in men with CAH, it is currently recommended that testicular ultrasonography be performed routinely in young men with this condition.

EDUCATIONAL OBJECTIVE

Diagnose adrenal myelolipomas as a complication of poorly controlled congenital adrenal hyperplasia.

REFERENCE(S)

German-Mena E, Zibari GB, Levine SN. Adrenal myelolipomas in patients with congenital adrenal hyperplasia: review of the literature and a case report. *Endocr Pract.* 2011;17(3):441-447. PMID: 21324823

Nermoen I, Rørvik J, Holmedal SH, et al. High frequency of adrenal myelolipomas and testicular adrenal rest tumours in adult Norwegian patients with classical congenital adrenal hyperplasia because of 21-hydroxylase deficiency. *Clin Endocrinol (Oxf).* 2011;75(6):753-759. PMID: 21689130

10 ANSWER: C) Ectopic ACTH-secreting small cell carcinoma of the lung

The presence of hypertension with hypokalemic metabolic alkalosis and edema suggests a state of mineralocorticoid excess. However, this patient has suppressed plasma renin activity and aldosterone, which suggests excess of some other mineralocorticoid-like steroid. Of course, the most likely steroid is cortisol. Neither primary aldosteronism (Answer B) (elevated aldosterone, suppressed plasma renin activity) nor 11-hydroxylase deficiency (Answer D) (suppressed plasma renin activity and aldosterone) is possible.

The most likely cause of hypercortisolism in a patient with a long history of cigarette smoking and a lung mass is an ectopic ACTH-secreting small cell lung cancer (Answer C). The prevalence of lung cancer in women is increasing. The prodigious hypercortisolism seen in these patients overwhelms intrarenal cortisol metabolism and results in a state of mineralocorticoid excess with suppressed plasma renin activity and aldosterone. Because of the catabolic nature of severe hypercortisolism and metastatic disease, patients with ectopic ACTH syndrome often present as cachectic and malnourished, with muscle weakness due to steroid-induced myopathy as a leading symptom.

Adrenocortical carcinoma (Answer A) may occasionally present with severe hypercortisolism and hypokalemia. However, adrenocortical carcinoma neoplasms are usually very large (>4 cm) and have an indeterminate attenuation value (Hounsfield units >20). In addition, one would not expect the contralateral adrenal gland to be enlarged due to the autonomous adrenal-dependent cortisol production from adrenocortical carcinoma.

Liddle syndrome (Answer E) is an autosomal dominant form of hypertension due to pathogenic variants in the genes encoding subunits of the amiloride-sensitive epithelial sodium channel (*SCNN1B* or *SCNN1G*). This syndrome usually presents in childhood or early adult life and is not associated with any adrenal enlargement.

The aldosterone-to-plasma renin activity ratio can provide useful clinical information in any patient with hypokalemia and hypertension. Of course, elevated ratios (ie, plasma aldosterone [PAC]/plasma renin activity [PRA] greater than or equal to 20 [555 in SI units]) suggest autonomous aldosterone secretion (primary aldosteronism). Elevations of both PAC and PRA (normal ratio) may be seen in all causes of renovascular hypertension, diuretic use, renin-secreting tumors (rare), malignant phase of hypertension, and coarctation of the aorta. However, low levels of PAC and PRA (normal ratio) may be caused by Liddle syndrome, Cushing syndrome, congenital adrenal hyperplasia (eg, 11β-hydroxylase deficiency), exogenous mineralocorticoid, syndrome of apparent mineralocorticoid excess (11β-hydroxysteroid dehydrogenase deficiency), or deoxycorticosterone-secreting adrenal tumors. Aldosterone (like cortisol) has a diurnal rhythm, so sampling should ideally be performed in the morning. Because the presence of marked hypokalemia may attenuate aldosterone secretion, potassium levels often need to be restored to normal (without a mineralocorticoid receptor antagonist) to accurately interpret the PAC.

EDUCATIONAL OBJECTIVE

Perform the differential diagnosis of hypertension, hypokalemia, and subnormal plasma renin and aldosterone.

REFERENCE(S)

Ejaz S, Vassilopoulou-Sellin R, Busaidy NL, et al. Cushing syndrome secondary to ectopic adreno-corticotropic hormone secretion the University of Texas MD Anderson Cancer Center Experience. *Cancer.* 2011;117(19):4381-4389. PMID: 21412758

Alexandraki KI, Grossman AB. The ectopic ACTH syndrome. *Rev Endocr Metab Disord.* 2010;11(2): 117-126. PMID: 20544290

11 ANSWER: C) Multiple endocrine neoplasia type 2B

This patient presents with a family history of bilateral pheochromocytoma indicating a genetic basis for his disorder. The presence of his marfanoid body habitus and mucosal neuromas (as observed in the photograph) are diagnostic of multiple endocrine neoplasia type 2B (MEN 2B) (Answer C). MEN 2B is an autosomal dominant disorder with variable penetrance, and it represents approximately 5% of all patients with MEN type 2. The MEN 2B phenotype includes pheochromocytoma (usually bilateral), medullary thyroid carcinoma, mucosal neuromas (involving the tongue, lips, and eyelids), thickened corneal nerves, intestinal ganglioneuromatosis, thin face, and marfanoid body habitus. MEN 2B is associated with pathogenic variants in codon 918 of the *RET* proto-oncogene in 95% of cases.

MEN 2A is an autosomal dominant disorder that is also associated with bilateral adrenal pheochromocytoma (which may be asynchronous), medullary thyroid carcinoma, and hyperparathyroidism. Medullary thyroid carcinoma is usually detected before pheochromocytoma. MEN 2A is also caused by pathogenic variants in the *RET* proto-oncogene, but these variants are distinct from those that cause MEN 2B.

Pheochromocytoma is reported in approximately 30% of patients with von Hippel–Lindau (VHL) syndrome (Answer E), an autosomal dominant disorder characterized by pheochromocytoma (frequently bilateral), retinal angiomas, cerebellar hemangioblastoma, epididymal cystadenoma, renal and pancreatic cysts, pancreatic islet-cell neoplasms, and renal carcinoma. The prevalence of VHL is approximately 1 in 35,000 persons. The *VHL* tumor suppressor gene encodes a protein that regulates hypoxia-induced proteins. More than 300 disease-causing *VHL* pathogenic variants have been identified that lead to loss of function of the VHL protein. Nearly 100% of patients affected with VHL have an identifiable pathogenic variant.

Neurofibromatosis type 1 (Answer D) is an autosomal dominant disorder characterized by neurofibromas, café-au-lait spots, axillary and inguinal freckling, and iris hamartomas. Approximately 2% of patients with neurofibromatosis type 1 develop catecholamine-secreting tumors; however, these are usually solitary benign lesions and are rarely bilateral.

Carney complex (Answer A) is the association of spotty facial pigmentation (involving the vermillion borders of the lips and eyelids), cardiac myxomas, cutaneous and mammary myxomas, Cushing syndrome due to primary pigmented nodular adrenal disease, testicular tumors, schwannomas, and pituitary GH hypersecretion. Carney complex is not associated with mucocutaneous neuromas or pheochromocytoma. Many cases of Carney complex are due to pathogenic variants in the gene encoding cyclic adenosine monophosphate-dependent protein kinase A regulatory subunit 1α (*PRKAR1A*).

MEN type 1 (Answer B) is characterized by pituitary tumors (~20%), primary hyperparathyroidism (>90%), and pancreatic neuroendocrine tumors. Pheochromocytomas have been reported, but they are unlikely to occur bilaterally. Skin lesions associated with MEN type 1 are angiofibromas and collagenomas.

EDUCATIONAL OBJECTIVE

Diagnose multiple endocrine neoplasia type 2B on the basis of clinical findings and differentiate among the familial syndromes associated with bilateral pheochromocytoma.

REFERENCE(S)

Gagel RF, Shefelbine S, Hayashi H, Cole G. Multiple endocrine neoplasia. In: Runge MS, Patterson C, eds. *Principles of Molecular Medicine*. 2nd ed. Humana Press; 2006:393-399.

Raue F, Frank-Raue K. Genotype-phenotype relationship in multiple endocrine neoplasia type 2. Implications for clinical management. *Hormones (Athens)*. 2009;8(1):23-28. PMID: 19269918

de Groot JW, Links TP, Plukker JT, Lips CJ, Hofstra RM. RET as a diagnostic and therapeutic target in sporadic and hereditary endocrine tumors. *Endocr Rev*. 2006;27(5):535-560. PMID: 16849421

12 ANSWER: E) Late-night salivary cortisol measurement

The loss of cortisol diurnal rhythm is a defining feature of Cushing disease. Saliva is an ultrafiltrate of plasma, and salivary cortisol concentrations roughly reflect plasma free cortisol concentrations. At night, plasma cortisol concentrations fall, and salivary cortisol decreases in parallel. Salivary cortisol testing has become routine and offers comparable diagnostic utility and greater convenience than late-night serum cortisol testing. In addition to its utility as a screening test for Cushing disease, late-night salivary cortisol measurement (Answer E) is more sensitive than other conventional tests in detecting recurrent disease. False-positive results with late-night salivary cortisol measurement occur in persons with gingival or tongue bleeding, with sleep disturbance, or who work night shifts. Also, contamination can influence test results, such as transfer of hydrocortisone cream from the hands to the device used to collect the saliva.

Measurement of 24-hour urinary free cortisol (Answer C) is relatively insensitive in detecting recurrent Cushing disease because only a small fraction (<1%) of cortisol is excreted unmetabolized, and only when the cortisol concentration exceeds the binding capacity of plasma.

Dexamethasone-suppression testing (Answers A and B) uses the empirically attenuated feedback inhibition of the pituitary adenoma to dexamethasone, compared with the normal pituitary. This distinction is not as reliable as the loss of diurnal rhythm in early, recurrent Cushing disease.

Inferior petrosal sinus sampling (Answer D) is only used to exclude ectopic ACTH syndrome *after* the diagnosis of ACTH-dependent hypercortisolism is established.

EDUCATIONAL OBJECTIVE

Compare the diagnostic performance of different testing approaches for recurrent Cushing disease.

REFERENCE(S)

Carrasco CA, Coste J, Guignat L, et al. Midnight salivary cortisol determination for assessing the outcome of transsphenoidal surgery in Cushing's disease. *J Clin Endocrinol Metab.* 2008;93(12):4728-4734. PMID: 18728161

Raff H, Auchus RJ, Findling JW, Niemann LK. Urine free cortisol in the diagnosis of Cushing's syndrome: is it worth doing and, if so, how? *J Clin Endocrinol Metab.* 2015;100(2):395-397. PMID: 25423573

13 ANSWER: C) Plasma very long-chain fatty acid measurement

The finding of primary adrenal insufficiency in a young man should always raise the suspicion of adrenoleukodystrophy (ALD), particularly when concurrent neurologic symptoms are present. ALD is an X-linked inherited metabolic storage disease associated with a defect in an ABC transporter that results in defective peroxisomal β-oxidation and accumulation of very long-chain fatty acids (C24, C26) in tissues, especially in the brain and the adrenal glands. The accumulation of very long-chain fatty acids causes demyelination associated with an intense inflammatory response in white matter. Neurologic manifestations include psychiatric symptoms, neuromuscular problems, slurred speech, and even dementia. When mild, the condition is often misdiagnosed as multiple sclerosis or another primary neurologic disease. ALD affects approximately 1 in 17,000 boys, and female carriers can be symptomatic neurologically, but rarely, if ever, develop adrenal insufficiency. Approximately 70% of boys with ALD develop adrenal insufficiency. Elevated plasma very long-chain fatty acids (Answer C) is a highly reliable test, and the diagnosis can be confirmed by genetic testing of the *ABCD1* gene. Adrenomyeloneuropathy is a milder form of this disorder that can coexist with ALD in the same family. Adrenomyeloneuropathy may present as primary adrenal insufficiency in young male patients, and the milder neurologic deficits portend a more favorable prognosis. Bone marrow transplant is curative if diagnosed before the cerebral disease has progressed beyond recovery.

Serum 21-hydroxylase antibodies (Answer D) are used to diagnose autoimmune adrenal insufficiency.

Lupus anticoagulant (Answer B) is often present with adrenal hemorrhage.

Occult corticosteroid use (Answer E) would suppress—not raise—ACTH.

Adrenal CT (Answer A) would show small adrenal glands in both ALD and autoimmune adrenalitis.

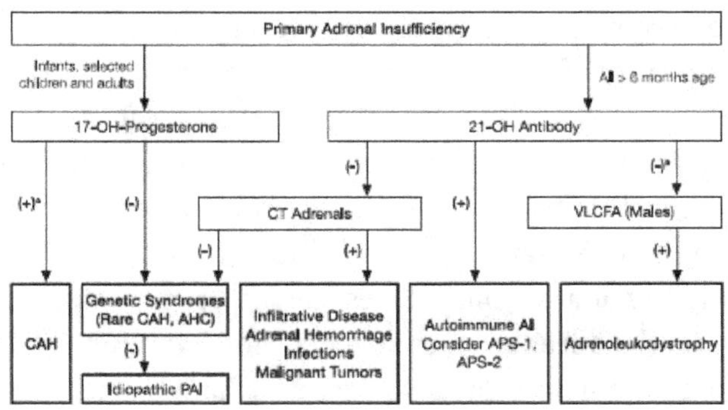

Reprinted from Bornstein SR et al. *J Clin Endocrinol Metab*, 2016; 101(2):364-389. © The Endocrine Society; Adapted with permission from E. S. Husebye ES et al. *J Intern Med.* 2014; 275(181): 104–115. © John Wiley & Sons, Inc.

EDUCATIONAL OBJECTIVE

Perform the differential diagnosis of adrenal insufficiency in a young man.

REFERENCE(S)

Dubey P, Raymond GV, Moser AB, Kharkar S, Bezman L, Moser HW. Adrenal insufficiency in asymptomatic adrenoleukodystrophy patients identified by very long-chain fatty acid screening. *J Pediatr.* 2005;146(4):528-532. PMID: 15812458

Mosser J, Douar AM, Sarde CO, et al. Putative X-linked adrenoleukodystrophy gene shares unexpected homology with ABC transporters. *Nature.* 1993;361(6414):726-730. PMID: 8441467

Bornstein SR, Allolio B, Arlt W, et al. Diagnosis and treatment of primary adrenal insufficiency: an Endocrine Society Clinical Practice Guideline. *J Clin Endocrinol Metab.* 2016;101(2):364-389. PMID: 26760044

14 ANSWER: A) Measure plasma metanephrines and perform a 1-mg overnight dexamethasone-suppression test

Because of hypertension and hypokalemia, this patient was evaluated for primary aldosteronism, and the screening aldosterone-to-renin ratio is marginally positive. Ordinarily, one would proceed to confirmatory testing, followed by CT, and then adrenal venous sampling to localize the source(s) of aldosterone. In this case, however, the weight gain, hyperglycemia, plethora, and dermal atrophy are suggestive of hypercortisolism as well. Proximal myopathy and striae are late manifestations in the development of Cushing syndrome and are insensitive findings. Because CT was performed, we know that she has a fairly large adrenal tumor—significantly larger than those that usually cause primary aldosteronism. On careful inspection, one can discern that the contralateral adrenal gland is somewhat atrophic, suggesting hypercortisolism from the adrenal tumor. When the diameter of adrenal cortical tumors is greater than 2.4 cm, the risk of hypercortisolism rises, and if the tumor is removed without testing cortisol dynamics, adrenal crisis might occur postoperatively. In addition, the CT scan in this vignette was done only with contrast, so one cannot use density to determine whether the tumor is lipid-rich and thus exclude pheochromocytoma.

Spironolactone (Answer D) would treat the mineralocorticoid excess but not glucocorticoid manifestations and this patient needs further evaluation.

Left adrenalectomy (Answer B) is incorrect because the possibilities of hypercortisolism and pheochromocytoma must be excluded before performing surgery for a tumor of that size.

Adrenal venous sampling (Answer E) and a saline infusion testing (Answer C) are routine in the evaluation of primary aldosteronism, but with the concern of hypercortisolism and the presence of a large adrenal tumor, measuring plasma metanephrines and performing a 1-mg overnight dexamethasone-suppression test (Answer A) is the correct next step.

In this case, the plasma metanephrines were normal, and the overnight dexamethasone-suppression test resulted in a cortisol concentration of 4.4 µg/dL (121.4 nmol/L). Subsequent testing documented an ACTH concentration of 6 pg/mL (1.3 pmol/L), DHEA-S concentration of 22 µg/dL (0.6 µmol/L), and normal urinary free cortisol excretion. Thus, the diagnosis of ACTH-independent hypercortisolism was established, which trumps the evaluation of primary aldosteronism and indicates that the adrenal tumor should be removed with perioperative glucocorticoid coverage. Coproduction of aldosterone and cortisol from adrenal cortical adenomas, particularly larger tumors, is well described. It is possible, although unlikely, that the primary aldosteronism is bilateral and unrelated to the adrenal tumor, so the patient should be rescreened for primary aldosteronism after adrenalectomy. If it persists, spironolactone would be an appropriate treatment.

EDUCATIONAL OBJECTIVE

Correlate the size of adrenal cortical adenomas with hormone production or coproduction and pursue appropriate evaluation and management.

REFERENCE(S)

Spath M, Korovkin S, Antke C, Anlauf M, Willenberg HS. Aldosterone- and cortisol-co-secreting adrenal tumors: the lost subtype of primary aldosteronism. *Eur J Endocrinol.* 2011;164(4):447-455. PMID: 21270113

Morelli V, Reimondo G, Giordano R, et al. Long-term follow-up in adrenal incidentalomas: an Italian multicenter study. *J Clin Endocrinol Metab.* 2014;99(3):827-834. PMID: 24423350

Fallo F, Bertello C, Tizzani D, et al. Concurrent primary aldosteronism and subclinical cortisol hypersecretion: a prospective study. *J Hypertens.* 2011;29(9):1773- 1777. PMID: 21720261

15 ANSWER: A) Perform adrenal CT

This patient has resistant hypertension and hypokalemia, and the index of suspicion for primary aldosteronism is very high. Case detection with the aldosterone-to-renin ratio is indicated and was indeed ordered. Of all medications, mineralocorticoid receptor antagonists are the most likely to interfere with screening because these drugs have a tendency to raise renin. However, if renin remains suppressed, the screen is valid despite the presence of any medications. The revised Endocrine Society guidelines (*see figure*) recommend eliminating confirmatory testing from the evaluation when renin is suppressed, hypokalemia is present, and the aldosterone concentration is greater than 20 ng/dL (>554.8 pmol/L), as is the case in this patient. Thus, the next step is adrenal CT (Answer A).

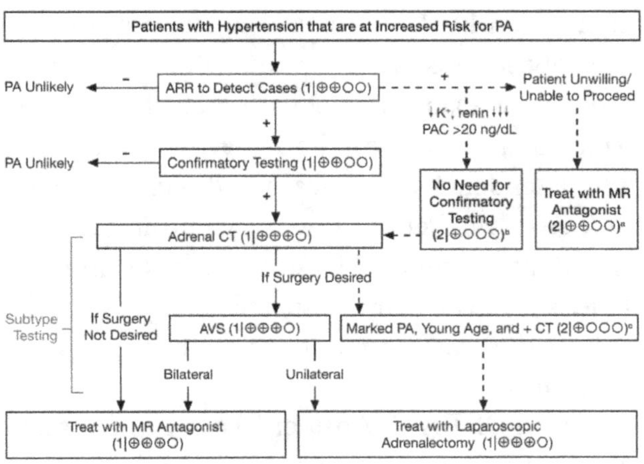

Reprinted from Funder JW et al. *J Clin Endocrinol Metab*, 2016; 101(5): 1889-1916. © The Endocrine Society; Adapted from Funder JW et al. *J Clin Endocrinol Metab*, 2008; 93(3): 3266–3281. © The Endocrine Society.

If the renin had not been low, the screen would not have been interpretable and would have required repeated testing. Volume and the renin-aldosterone axis might take up to 6 weeks (but typically only 2 weeks) to re-equilibrate after stopping spironolactone (Answer D), and in this case it is not required.

Similarly, discontinuation of other antihypertensive agents (Answer C) is not required for diagnosis if the renin is suppressed.

MRI (Answer B) is inferior to CT due to low resolution.

The patient is tolerating spironolactone, so changing to eplerenone (Answer E), which is more expensive, is not necessary. In fact, all of the subsequent steps of the evaluation can be performed without stopping spironolactone, as long as the renin remains suppressed on that dosage. If the patient cannot or does not wish to pursue surgical management, one should continue medical therapy with a mineralocorticoid receptor antagonist. If he develops gynecomastia and/or erectile dysfunction from spironolactone, then substitution of eplerenone would be appropriate.

EDUCATIONAL OBJECTIVE

Guide screening and evaluation for primary aldosteronism.

REFERENCE(S)

Funder JW, Carey RM, Mantero F, et al. The management of primary aldosteronism: case detection, diagnosis, and treatment: an Endocrine Society clinical practice guideline. *J Clin Endocrinol Metab.* 2016;101(5):1889-1916. PMID: 26934393

Haase M, Riester A, Kropil P, et al. Outcome of adrenal vein sampling performed during concurrent mineralocorticoid receptor antagonist therapy. *J Clin Endocrinol Metab.* 2014;99(12):4397-4402. PMID: 25222758

Vaidya A, Malchoff CD, Auchus RJ; AACE Adrenal Scientific Committee. An individualized approach to the evaluation and management of primary aldosteronism. *Endocr Pract.* 2017;23(6):680-689. PMID: 28332881

16 ANSWER: C) Change hydrocortisone dosage to 30 mg in the morning and 20 mg in the afternoon and evening

Mitotane therapy is typically prescribed for residual adrenal cancer following debulking surgery or as adjuvant therapy for high-risk disease. Mitotane has a number of adverse effects and alters endocrine laboratory tests through a variety of mechanisms, including direct adrenal cytotoxicity. This patient had Cushing syndrome before surgery, and debulking has left him with adrenal insufficiency due to a temporarily suppressed hypothalamic-pituitary-adrenal axis, as evidenced by the undetectable plasma ACTH. At the same time, mitotane markedly increases corticosteroid-binding globulin and potently induces expression of CYP3A4, a major enzyme in cortisol catabolism. As a consequence, the dosage requirement and frequency of oral hydrocortisone increases markedly with concomitant mitotane therapy, and this patient's symptoms of adrenal insufficiency are due to inadequate cortisol exposure (thus, Answer C is correct).

Switching to methylprednisolone (Answer D) would require higher equivalent doses. Although methylprednisolone does not depend on activation through 11β-hydroxysteroid dehydrogenase, it is still (like all other glucocorticoids) metabolized and inactivated by CYP3A4.

Mitotane rarely causes aldosterone deficiency, and this patient is not volume depleted, so fludrocortisone at the dosage of 0.1 mg daily (Answer A) will not provide benefit.

He is at high risk of cancer recurrence, and reducing the mitotane dosage (Answer E) would result in subtherapeutic drug levels, which is unwise.

Hypogonadism and gynecomastia can occur with mitotane therapy, due to a rise in SHBG and some inhibition of testosterone synthesis, but his testosterone and inferred bioavailable testosterone are normal and do not account for his symptoms. Thus, adding testosterone enanthate (Answer B) is incorrect.

EDUCATIONAL OBJECTIVE

Adjust the dosage of hydrocortisone during mitotane therapy for adrenal carcinoma.

REFERENCE(S)

Chortis V, Taylor AE, Schneider P, et al. Mitotane therapy in adrenocortical cancer induces CYP3A4 and inhibits 5α-reductase, explaining the need for personalized glucocorticoid and androgen replacement. *J Clin Endocrinol Metab.* 2013;98(1):161-171. PMID: 23162091

Kroiss M, Quinkler M, Lutz WK, Allolio B, Fassnacht M. Drug interactions with mitotane by induction of CYP3A4 metabolism in the clinical management of adrenocortical carcinoma. *Clin Endocrinol (Oxf).* 2011;75(5):585-591. PMID: 21883349

Else T, Kim AC, Sabolch A, et al. Adrenocortical carcinoma. *Endocr Rev.* 2014;35(2):282-326. PMID: 24423978

17 ANSWER: D) Serum cortisol and 11-deoxycortisol measurements by tandem mass spectrometry

Metyrapone inhibits several enzymes in cortisol biosynthesis, most importantly 11β-hydroxylase (P450 11B1). As a result, 11-deoxycortisol rises. In addition, steroids more proximal to the block in the pathway increase, including mineralocorticoids such as 11-deoxycorticosterone and androgen precursors. The cortisol immunoassays used in most hospital laboratories show significant cross-reactivity with 11-deoxycortisol. Consequently, when serum 11-deoxycortisol concentrations are markedly elevated as in patients with Cushing syndrome who are treated with metyrapone, the serum cortisol value can be artifactually elevated, and the tendency to increase the dosage to lower the cortisol further can lead to symptoms of adrenal insufficiency. Measuring cortisol and 11-deoxycortisol by mass spectrometry (Answer D) obviates the cross-reactivity and affords true values.

Serum DHEA-S (Answer E) can be increased with metyrapone, but it is not used in dosage adjustment.

Likewise, the accumulation of 11-deoxycorticosterone can cause volume expansion and suppress plasma renin activity (Answer C), but this parameter is also not used to monitor therapy.

A cosyntropin-stimulation test (Answer A) is of no value in diagnosing or monitoring Cushing syndrome.

Measurement of late-night salivary cortisol (Answer B) is not useful to assess for cortisol deficiency.

EDUCATIONAL OBJECTIVE

Interpret results of serum cortisol testing in patients taking metyrapone.

REFERENCE(S)

Valassi E, Crespo I, Gich I, Rodriguez J, Webb SM. A reappraisal of the medical therapy with steroidogenesis inhibitors in Cushing's syndrome. *Clin Endocrinol (Oxf).* 2012;77(5):735-742. PMID: 22533782

Monaghan PJ, Owen LJ, Trainer PJ, Brabant G, Keevil BG, Darby D. Comparison of serum cortisol measurement by immunoassay and liquid chromatography-tandem mass spectrometry in patients receiving the 11β-hydroxylase inhibitor metyrapone. *Ann Clin Biochem.* 2011;48(Pt 5):441-446. PMID: 21813575

18 ANSWER: A) Add fludrocortisone acetate, 0.1 mg daily

Adrenal replacement therapy is guided primarily on clinical grounds with limited laboratory testing. In particular, plasma ACTH does not normalize with physiologic replacement doses and should not be used to titrate glucocorticoid in the same way that the TSH is used to guide thyroxine replacement. Weight regain is a good sign that glucocorticoid dosing is adequate, and lack of cushingoid stigmata suggests that he is not overtreated. Fatigue persists in some patients, and if it is due to glucocorticoid deficiency, this will transiently improve following each dose, which is not the case in this man. Consequently, a more distributed dose of methylprednisolone (Answer B) is not going to help, and a bedtime dose of glucocorticoid is generally unnecessary for patients with adrenal insufficiency—other than in congenital adrenal hyperplasia to lower cortisol precursor production. A single morning dose of hydrocortisone (Answer E) is sometimes sufficient for partial secondary adrenal insufficiency, but it is most likely not going to provide adequate exposure through the day in a patient with primary adrenal insufficiency.

Chronic volume depletion is another cause of fatigue in patients with adrenal insufficiency. This patient has constant fatigue, a mild increase in heart rate, and borderline-low blood pressure. More importantly, the plasma renin activity is quite elevated and the serum potassium value is high-normal. The patient was asked to stand for 2 minutes, and his blood pressure fell to 88/66 mm Hg and pulse rate rose to 115 beats/min. Hydrocortisone (cortisol) is a mineralocorticoid, but the enzyme 11β-hydroxysteroid dehydrogenase type 2 inactivates most of the cortisol before it binds to the mineralocorticoid receptor. Hydrocortisone dosages of roughly 25 mg daily or more provide a variable amount of mineralocorticoid activity. In this patient, 30 mg daily was sufficient to maintain his volume status. In contrast, neither methylprednisolone nor dexamethasone (Answer D) provides much mineralocorticoid activity.

With the switch from hydrocortisone to methylprednisolone, he has become volume depleted (thus, recommending no changes [Answer C] is incorrect), and he now needs fludrocortisone acetate therapy (Answer A). This scenario is often encountered in the setting of congenital adrenal hyperplasia, where the use of glucocorticoids other than hydrocortisone is common. For many patients with primary adrenal insufficiency, the "standard" fludrocortisone dosage of 0.1 mg daily is inadequate, and he might require a higher dosage to restore volume status and normalize plasma renin activity and serum potassium.

EDUCATIONAL OBJECTIVE

Characterize the differences in mineralocorticoid activity of cortisol replacement therapies.

REFERENCE(S)

Bornstein SR, Allolio B, Arlt W, et al. Diagnosis and treatment of primary adrenal insufficiency: an Endocrine Society Clinical Practice Guideline. *J Clin Endocrinol Metab.* 2016;101(2):364-389. PMID: 26760044

Bancos I, Hahner S, Tomlinson J, Arlt W. Diagnosis and management of adrenal insufficiency. *Lancet Diabetes Endocrinol.* 2015;3(3):216-226. PMID: 25098712

Esposito D, Pasquali D, Johannsson G. Primary adrenal insufficiency: managing mineralocorticoid replacement therapy. *J Clin Endocrinol Metab.* 2018;103(2):376-387. PMID: 29156052

19 ANSWER: B) Left adrenal gland is the source (left adenoma)

For adrenal venous sampling, the cortisol concentrations in the adrenal vein samples are used to determine whether the adrenal veins were accessed and to correct for the fractional dilution of the adrenal vein blood with mixed venous blood.

This ratio of cortisol in the adrenal vein blood to cortisol in the mixed venous blood is often called the selectivity index. The selectivity index on both sides should be greater than 2 if adrenal venous sampling is performed without cosyntropin infusion and greater than 4 if performed with cosyntropin. Otherwise, the sample does not contain sufficient adrenal vein blood to interpret the results, and the study should not be interpreted unless both selectivity indices are greater than these minimum values. Usually, the right side, which is more difficult to access, is more likely to fail the selectivity index test. In this case, although the cortisol in the right adrenal vein is much lower than the left, the selectivity index is 300/22 = 13.6 (more than adequate). Thus, the study is successful, and all the information is available for interpretation (thus, Answer E is incorrect).

Next, the lateralization indices are calculated, dividing aldosterone by cortisol to obtain aldosterone-to-cortisol (A/C) ratios or cortisol-corrected aldosterone values (*see table*). If the adrenal vein A/C ratios differ by a factor of 4 or more for a cosyntropin-stimulated study (>2 without cosyntropin), the study is interpreted as lateralization to the higher (dominant) adrenal vein. When the A/C ratio in the lower (nondominant) adrenal vein is lower than in the inferior vena cava, also called "contralateral suppression," there is even greater confidence that aldosterone production is lateralized to the dominant adrenal. Note that contralateral suppression is not always observed in studies with convincing lateralization, so lack of contralateral suppression does not equate to bilateral aldosterone production. Contralateral suppression can also be used to lateralize aldosterone production to the other adrenal when only one adrenal vein is accessed successfully. In this case, the quotient of A/C ratios is 10/1 = 10, favoring the left adrenal, and contralateral suppression (1 < 2) is observed for the right adrenal. Thus, aldosterone production lateralizes to the left (thus, Answer B is correct and Answers C and D are incorrect).

Guidelines for performing adrenal venous sampling recommend discontinuing mineralocorticoid receptor antagonists for several weeks before performing the study. The concern is that if the dose is sufficient to antagonize the aldosterone, volume depletion will occur and renin will rise. Renin will stimulate aldosterone production from both adrenal glands and could obscure a lateralizing gradient. Thus, if the results showed bilateral aldosterone production, the study might be invalid because of spironolactone exposure. However, lateralization in the presence of spironolactone or eplerenone can still be interpreted with confidence (thus, Answer A is incorrect).

EDUCATIONAL OBJECTIVE

Interpret results of adrenal venous sampling.

REFERENCE(S)

Haase M, Riester A, Kröpil P, et al. Outcome of adrenal vein sampling performed during concurrent mineralocorticoid receptor antagonist therapy. *J Clin Endocrinol Metab.* 2014;99(12):4397-4402. PMID: 25222758

Nanba AT, Wannachalee T, Shields JJ, et al. Adrenal vein sampling lateralization despite mineralocorticoid receptor antagonists exposure in primary aldosteronism. *J Clin Endocrinol Metab.* 2019;104(2): 487-492. PMID: 30239792

Funder JW, Carey RM, Mantero F, et al. The management of primary aldosteronism: case detection, diagnosis, and treatment: an Endocrine Society clinical practice guideline. *J Clin Endocrinol Metab.* 2016;101(5):1889-1916. PMID: 26934393

Rossi GP, Auchus RJ, Brown M, et al. An expert consensus statement on the use of adrenal vein sampling for the subtyping of primary aldosteronism. *Hypertension.* 2014;63(1):151-160. PMID: 24218436

20 ANSWER: E) Testicular ultrasonography

An alarming number of young adults with classic 21-hydroxylase deficiency, especially men, become partially or completely nonadherent to their adrenal replacement therapy after leaving pediatric endocrinology care. This patient's story is not unusual, and the consequences of prolonged suboptimal disease control should be assessed. His mineralocorticoid replacement is adequate, and serum aldosterone measurement (Answer B) is uninformative and will not change his treatment. Although his serum testosterone value is in the normal male range, most is derived from his adrenals, because his androstenedione is much higher than his testosterone. On the basis of these 2 tests alone, his disease control is poor despite resuming treatment after a lapse of 3.5 years, and his treatment should be intensified. His 17-hydroxyprogesterone level (Answer C) would be predictably high, and his semen analysis (Answer D) would be expected to show azoospermia.

About half of young men with classic 21-hydroxylase deficiency develop testicular adrenal rest tumors (TARTs). These are ACTH-responsive masses that are either ectopic adrenal tissue or reprogrammed steroidogenic stem cells in the testes that grow and produce a pattern of steroids similar to that of the adrenal cortex of these patients. TARTs are firm, irregular masses arising from the rete testis posteriorly and are typically bilateral. In 21-hydroxylase deficiency, the adrenals produce abundant androstenedione and inefficiently convert this precursor to testosterone, so the major laboratory feature is elevated androstenedione, disproportionate to the testosterone, which is typically "normal," but not derived from the normal testicular Leydig cells. The high adrenal androgen production suppresses LH. Initially, FSH is also low, but with time the masses compromise blood flow to the normal testis and cause irreversible damage to the Sertoli and germ cells, and FSH rises. The presence of TARTs and high FSH are poor prognostic factors for fertility in men with classic 21-hydroxylase deficiency. Intensification of glucocorticoid therapy can allow regression of the rests and restoration of fertility, but this can take many months. Surgical removal of TARTs often provides long-term control of the tumors, but it does not restore testicular function. Thus, testicular ultrasonography (Answer E) is indicated. A physical examination should be performed first, but this was not given as an option.

Although adrenal enlargement, nodular hyperplasia, and myelolipomas are common in adults with classic 21-hydroxylase deficiency, routine adrenal imaging (Answer A) is not recommended and will not assess his more pressing issue of testicular dysfunction.

EDUCATIONAL OBJECTIVE

Evaluate testicular adrenal rest tumors in men with congenital adrenal hyperplasia.

REFERENCE(S)

Speiser PW, Arlt W, Auchus RJ, et al. Congenital adrenal hyperplasia due to steroid 21-hydroxylase deficiency: an Endocrine Society clinical practice guideline. *J Clin Endocrinol Metab.* 2018;103(11): 4043-4088. PMID: 30272171

Auchus RJ, Arlt W. Approach to the patient: the adult with congenital adrenal hyperplasia. *J Clin Endocrinol Metab.* 2013;98(7):2645-2655. PMID: 23837188

Reisch N, Rottenkolber M, Greifenstein A, et al. Testicular adrenal rest tumors develop independently of long-term disease control: a longitudinal analysis of 50 adult men with congenital adrenal hyperplasia due to classic 21-hydroxylase deficiency. *J Clin Endocrinol Metab.* 2013;98(11):E1820-E1826. PMID: 23969190

Claahsen-van der Grinten HL, Otten BJ, Takahashi S, et al. Testicular adrenal rest tumors in adult males with congenital adrenal hyperplasia: evaluation of pituitary-gonadal function before and after successful testis-sparing surgery in eight patients. *J Clin Endocrinol Metab.* 2007;92(2):612-615. PMID: 17090637

King TF, Lee MC, Williamson EE, Conway GS. Experience in optimizing fertility outcomes in men with congenital adrenal hyperplasia due to 21 hydroxylase deficiency. *Clin Endocrinol (Oxf).* 2016;84(6):830-836. PMID: 26666213

21 ANSWER: D) Lynch syndrome (hereditary nonpolyposis colon cancer)

This patient has adrenocortical cancer and a classic family history of Lynch syndrome (Answer D), which includes colon cancer and uterine cancer, often diagnosed at a young age (<50 years), as core syndromic expression. Individuals with Lynch syndrome are also predisposed to developing pancreatic cancer, ovarian cancer, prostate cancer, and sebaceous gland cancers. Lynch syndrome is caused by germline pathogenic variants in *MSH2, MSH6, PMS2,* or *MLH1,* and immunohistochemical staining for the gene products can be used to screen the pathologic specimen. Adrenal cancer occurs in a minority of patients with Lynch syndrome, but the prevalence of Lynch syndrome among patients with adrenocortical cancer is the same as in patients with colon or uterine cancer (3%-5%), making evaluation for this familial cancer syndrome worthwhile in patients with adrenal cancer.

Li-Fraumeni syndrome (Answer C) is a cancer syndrome predisposing to young-onset breast cancer, lung cancer, sarcomas, brain cancer, and adrenal cancer. Up to 80% of all children with adrenal cancer have a germline pathogenic variant in the *TP53* gene, and *TP53* pathogenic variants can be found in adult patients with adrenal cancer (up to 2%-3%). However, the family history in this case is not typical of Li-Fraumeni syndrome. In a significant number of cases, the family history will be negative, as up to 20% of all pathogenic *TP53* variants are de novo.

Familial adenomatous polyposis (Answer B) predisposes to colon polyps and colon cancer (usually age 20-40 years), as well as to some other tumors. Adrenal adenomas are more common in patients with familial adenomatous polyposis, but adrenal cancer is rare.

The adrenal phenotype in Carney complex (Answer A), with the main manifestations of GH hypersecretion, cardiac myxomas, and testicular large-cell calcifying Sertoli-cell tumors, is primary pigmented nodular adrenal disease, with hypercortisolism and normal-sized adrenal glands. Adrenal cancer has been described, but it is rare among patients with Carney complex/primary pigmented nodular adrenal disease due to germline pathogenic *PRKAR1A* variants.

Multiple endocrine neoplasia type 1 (Answer E) predisposes to primary hyperparathyroidism (usually before age 40 years), pituitary adenomas, and foregut neuroendocrine tumors. Cushing syndrome can be due to adrenal tumors, pituitary tumors, or ectopic ACTH or corticotropin-releasing hormone production by neuroendocrine tumors. There is an increased incidence of adrenal tumors in multiple endocrine neoplasia type 1. Up to 40% of affected patients have at least 1 adrenal nodule, but they are usually benign. Although the relative risk for adrenal cancer is increased in patients with multiple endocrine neoplasia, the personal and family history in this patient is not suggestive of this syndrome.

EDUCATIONAL OBJECTIVE

Describe the hereditary predisposition to adrenocortical carcinoma.

REFERENCE(S)

Fassnacht M, Dekkers OM, Else T, et al. European Society of Endocrinology clinical practice guidelines on the management of adrenocortical carcinoma in adults, in collaboration with the European Network for the Study of Adrenal Tumors. *Eur J Endocrinol.* 2018;179(4):G1-G46. PMID: 30299884

Raymond VM, Everett JN, Furtado LV, et al. Adrenocortical carcinoma is a lynch syndrome-associated cancer [*J Clin Oncol.* 2013;31(28):3612]. *J Clin Oncol.* 2013;31(24):3012-3018. PMID: 23752102

22 ANSWER: C) Serum 11-deoxycortisol measurement

The elevated ACTH and low cortisol values indicate a primary adrenal problem, which manifests as hypertension and hypokalemia. The differential diagnosis for ACTH-dependent mineralocorticoid excess is best approached considering the pathologic mineralocorticoid in each case:

- Aldosterone
  - Glucocorticoid-remediable aldosteronism (familial hyperaldosteronism type 1)
- Cortisol
  - Cushing syndrome; apparent mineralocorticoid excess (genetic or licorice)
- 11-Deoxycorticosterone
  - 17α-hydroxylase deficiency, 11β-hydroxylase deficiency

In this case, the cortisol and aldosterone are both suppressed, which excludes apparent mineralocorticoid excess and glucocorticoid-remediable aldosteronism (thus, Answers A and E are incorrect).

Although 17-hydroxyprogesterone is elevated, 21-hydroxylase deficiency causes hypotension rather than hypertension. Thus, genotyping the *CYP21A2* gene (Answer B) is incorrect.

Measurement of serum 17-hydroxypregnenolone (Answer D) assesses for 3β-hydroxysteroid dehydrogenase deficiency, which also causes hypotension.

Given the patient's normal virilization and Middle Eastern ancestry, he has 11β-hydroxylase deficiency, which is diagnosed by documenting an elevated 11-deoxycortisol concentration (Answer C). Note that 17-hydroxyprogesterone also accumulates behind the block at 11-hydroxylase, but it is not as high as it is in 21-hydroxylase deficiency. The remaining etiology is 17α-hydroxylase deficiency, but this defect also causes androgen deficiency, which is inconsistent with the clinical picture. Serum 11-deoxycorticosterone is elevated in both 11β- and 17α-hydroxylase deficiency, but 11-deoxycortisol is elevated in only 11β-hydroxylase deficiency. In 17α-hydroxylase deficiency, corticosterone is also elevated. In both conditions, the mineralocorticoids defend against adrenal crises, despite cortisol deficiency.

EDUCATIONAL OBJECTIVE

Construct the differential diagnosis of ACTH-dependent mineralocorticoid excess and diagnose 11β-hydroxylase deficiency.

REFERENCE(S)

Parajes S, Loidi L, Reisch N, et al. Functional consequences of seven novel mutations in the CYP11B1 gene: four mutations associated with nonclassic and three mutations causing classic 11β-hydroxylase deficiency. *J Clin Endocrinol Metab.* 2010;95(2):779-788. PMID: 20089618

Zachmann M, Tassinari D, Prader A. Clinical and biochemical variability of congenital adrenal hyperplasia due to 11 beta-hydroxylase deficiency. A study of 25 patients. *J Clin Endocrinol Metab.* 1983;56(2):222-229. PMID: 6296182

Miller WL, Auchus RJ. The molecular biology, biochemistry, and physiology of human steroidogenesis and its disorders [published correction appears in *Endocr Rev.* 2011;32(4):579]. *Endocr Rev.* 2011;32(1):81-151. PMID: 21051590

Bone Board Review

Natalie E. Cusano, MD, MS

1 ANSWER: D) Teriparatide

Of the listed medications, teriparatide (Answer D) is the only agent approved by the US FDA for management of osteoporosis in men. Teriparatide is indicated for: "Treatment of osteoporosis in postmenopausal females who are at high risk for fracture (defined as history of osteoporotic fracture or multiple risk factors for fracture); treatment to increase bone mass in males with primary or hypogonadal osteoporosis who are high risk for fracture; and treatment of males and females with glucocorticoid-induced osteoporosis." This patient has a history of atraumatic vertebral fracture and is at high risk for future fracture, with a clear indication for osteoanabolic therapy. The osteoanabolic agent abaloparatide was recently approved for treatment to increase bone density in men who are high risk for fracture (defined as history of osteoporotic fracture or multiple risk factors for fracture). Romosozumab (Answer C) is an effective osteoanabolic therapy for postmenopausal osteoporosis, and it can be considered off-label for select men who are at high fracture risk.

Because there are no large randomized controlled trials showing antifracture efficacy for testosterone in men with osteoporosis, testosterone therapy (Answer E) should be considered only for hypogonadal men who are symptomatic, have an organic cause for the hypogonadism, have testosterone levels less than 200 ng/dL (<6.9 nmol/L), and/or are not candidates for other therapies.

While alendronate, risedronate, zoledronic acid, and denosumab have been approved for therapy to reduce fracture risk in men, ibandronate (Answer A) has not. Of note, ibandronate has not been demonstrated to decrease the risk of nonvertebral fractures and is not generally a first-line agent for treatment of postmenopausal osteoporosis as per most guidelines.

Calcitonin (Answer B) is a relatively weak antiresorptive agent with a limitation of use statement in postmenopausal osteoporosis due to possible association with malignancy.

EDUCATIONAL OBJECTIVE

Manage osteoporosis in men at high fracture risk.

REFERENCE(S)

Porcelli T, Maffezzoni F, Pezzaioli LC, et al. Management of endocrine disease: male osteoporosis: diagnosis and management - should the treatment and the target be the same as for female osteoporosis? *Eur J Endocrinol.* 2020;183(3): R75-R93. PMID: 32544873

2 ANSWER: D) +12% improvement in lumbar spine bone density and 70% vertebral fracture risk reduction

Romosozumab is a monoclonal antibody against sclerostin that has been approved for treatment of postmenopausal women with osteoporosis at high fracture risk. In the pivotal clinical trial, treatment with romosozumab resulted in improvements in bone density of 13.3% (95% CI, 11.9-14.7) at the lumbar spine, 6.9% at the total hip (95% CI, 5.6-8.1), and 5.9% at the femoral neck (95% CI, 4.3-7.4) compared with placebo at 12 months (*P* < .001 for all comparisons). Vertebral fracture risk was 73% lower in the romosozumab arm than in the placebo arm (incidence, 0.5% [16 of 3321 patients]) in the romosozumab group vs 1.8% (59 of 3322) in the placebo group. The risk ratio was 0.27 (95% CI, 0.16-0.47) (*P* < .001). Answer D correctly gives the correct approximate expected changes for improvement in bone density and vertebral fracture risk reduction.

Romosozumab has been approved by the US FDA with a boxed warning that therapy should not be initiated in patients who have had a myocardial infarction or stroke within the preceding year.

EDUCATIONAL OBJECTIVE

Describe the densitometric changes and vertebral fracture risk reduction with romosozumab therapy.

REFERENCE(S):

Cosman F, Crittenden DB, Adachi JD, et al. Romosozumab treatment in postmenopausal women with osteoporosis. *N Engl J Med.* 2016;375(16):1532-1543. PMID: 27641143

3 ANSWER: B) Hypophosphatasia

The differential diagnosis for low alkaline phosphatase is presented in the *box.* Hypophosphatasia (Answer B) is a rare genetic disease caused by loss-of-function pathogenic variants in the *ALPL* gene, which encodes the tissue-nonspecific isoenzyme of alkaline phosphatase (TNSALP). TNSALP is particularly abundant in the bone, liver, and kidneys but is also expressed in other tissues, including cartilage and teeth. The main physiologic substrates of TNSALP are inorganic pyrophosphate and pyridoxal-5′-phosphate (the active metabolite of vitamin B_6). Loss of function of TNSALP in patients with hypophosphatasia results in a generalized reduction in alkaline phosphatase activity and accumulation of TNSALP substrates, including inorganic pyrophosphate and vitamin B_6. The prevalence of severe hypophosphatasia is approximately 1 in 100,000 among Anglo-Saxon populations and is more prevalent among the Mennonites in Manitoba, Canada, where 1 in every 25 persons is a carrier. Inheritance is autosomal recessive for the infantile forms but either autosomal recessive or autosomal dominant for the milder adult forms, with variable penetrance. The clinical presentation and severity of hypophosphatasia are variable due to the large number of described variants in the *ALPL* gene. This patient has a history of chronic dental issues, fracture, and other symptoms dating from childhood, as well as a low alkaline phosphatase level. She was diagnosed with hypophosphatasia after measurement of vitamin B_6 and genetic testing for *ALPL* pathogenic variants was pursued. A diagnosis of hypophosphatasia was confirmed, and enzyme replacement therapy with asfotase alfa has improved her symptoms.

While profound hypothyroidism (Answer C) can cause low alkaline phosphatase, this patient's slight TSH elevation is unlikely to result in a significant lowering of alkaline phosphatase.

Celiac disease (Answer A) is another cause of low alkaline phosphatase; however, this patient does not have anemia or vitamin D deficiency to suggest malabsorption.

Pathogenic variants in the *PHEX* gene (Answer E) cause X-linked hypophosphatemic rickets, which presents with low phosphate, not low alkaline phosphatase.

Recent fracture (Answer D) can result in elevated, not decreased, alkaline phosphatase.

Box. Differential Diagnosis of Low Alkaline Phosphatase

Hypophosphatasia
Renal adynamic bone disease
Treatment with antiresorptive agents (ie, bisphosphonates, denosumab)
Hypoparathyroidism
Profound hypothyroidism
Vitamin D intoxication (perhaps via hypercalcemia and PTH suppression)
Celiac disease
Wilson disease
Cardiac bypass surgery
Sepsis/multiorgan system failure

Adapted from Lewiecki EM et al. *J Clin Densitom*, 2017; 20(2):134-152. © 2017 Elsevier Inc., on behalf of International Society for Clinical Densitometry.

EDUCATIONAL OBJECTIVE

Construct the differential diagnosis of low alkaline phosphatase.

REFERENCE(S)

Bianchi ML, Bishop NJ, Guañabens N, et al; Rare Bone Disease Action Group of the European Calcified Tissue Society. Hypophosphatasia in adolescents and adults: overview of diagnosis and treatment. *Osteoporos Int.* 2020;31(8):1445-1460. PMID: 32162014

Lewiecki EM. New and emerging concepts in the use of denosumab for the treatment of osteoporosis. *Ther Adv Musculoskelet Dis.* 2018;10(11):209-223. PMID: 30386439

4 ANSWER: B) Patients who have completed 24 months of teriparatide can continue or restart therapy

Teriparatide is the biologically active 1-34 amino-acid fragment from the intact PTH 1-84 molecule. There was a boxed warning from the US FDA based on studies in Fischer 344 rats demonstrating that high doses of teriparatide, approximately 3 times greater than the approved human dosing based on milligrams per kilogram of body weight, administered over the majority of the lifespan of a rat, were associated with the development of osteosarcoma. The lifetime limitation had been established because 24 months was the longest that any individual had been treated with teriparatide in the labeling clinical trial. Since drug approval, there has been no adverse signal of osteosarcoma in humans treated with teriparatide. A 15-year postmarketing surveillance study showed no difference in the observed incidence of osteosarcoma compared with the background incidence rate for individuals not treated with teriparatide. In November 2020, the FDA removed the 2-year lifetime treatment limitation and the boxed warning about the potential risk of osteosarcoma. Thus, patients who have completed 24 months of teriparatide can continue or restart therapy (Answer B).

Patients at higher baseline risk of osteosarcoma, including children with open epiphyses (Answer D), patients with history of radiation therapy (Answer C), and patients with Paget disease (Answer E), should still not be prescribed teriparatide. It is important to follow an osteoanabolic agent with an antiresorptive therapy (Answer A) to maintain densitometric gains.

EDUCATIONAL OBJECTIVE

Review treatment updates with teriparatide.

REFERENCE(S)

Gilsenan A, Midkiff K, Harris D, Kellier-Steele N, McSorley D, Andrews EB. Teriparatide did not increase adult osteosarcoma incidence in a 15-year us postmarketing surveillance study. *J Bone Miner Res.* 2021;36(2):244-251. PMID: 32990990

5 ANSWER: C) Incipient primary hyperparathyroidism

Primary hyperparathyroidism is one of the most common endocrine disorders and is classically diagnosed in the setting of hypercalcemia with an elevated or inappropriately normal PTH. Serum calcium values can occasionally be normal as part of the disease course. This patient has a history of 2 elevated calcium values. Serum calcium on his current laboratory evaluation is at the upper end of normal with an elevated PTH concentration. He was presumptively diagnosed with incipient primary hyperparathyroidism (Answer C) and has subsequently had laboratory results demonstrating elevations in both serum calcium and PTH.

In primary hyperparathyroidism, PTH facilitates the conversion of 25-hydroxyvitamin D to 1,25-dihydroxyvitamin D, and up to 25% of patients have frankly elevated 1,25-dihydroxyvitamin D levels. In sarcoidosis (Answer E) and other granulomatous diseases, while 1,25-dihydroxyvitamin D is typically elevated because macrophages in the granulomas synthesize the active metabolite of vitamin D, PTH levels are also suppressed. 25-Hydroxyvitamin D levels would be elevated, typically above 150 ng/mL (>374.3 nmol/L), and PTH levels would also be suppressed in the case of vitamin D toxicity (Answer A).

Lithium alters feedback mechanisms within the parathyroid gland, increasing the set point at which calcium suppresses PTH secretion. It also increases calcium reabsorption within the loop of Henle, decreasing urinary calcium excretion. Serum calcium remains within the normal range for most patients. While estimates vary, up to 20% of patients on lithium develop hypercalcemia. If lithium can be discontinued safely, serum calcium may normalize after 1 to 4 weeks in patients taking lithium for up to a few years. Normalization of serum calcium is less likely in patients who have been taking lithium for more than 10 years (thus, Answer D is incorrect).

Familial hypocalciuric hypercalcemia (FHH) (Answer B) is a rare, benign disorder caused by loss-of-function pathogenic variants in the gene encoding the calcium-sensing receptor. Patients with FHH usually have a positive family history, although a given patient could represent an index case. The extremely high penetrance of FHH ensures that virtually all patients develop hypercalcemia by their third decade. Thus, FHH is not of concern in this patient despite a low urinary calcium value. In FHH, 24-hour urinary calcium excretion is typically less than 100 mg with a calcium-to-creatinine clearance ratio less than 0.01, while typically the ratio is greater than 0.02 in patients with primary hyperparathyroidism. It can be difficult to distinguish between FHH and primary hyperparathyroidism when the ratio is between 0.01 and 0.02; however, patients must be vitamin D replete (>20 ng/mL [>49.9 mmol/L]) with good kidney function for the collection to be interpretable. In younger patients, genetic testing may assist with making the diagnosis.

EDUCATIONAL OBJECTIVE

Diagnose primary hyperparathyroidism.

REFERENCE(S)

Cusano NE, Bilezikian JP. Parathyroid hormone in the evaluation of hypercalcemia. *JAMA*. 2014;312(24):2680-2681. PMID: 25536261

Bilezikian JP, Khan AA, Silverberg SJ, et al; International Workshop on Primary Hyperparathyroidism. Evaluation and management of primary hyperparathyroidism: summary statement and guidelines from the Fifth International Workshop. *J Bone Miner Res*. 2022;37(11):2293-2314. PMID: 36245251

6 ANSWER: C) +8% improvement in lumbar spine bone density and 50% vertebral fracture risk reduction

The efficacy of alendronate to improve bone density was evaluated in two 3-year, multicenter studies of virtually identical design, one performed in the United States and the other in 15 different countries (multinational). In the US study, after 3 years, alendronate at the approved treatment dosage induced bone density increases of 9.6 ± 0.4% at the lumbar spine, 4.7 ± 0.7% at the femoral neck, and 5.0 ± 0.4% at the total hip (mean ± SE; each $P \leq .001$) vs decreases of 0.8 to 1.6% with placebo. In the multinational study, after 3 years, alendronate induced bone density increases of 6.8 ± 0.6% at the lumbar spine and 4.8 ± 0.6% at the femoral neck (mean ± SE; each $P \leq .001$) vs decreases of 0.6 to 0.7% with placebo.

The efficacy of alendronate on vertebral fracture risk was evaluated in multiple trials prior to approval, including: (1) the combined US/multinational data of women with a bone density T-score at or below −2.5 with or without prior vertebral fracture; (2) the 3-year Fracture Intervention Trial (FIT) of women with a history of at least 1 baseline vertebral fracture; and (3) the 4-year FIT of women with low bone density but no history of vertebral fracture. Alendronate reduced the percentage of women experiencing at least 1 new radiographic vertebral fracture from 6.2% to 3.2% (48% relative risk reduction, $P = .034$) in the combined US/multinational studies; from 15.0% to 7.9% (47% relative risk reduction, $P < .001$) in the 3-year FIT; and from 3.8% to 2.1% (44% relative risk reduction, $P = .001$) in the 4-year FIT.

Thus, of the answer choices, this patient is most likely to experience +8% improvement in lumbar spine bone density and 50% vertebral fracture risk reduction (Answer C) after 36 months of alendronate therapy.

EDUCATIONAL OBJECTIVE

Describe the densitometric changes and vertebral fracture risk reduction with alendronate therapy.

REFERENCE(S)

Devogelaer JP, Broll H, Correa-Rotter R, et al. Oral alendronate induces progressive increases in bone mass of the spine, hip, and total body over 3 years in postmenopausal women with osteoporosis. *Bone.* 1996;18(2):141-150. PMID: 8833208

Tucci JR, Tonino RP, Emkey RD, Peverly CA, Kher U, Santora AC 2nd. Effect of three years of oral alendronate treatment in postmenopausal women with osteoporosis. *Am J Med.* 1996;101(5):488-501. PMID: 8948272

Black DM, Cummings SR, Karpf DB, et al. Randomised trial of effect of alendronate on risk of fracture in women with existing vertebral fractures. Fracture Intervention Trial Research Group. *Lancet.* 1996;348(9041):1535-1541. PMID: 8950879

Cummings SR, Black DM, Thompson DE, et al. Effect of alendronate on risk of fracture in women with low bone density but without vertebral fractures: results from the Fracture Intervention Trial. *JAMA.* 1998;280(24):2077-2082. PMID: 9875874

7 ANSWER: D) Intravenous bolus of 150 mg calcium gluconate followed by a continuous calcium gluconate infusion of 1 mg/kg per h

This patient has developed hypocalcemia in the setting of hungry bone syndrome after parathyroidectomy. Intravenous calcium should be considered for patients presenting with clinical features of hypocalcemia from any etiology, including symptoms of paresthesias, carpopedal spasm, bronchospasm or laryngospasm, tetany, seizures, mental status changes, positive Chvostek or Trousseau signs, bradycardia, impaired cardiac contractility, and prolonged QT interval. While some patients with marked hypocalcemia (ie, corrected calcium <7.0 mg/dL [<1.8 mmol/L]) may not be symptomatic, intravenous therapy may be indicated because at those levels, life-threatening features such as laryngeal spasm and seizures can appear acutely (thus, Answer A is incorrect). This patient needs rapid correction of hypocalcemia. Calcium gluconate is preferred over calcium chloride because the latter is more likely to cause vein sclerosis and tissue necrosis if extravasated (thus, Answers B and C are incorrect). Dosing at 1 mg/kg per h would be a total dose of 1680 mg daily for a 70-kg patient (thus, Answer D is correct); a higher rate might be required for patients with a profound calcium deficiency. The dose of intravenous calcium is dangerously high in Answer E.

Ordering intravenous calcium can be potentially confusing. For intravenous use, a 10-mL ampule of calcium gluconate contains 93 mg of calcium; a 10-mL ampule of 10% calcium chloride contains 272 mg of calcium. In some situations, adding a calcium salt to an intravenous liter bag of 0.9% saline or 5% dextrose requires removing some of the fluid to allow space for the added calcium salt.

Hungry bone syndrome was first described by Albright and Reifenstein in 1950 in patients with hyperparathyroidism who presented with severe and prolonged hypocalcemia after parathyroidectomy. Typically, hungry bone syndrome is characterized by postoperative hypocalcemia (<8.5 mg/dL [<2.1 mmol/L]), a simultaneous inorganic phosphate value less than 3.0 mg/dL (<10.0 mmol/L), and hypocalcemia lasting longer than 4 days requiring high dosages of calcium supplementation despite optimization of vitamin D. In the case of patients with end-stage kidney disease, treatment with activated vitamin D (calcitriol) is always necessary.

PTH and calcitriol (1α,25[OH]2D3) regulate calcium and phosphate homeostasis. PTH is secreted in response to hypocalcemia after being sensed by the parathyroid calcium-sensing receptor. PTH receptors are mainly present in kidney and bone tissue, and when activated, they increase calcium efflux from bone and decrease renal excretion of calcium to restore normal serum calcium concentrations. Hungry bone syndrome pathophysiology begins with elevated PTH production (primary, secondary, or tertiary hyperparathyroidism), which augments bone and calcium turnover. Surgical treatment of primary or tertiary hyperparathyroidism with resection of 1 or more overactive parathyroid glands causes a sudden cessation of bone resorption. Consequently, a marked depletion of serum circulating calcium, phosphate, and magnesium is seen as the "hungry bones" remineralize.

Patients at highest risk for hungry bone syndrome are those with the most severe hyperparathyroidism preoperatively, and they often have elevated alkaline phosphatase levels and areas of osteitis fibrosa cystica ("brown tumors") visible on skeletal radiographs. Some have advocated use of intravenous bisphosphonates preoperatively to prevent hungry bone syndrome even though this could also delay skeletal remineralization. In severe cases of hungry bone syndrome, intravenous or high-dosage oral calcium and vitamin D may be needed for many weeks or months.

EDUCATIONAL OBJECTIVE

Manage acute, symptomatic hypocalcemia in the setting of hungry bone syndrome.

REFERENCE(S):

Zalonga GP, Chernow B. Hypocalcemia in critical illness. *JAMA*. 1986;256(14):1924-1929. PMID: 3531557

Juárez-León ÓA, Gómez-Sámano MÁ, Cuevas-Ramos D, et al. Atypical parathyroid adenoma complicated with protracted hungry bone syndrome after surgery: a case report and literature review. *Case Rep Endocrinol.* 2015;2015:757951. PMID: 26640724

Witteveen JE, van Thiel S, Romijn JA, Hamdy NA. Hungry bone syndrome: still a challenge in the post-operative management of primary hyperparathyroidism: a systematic review of the literature. *Eur J Endocrinol.* 2013;168(3):R45-R53. PMID: 23152439

8 ANSWER: E) Paget disease

This patient has an elevated bone-specific alkaline phosphatase; periosteal thickening on imaging; scintigraphy demonstrating increased uptake; and a bone biopsy showing active osteoclasts, reactive woven bone, and cement lines (indicative of past bone remodeling)—all consistent with Paget disease (Answer E).

In recent years, the prevalence and severity of Paget disease have appeared to decrease. The disease is easily diagnosed and effectively treated, but its pathogenesis remains incompletely understood. It can affect one (monostotic) or multiple (polyostotic) bones, most commonly the pelvis, femur, lumbar vertebrae, and skull. Paget disease near a weight-bearing joint changes the properties of subchondral bone, leading to progressive joint destruction, even though the joint itself is not directly involved. Paget disease does not extend across joint spaces, and rarely, if ever, shows up at new locations that were not involved at the time of initial diagnosis. Fractures of involved bones may occur (the femur is a frequent site). Rarely, Paget disease can transform into osteosarcoma.

Monostotic Paget disease can present with normal total and/or bone-specific alkaline phosphatase levels, in which case scintigraphy is used to determine disease activity. A bone biopsy is not needed to diagnose Paget disease when the radiographic and laboratory findings are consistent, although it was performed in this patient due to the possible concern for osteomyelitis.

Indications for treatment in an asymptomatic patient include the following:

- Involvement of a weight-bearing bone (eg, spine or leg)
- Involvement near a joint
- Involvement of the skull
- Serum alkaline phosphatase level greater than 3 times the upper normal limit

Zoledronic acid is clearly the most effective treatment. It normalizes bone turnover markers and maintains normal values for the longest duration of any medication. Normal turnover markers are associated with the normalization of pagetic woven bone to lamellar bone and can eliminate pain arising from pagetic bone. A single dose of zoledronic acid results in many years of disease inactivity in most patients.

Multiple myeloma (Answer C) presents with lytic lesions that are not active on scintigraphy.

Metastatic prostate cancer (Answer B) is osteoblastic and lesions would be active on scintigraphy; however, commonly affected bones are the spine, hips, and ribs. Sclerotic bone lesions can be challenging to biopsy, but this would demonstrate prostate cancer in experienced hands. This patient's elevated PSA is consistent with his diagnosis of benign prostatic hypertrophy.

Osteomyelitis (Answer D) can present with similar findings on imaging and scintigraphy; however, biopsy demonstrates an infectious etiology, with staphylococci being the most common isolate.

The classic radiographic findings in fibrous dysplasia (Answer A) include irregular, marginated, ground-glass lucencies surrounded by reactive bone. The shaft has an appearance that has been described as a soap bubble.

This patient received a single dose of zoledronic acid, 5 mg intravenously, with subsequent normalization of bone-specific alkaline phosphatase and continued remission of disease after 2 years.

EDUCATIONAL OBJECTIVE

Diagnose Paget disease.

REFERENCE(S)

Reid IR, Lyles K, Su G, et al. A single infusion of zoledronic acid produces sustained remissions in Paget disease: data to 6.5 years. *J Bone Miner Res.* 2011;26(9):2261-2270. PMID: 21638319

Ralston SH. Clinical practice. Paget's disease of bone. *N Engl J Med.* 2013;368(7):644-650. PMID: 23406029

Singer FR, Bone HG 3rd, Hosking DJ, et al. Paget's disease of bone: an endocrine society clinical practice guideline. *J Clin Endocrinol Metab.* 2014;99(12):4408-4422. PMID: 25406796

9 ANSWER: A) Inquire about the calibration of the densitometer

Reviewing the images and numbers from a DXA study is always important, particularly when the results do not make sense. In this case, the increases in bone density are above the expected results after a single dose of zoledronic acid.

This patient's bone density images do not have any obvious inconsistencies (thus, Answers C and D are incorrect).

A mistake in DXA measurement can occur if the spine analysis bars are placed incorrectly. In *figure 2B*, the analysis bar is one level higher than the previous study in *figure 2A* (ie, L4 on the current study is actually L3). The ribs can provide a helpful landmark, as the last ribs generally articulate with T12. While the second lumbar spine DXA image for the patient in the vignette shows more of the sacrum and less of T12, one can see the analyzed vertebra are the same, and the outlining of the vertebrae is similar to the previous image. Another mistake in DXA measurement can be differences in positioning from year to year or incorrect placement of the region of interest of the femoral neck or total hip. The lower edge of the hip region of interest should be approximately 2.5 cm below the lesser trochanter (correct in *figure 3A* and incorrect in *figure 3B*).

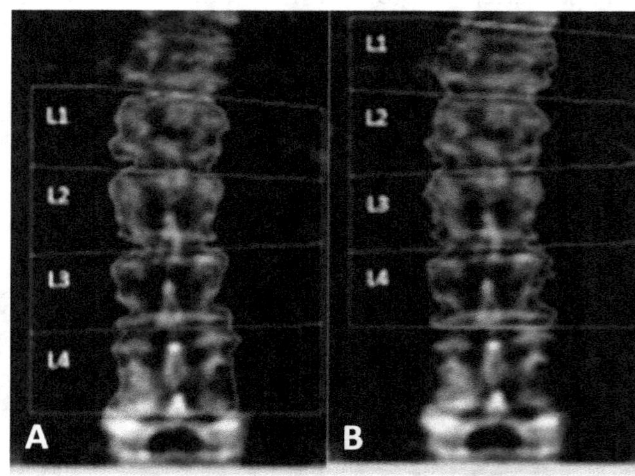

Figure 2.

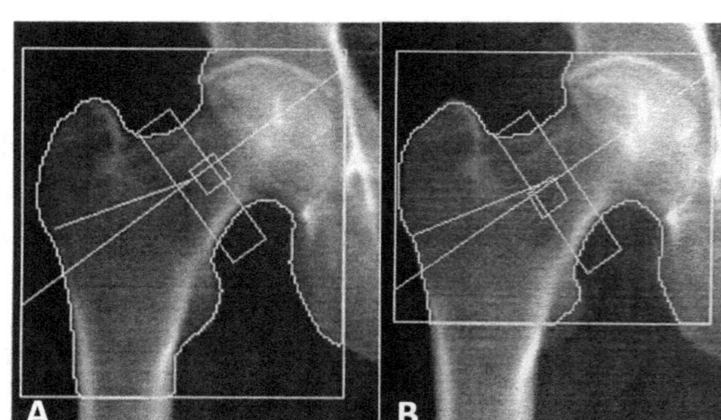

Figure 3.

Since both the spine and hip sites have increased without apparent errors in measurement, the next step would be to inquire into a systemic issue with the measurement. In this case, the bone densitometer had recently been miscalibrated (Answer A). Her bone density demonstrated improvements of 4% at the lumbar spine and 3% at the total hip when the machine was recalibrated.

While breast cancer can metastasize to bone (Answer B), this is unlikely in the setting of ductal carcinoma in situ. Metastatic disease to the bone in breast cancer is typically lytic (and thus would not be picked up as increased bone density), although some patients can have blastic or mixed lesions appearing as discrete areas of sclerosis.

This patient is on aromatase inhibitor therapy, which is a known contributor to bone loss. Treatment should not be discontinued at this time despite improvement in bone density into the osteopenic range (thus, Answer E is incorrect). International guidelines recommend antiresorptive treatment for patients initiating aromatase inhibitor therapy who have a T-score of –2.0 or less regardless of additional risk factors, for the duration of aromatase inhibitor treatment.

EDUCATIONAL OBJECTIVE

Carefully review DXA images to identify common technical errors and consider when results are discordant with clinical expectations.

REFERENCE(S)

Watts NB. Fundamentals and pitfalls of bone densitometry using dual-energy X-ray absorptiometry (DXA). *Osteoporos Int.* 2004;15(11):847-854. PMID: 15322740

Hadji P, Aapro MS, Body J-J, et al. Management of aromatase inhibitor-associated bone loss (AIBL) in postmenopausal women with hormone sensitive breast cancer: joint position statement of the IOF, CABS, ECTS, IEG, ESCEO IMS, and SIOG. *J Bone Oncol.* 2017;7:1-12. PMID: 28413771

Schousboe JT, Shepherd JA, Bilezikian JP, Baim S. Executive summary of the 2013 international society for clinical densitometry position development conference on bone densitometry. *J Clin Densitom.* 2013;16(4):455-466. PMID: 24183638

10 ANSWER: A) Alendronate, 70 mg weekly for 1 year

This patient has been treated with denosumab therapy for 5 years with significant improvements in bone density. Her most recent bone density values are within the osteopenic range at all sites. It is reasonable to plan for an upcoming "drug holiday" due to the rare adverse effects of osteonecrosis of the jaw and atypical femoral fracture associated with antiresorptive therapy. However, cessation of denosumab results in an increase in bone resorption markers above pretreatment values for approximately 24 months after the last dose. Bone mineral density returns to pretreatment values within 18 months of the last denosumab injection. Abrupt discontinuation of denosumab therapy has been associated with increased risk of multiple vertebral fractures, as early as 7 months from the last dose. Thus, a drug holiday from antiresorptive therapy (Answer B) is not the best option at this time. The US FDA insert for denosumab recommends considering transition to another antiresorptive agent if denosumab is discontinued. Therapy with alendronate for 1 year (Answer A) before a drug holiday is reasonable, and studies have demonstrated that alendronate is able to maintain bone density after denosumab therapy in most patients.

Zoledronic acid can be considered for patients who have an intolerance to oral bisphosphonate therapy, however, studies of small cohorts of patients have shown that a single dose of zoledronic acid, 5 mg intravenously, administered 6 months from the last dose of denosumab results in declines in bone density in many patients. A second dose of zoledronic acid may be needed for patients who experience significant declines in bone density. Zoledronic acid, 5 mg intravenously in 6 months (Answer E) (ie, 12 months from her last denosumab dose), is not appropriate due to the risk of multiple vertebral fractures described above.

In small studies, raloxifene (Answer D) was able to partially attenuate losses in bone density in patients discontinuing denosumab compared with patients who do not take subsequent therapy. However, significant declines were noted at the spine and hip sites.

Ibandronate (Answer C) has not been studied after denosumab therapy. In addition, a drug holiday should be considered for this patient at some point, and therapy with ibandronate indefinitely is incorrect.

Of note, the Fracture Reduction Evaluation of Denosumab in Osteoporosis Every 6 Months (FREEDOM) extension trial demonstrated improvement/maintenance of bone density with continued use for 10 years; there are no data beyond 10 years of treatment. Denosumab therapy can be continued for patients with uninterrupted insurance coverage with discussion of risks and benefits.

EDUCATIONAL OBJECTIVE

Transition from denosumab to another antiresorptive agent prior to drug discontinuation.

REFERENCE(S)

Cummings SR, Ferrari S, Eastell R, et al. Vertebral fractures after discontinuation of denosumab: a post hoc analysis of the randomized placebo-controlled FREEDOM trial and its extension. *J Bone Miner Res.* 2018;33(2):190-198. PMID: 29105841

Lewiecki EM. New and emerging concepts in the use of denosumab for the treatment of osteoporosis. *Ther Adv Musculoskelet Dis.* 2018;10(11):209-223. PMID: 30386439

Freemantle N, Satram-Hoang S, Tang ET, et al. Final results of the DAPS (Denosumab Adherence Preference Satisfaction) study: a 24-month, randomized, crossover comparison with alendronate in postmenopausal women. *Osteoporos Int.* 2012;23(1):317-326. PMID: 21927922

Sølling AS, Harsløf T, Langdahl B. Treatment With Zoledronate Subsequent to Denosumab in Osteoporosis: A 2-Year Randomized Study. *J Bone Miner Res.* 2021;36(7):1245-1254. PMID: 33813753

11 ANSWER: D) No treatment necessary

Fifty percent of circulating calcium is bound to serum proteins, primarily to albumin. In this patient with multiple myeloma, the serum albumin is normal. However, in some patients with multiple myeloma, high circulating levels of serum immunoglobulins can also bind calcium, leading to "pseudohypercalcemia." The key to recognizing this condition is to note the marked discordance between the serum calcium (very high) and the patient's symptoms (almost none). No therapy is needed (Answer D).

Normal saline intravenously (Answer C), cinacalcet therapy (Answer A), pamidronate therapy (Answer E), and emergency plasmapheresis (Answer B) are reasonable steps in the treatment of true, severe hypercalcemia, but they are not needed in this case.

EDUCATIONAL OBJECTIVE

Diagnose "pseudohypercalcemia" and guide management.

REFERENCE(S)

Jacobs TP, Bilezikian JP. Clinical review: rare causes of hypercalcemia. *J Clin Endocrinol Metab.* 2005;90(11):6316-6322. PMID: 16131579

Schwab JD, Strack MA, Hughes LD, Shaker JL. Pseudohypercalcemia in an elderly patient with multiple myeloma: report of a case and review of literature. *Endocr Pract.* 1995;1(6):390-392. PMID: 15251564

12 ANSWER: C) 21-Hydroxylase antibodies

This patient has autoimmune polyendocrine syndrome type 1 (APS type 1) due to a pathogenic variant in the autoimmune regulator gene (*AIRE*). APS type 1 is also known by the acronym APECED (autoimmune polyendocrinopathy-candidiasis-ectodermal dystrophy). The classic presentation includes at least 2 of the following 3 major clinical components: chronic mucocutaneous candidiasis, primary hypoparathyroidism, and autoimmune adrenal insufficiency. Premature ovarian insufficiency occurs in about 60% of patients. Malabsorption and other gastrointestinal issues occur in 25% of patients with APS type 1. Studies have shown that primary adrenal insufficiency may be diagnosed before clinical symptoms by checking for antibodies against the 21-hydroxylase enzyme (Answer C). Note that screening with an 8-AM serum cortisol level is not sensitive enough to detect preclinical disease, although inclusion of an

ACTH measurement with the morning cortisol might show early adrenal insufficiency.

Antiphospholipid antibodies (Answer A) are found in the setting of antiphospholipid antibody syndrome, an autoimmune disorder occurring mainly in young women. Clinical presentations include deep vein thrombosis, stroke, pregnancy complications, and recurrent miscarriage.

Glutamic acid decarboxylase (GAD-65) antibodies (Answer B) are often present in individuals with APS type 1, but they have not been shown to predict the development of type 1 diabetes, which occurs in about 18% of those with the syndrome. Islet-cell antibodies are a better predictor.

Tissue transglutaminase antibodies (Answer D) are used to diagnose celiac disease, which is not a feature of APS type 1.

TPO antibodies (Answer E) as a predictor of autoimmune thyroid disease is not the best answer. About 12% of patients with APS type 1 develop hypothyroidism in contrast to 60% who develop Addison disease. Screening for adrenal insufficiency is much more critical.

EDUCATIONAL OBJECTIVE

Diagnose autoimmune polyendocrine syndrome type 1 as a cause of hypoparathyroidism and recommend appropriate adrenal screening.

REFERENCE(S)

Weiler FG, Dias-da-Silva MR, Lazaretti-Castro M. Autoimmune polyendocrine syndrome type 1: case report and review of literature. *Arq Bras Endocrinol Metabol.* 2012;56(1):54-66. PMID: 22460196

Akirav EM, Ruddle NH, Herold KC. The role of AIRE in human autoimmune disease. *Nat Rev Endocrinol.* 2011;7(1):25-33. PMID: 21102544

Eisenbarth GS, Gottlieb PA. Autoimmune polyendocrine syndromes. *N Engl J Med.* 2004;350(20):2068-2079. PMID: 15141045

13 ANSWER: E) Tissue transglutaminase antibody assessment

When a patient on potent antiosteoporosis therapy shows a poor response, such as a significant decline in bone mineral density, it is important to review the history, physical examination findings, medications, and laboratory results to look for any secondary causes that may have been missed or developed in the interim. The most common cause for a poor outcome, particularly with self-administered medications, is nonadherence. It is estimated that 50% of patients starting on oral bisphosphonates stop the drugs within 3 to 6 months. Many others take the drugs intermittently or improperly. Consequences of nonadherence include loss of bone mineral density, increased fracture risk, and higher health care costs. Other etiologies of nonresponse include calcium and/or vitamin D deficiencies, poor absorption of oral bisphosphonates, errors in DXA measurements, or underlying diseases that remain undiagnosed or untreated.

This patient has laboratory evidence of inadequate calcium and vitamin D with a low 25-hydroxyvitamin level and secondary hyperparathyroidism. Additionally, she notes unexplained weight loss, fatigue, and gastrointestinal upset. The single best explanation for this clinical scenario would be celiac disease with positive tissue transglutaminase antibodies (Answer E). While some patients with celiac disease present with severe symptoms such as diarrhea, abdominal gas, and cramping, others have more subtle presentations as in this case. Multiple myeloma should always be ruled out in cases of unexplained bone loss, osteoporosis, or fractures, but the clinical presentation and laboratory findings would be different, so serum protein electrophoresis (Answer D) is incorrect.

While it is not wrong to measure 24-hour urinary calcium excretion (Answer C), this would not provide a definitive diagnosis. In celiac disease, the urinary calcium excretion would be low as a result of calcium malabsorption and secondary hyperparathyroidism.

A cosyntropin-stimulation test (Answer A) to diagnose adrenal insufficiency could explain weight loss and gastrointestinal upset, but it would not explain findings consistent with malabsorption or bone loss; serum calcium would usually be normal or elevated in Addison disease.

Finally, a marker of bone resorption (Answer B) could be elevated in a case of oral bisphosphonate nonadherence/malabsorption, but again, this would not point to a specific diagnosis.

EDUCATIONAL OBJECTIVE

Identify a secondary cause for nonresponse to osteoporosis therapy (celiac disease).

REFERENCE(S)

Modi A, Siris ES, Tang J, Sen S. Cost and consequences of noncompliance with osteoporosis treatment among women initiating therapy. *Curr Med Res Opin.* 2015;31(4):757-765. PMID: 25661017

Mirza F, Canalis E. Management of endocrine disease: secondary osteoporosis: pathophysiology and management. *Eur J Endocrinol.* 2015;173(3): R131-R151. PMID: 25971649

Heikkilä K, Pearce J, Mäki M, Kaukinen K. Celiac disease and bone fractures: a systematic review and meta-analysis. *J Clin Endocrinol Metab.* 2015; 100(1):25-34. PMID: 25279497

Painter SE, Kleerekoper M, Camacho PM. Secondary osteoporosis: a review of the recent evidence. *Endocr Pract.* 2006;12(4):436-445. PMID: 16901802

Lewiecki EM, Watts NB. Assessing response to osteoporosis therapy. *Osteoporos Int.* 2008;19(10): 1363-1368. PMID: 18546030

14 ANSWER: C) Foreign-body granulomas

This patient has non–PTH-mediated hypercalcemia. In the setting of hypercalcemia and low PTH, 1,25-dihydroxyvitamin D should be suppressed, not elevated. Calciphylaxis (Answer A) is an incorrect diagnosis because it occurs in cases where calcium, phosphate, and PTH are all high and it is associated with necrosis of the skin. Calciphylaxis typically occurs in patients with end-stage kidney disease.

Fibrodysplasia ossificans progressiva (Answer B) is an inherited disorder that does not present with hypercalcemia.

Sarcoidosis (Answer D) and T-cell lymphoma (Answer E) can result in 1,25-dihydroxyvitamin D–mediated hypercalcemia, but this patient's history, physical examination findings, and imaging all point to foreign-body granulomas (Answer C) due to silicone injections as the cause of her hypercalcemia. This suspicion was confirmed by biopsy of one of the nodular masses. Certain lymphomas and granulomas with activated macrophages contain the 1α-hydroxylase enzyme that converts 25-hydroxyvitamin D to 1,25-dihydroxyvitamin D. This activated vitamin D causes hypercalcemia primarily by increasing the gut absorption of calcium (and phosphate), but also by directly causing bone resorption.

EDUCATIONAL OBJECTIVE

Diagnose 1,25-dihydroxyvitamin D–mediated hypercalcemia due to foreign-body granulomas.

REFERENCE(S)

Agrawal N, Altiner S, Mezitis NH, Helbig S. Silicone-induced granuloma after injection for cosmetic purposes: a rare entity of calcitriol-mediated hypercalcemia. *Case Rep Med.* 2013;2013:807292. PMID: 24363673

Visnyei K, Samuel M, Heacock L, Cortes JA. Hypercalcemia in a male-to-female transgender patient after body contouring injections: a case report. *J Med Case Rep.* 2014;8:71. PMID: 24572248

Camuzard O, Dumas P, Foissac R, et al. Severe granulomatous reaction associated with hypercalcemia occurring after silicone soft tissue augmentation of the buttocks: a case report. *Aesthetic Plast Surg.* 2014;38(1):95-99. PMID: 24281899

Loke SC, Leow MK-S. Calcinosis cutis with siliconomas complicated by hypercalcemia. *Endocr Pract.* 2005;11(5):341-345. PMID: 16191496

15 ANSWER: A) Continue calcium and vitamin D and repeat DXA in 2 years

According to the Bone Health & Osteoporosis Foundation (formerly the National Osteoporosis Foundation), as well as guidelines from the Endocrine Society and the American Association of Clinical Endocrinology, osteoporosis can be diagnosed by a T-score in the hip or spine of less than or equal to –2.5 or by a low-trauma fracture of the hip or spine. A low-trauma or fragility fracture is defined as a fracture from standing height or less. This patient has a history of traumatic rib fractures, but no low-trauma fractures meeting the criteria for osteoporosis. Therefore, she has low bone mass (osteopenia), and the best tool to determine whether she should be treated pharmacologically is the FRAX calculator. Relying on FRAX results, patients who have an absolute 10-year fracture risk of 20% or higher for any major fracture or 3% or higher for hip fracture should be treated pharmacologically. This patient's fracture risk is well below the treatment threshold, and she should therefore continue with her dietary calcium and vitamin D for now and undergo DXA again in 2 years (Answer A).

Treating her with a bisphosphonate (Answer B), denosumab (Answer C), or the selective estrogen receptor modulator raloxifene (Answer E), is incorrect. Estrogen replacement therapy (Answer D) is not approved by the US FDA for treatment of osteoporosis and is only given to postmenopausal women with significant menopausal symptoms, which she does not have.

EDUCATIONAL OBJECTIVE

Use the FRAX tool to determine treatment of patients with low bone mass.

REFERENCE(S)

Eastell R, Rosen CJ, Black DM, Cheung AM, Murad MH, Shoback D. Pharmacologic management of osteoporosis in postmenopausal women: an Endocrine Society clinical practice guideline. *J Clin Endocrinol Metab.* 2019;104(5):1595-1622. PMID: 30907953

Camacho PM, Petak SM, Binkley N, et al. American Association of Clinical Endocrinologists/American College of Endocrinology clinical practice guidelines for the diagnosis and treatment of postmenopausal osteoporosis-2020 update. *Endocr Pract.* 2020;26(5):564-570. PMID: 32427503

LeBoff MS, Greenspan SL, Insogna KL, et al. The clinician's guide to prevention and treatment of osteoporosis. *Osteoporos Int.* 2022;33(10):2049-2102. PMID: 35478046

16 ANSWER: E) Zoledronate, 5 mg intravenously

This patient has Paget disease of the pelvis with symptomatic extension into the left hip joint, and he therefore needs treatment. Historically known as "osteitis deformans," Paget disease is a localized disorder of bone remodeling that progresses slowly and leads to deformities of affected bones, as well as skeletal, joint, neurologic, and vascular complications. Microscopic studies show signs of excessive bone resorption and disorganized, dysregulated bone formation. This weakens the bone, leading to deformity, pain, fracture, neurologic impingement, and/or joint complications. In mild cases, there are no symptoms, and the disease is detected incidentally on radiographs or by an elevated alkaline phosphatase level.

In some parts of the world, Paget disease is the second most common bone disorder after osteoporosis, although in recent years, its prevalence and severity appear to be decreasing. The disease is easily diagnosed and effectively treated, but its pathogenesis remains incompletely understood. It can affect one (monostotic) or multiple (polyostotic) bones, most commonly the pelvis, femur, lumbar vertebrae, and skull, but it never affects the entire skeleton and does not spread from one bone to another. Rarely, Paget disease can transform into osteosarcoma.

Symptoms of Paget disease include bone pain, bone deformity, loss of hearing, tinnitus, cranial nerve dysfunction, osteoarthritis, high-output heart failure, fracture, and hypercalcemia. Some patients have no symptoms at all. The diagnosis is made by documenting an elevated serum alkaline phosphatase concentration, along with normal levels of calcium, phosphate, and liver transaminases. Characteristic radiographic findings on skeletal survey and bone scans can be helpful to diagnose the disease and determine the extent of the condition. Treatment includes oral or intravenous bisphosphonates. The best recommendation for this patient is zoledronate, 5 mg intravenously (1 dose) (Answer E). The listed doses of alendronate (Answer A) and risedronate (Answer D) are not appropriate for Paget disease.

Calcitonin nasal spray (Answer B) is considered to be a much less effective therapy for Paget disease compared with bisphosphonates.

Physical therapy alone (Answer C) is not appropriate for a patient with active, symptomatic Paget disease and would not alleviate his bone pain.

The 2014 Endocrine Society clinical practice guideline recommends treatment with a bisphosphonate for "most patients with active Paget's disease who are at risk for future complications," but this has been challenged by others who contend that the only symptom proven to be ameliorated by bisphosphonate treatment is bone pain. Studies suggest that a single dose of zoledronate can control pain and sustain reductions in bone resorption for several years. The Endocrine Society guideline suggests that the definition of "remission" with any given treatment should include: (1) symptom control and (2) reduction of bone turnover to below the midpoint of the reference range.

Table 2. Recommended Bisphosphonate Dosing Regimens

Drug	Dosage
Zoledronate	5 mg given as a single infusion over 15 min, Retreatment is seldom required within 5 y.
Alendronate	40 mg/dL for 6 mo. Retreatment may be required between 2 and 6 y.
Risedronate	30 mg/dL for 2 mo. Retreatment may be required between 1 and 5 y.

Reprinted from Singer FR et al. *J Clin Endocrinol Metab*, 2014; 99(12):4408-4422. © The Endocrine Society.

EDUCATIONAL OBJECTIVE

Apply treatment guidelines for Paget disease.

REFERENCE(S)

Reid IR, Miller P, Lyles K, et al. Comparison of a single infusion of zoledronic acid with risedronate for Paget's disease. *N Engl J Med.* 2005;353(9):898-908. PMID: 16135834

Singer FR, Bone HG 3rd, Hosking DJ, et al; Endocrine Society. Paget's disease of bone: an Endocrine Society clinical practice guideline. *J Clin Endocrinol Metab.* 2014;99(12):4408-4422. PMID: 25406796

Ralston SH. Clinical practice. Paget's disease of bone. *N Engl J Med.* 2013;368(7):644-650. PMID: 23406029

Genuth SM, Klein L. Hypoparathyroidism and Paget's disease: the effect of parathyroid hormone administration. *J Clin Endocrinol Metab.* 1972;35(5):693-699. PMID: 4262771

17 ANSWER: E) X-linked hypophosphatemic rickets

X-linked hypophosphatemic rickets (Answer E) is an X-linked dominant form of rickets that is relatively unresponsive to vitamin D. The hypophosphatemia arises as a consequence of a defective *PHEX* gene product (phosphate-regulating gene with homology to endopeptidases on the X chromosome), which ultimately results in elevated FGF-23 levels and impaired renal proximal tubule phosphate reabsorption. In addition, despite severe hypophosphatemia, 1,25-dihydroxyvitamin D_3 production is not appropriately enhanced due to FGF-23–mediated suppression of 1α-hydroxylase activity. Thus, the "normal" level of 1,25-dihydroxyvitamin D_3 is inappropriate in the setting of elevated PTH and low serum phosphate.

Vitamin D–resistant rickets (Answer D) is characterized by low serum calcium, low serum phosphate, high PTH, and normal 25-hydroxyvitamin D levels. The key to distinguishing vitamin D–resistant rickets from other forms of rickets is to measure the 1,25-dihydroxyvitamin D level. There are 2 different types of "vitamin D–resistant rickets." Persons with the first type have inactivating pathogenic variants in the gene encoding the 1α-hydroxylase enzyme. They are unable to synthesize 1,25-dihydroxyvitamin D, and they present with very low or undetectable 1,25-dihydroxyvitamin D levels. These patients respond quite well to treatment with exogenous activated vitamin D metabolites but not as well to the usual vitamin D supplementation (hence, they were considered "resistant" to vitamin D in the era before activated vitamin D supplements were available). In contrast, patients with true vitamin D–resistant rickets have inactivating pathogenic variants in the gene encoding the vitamin D receptor, resulting in high 1,25-dihydroxyvitamin D levels and generally poor response to exogenous activated vitamin D metabolites. This patient does not have vitamin D–resistant rickets in view of his normal serum calcium level and lack of an elevated 1,25-dihydroxyvitamin D level.

Tumor-induced osteomalacia (Answer B) is highly unlikely given the childhood presentation in this case. In the setting of oncogenic osteomalacia, 1,25-dihydroxyvitamin D levels are severely reduced due to suppression by high FGF-23 levels from these often small mesenchymal tumors.

McCune-Albright syndrome (Answer A) can be associated with rickets and osteomalacia due to hyperphosphaturic hypophosphatemia, but one would expect polyostotic fibrous dysplasia, café-au-lait macules, and other endocrine disorders.

Finally, this patient's 25-hydroxyvitamin D concentration of 24 ng/mL (59.9 nmol/L) is not low enough to result in such severe rickets/osteomalacia. In true vitamin D–deficient rickets (Answer C), 25-hydroxyvitamin D levels are often too low to be measured.

EDUCATIONAL OBJECTIVE

Diagnose X-linked hypophosphatemic rickets.

REFERENCE(S)

Connor J, Olear EA, Insogna KL, et al. Conventional therapy in adults with X-linked hypophosphatemia: effects on enthesopathy and dental disease. *J Clin Endocrinol Metab.* 2015;100(10):3625-3632. PMID: 26176801

Dahir K, Roberts MS, Krolczyk S, Simmons JH. X-linked hypophosphatemia: a new era in management. *J Endocr Soc.* 2020;4(12):bvaa151. PMID: 33204932

18 ANSWER: E) Stop calcitonin and continue current hydration and monitoring

This is a classic case of humoral hypercalcemia of malignancy leading to a hypercalcemic crisis. The underlying etiology is secretion of PTHrP from squamous cell carcinoma of the lung. Hypercalcemic crisis is defined as a corrected serum calcium value of 14 mg/dL (3.5 mmol/L) or higher with rapid deterioration of multiple organs (eg, central nervous system, cardiac, gastrointestinal, and kidney). Acute management of hypercalcemic crisis involves saline hydration, subcutaneous calcitonin for 24 to 48 hours, intravenous bisphosphonate (or subcutaneous denosumab in selected cases), and treatment of the underlying disease.

Furosemide (Answer D) should be added only when there is clinical evidence of volume overload or congestive heart failure. In cases of vitamin D–mediated hypercalcemia, prednisone 40 to 60 mg daily, or another glucocorticoid equivalent (Answer C) may be useful, but it should not be given without biochemical evidence of inappropriate vitamin D levels. Finally, in patients with hypercalcemic crisis due to primary hyperparathyroidism, cinacalcet can be a "bridge" to parathyroidectomy.

The peak hypocalcemic action of intravenous bisphosphonate starts around 48 hours after administration and peaks around day 6. Because this patient is clinically improving after only 48 hours, the best next step is to stop calcitonin and continue current hydration and monitoring (Answer E).

To give another dose of zoledronic acid (Answer A) so quickly would be unnecessary and could potentially lead to prolonged hypocalcemia.

Denosumab (Answer B) is also approved for treatment of hypercalcemia from solid tumors, but it would not be needed now for the same reason. Ultimately, the key to treating malignant hypercalcemia is to treat the underlying cancer with surgery, chemotherapy, and other modalities.

EDUCATIONAL OBJECTIVE

Manage hypercalcemic crisis in a patient with humoral hypercalcemia of malignancy.

REFERENCE(S)

Hu MI, Glezerman IG, Leboulleux S, et al. Denosumab for treatment of hypercalcemia of malignancy. *J Clin Endocrinol Metab.* 2014;99(9): 3144-3152. PMID: 24915117

Stewart AF. Clinical practice. Hypercalcemia associated with cancer. *N Engl J Med.* 2005;352(4):373-379. PMID: 15673803

Ahmad S, Kuraganti G, Steenkamp D. Hypercalcemic crisis: a clinical review. *Am J Med.* 2015;128(3):239-245. PMID: 25447624

19 ANSWER: B) Hydrochlorothiazide, 25 mg once daily

According to the 2013 American College of Physicians guidelines, in patients who had a single kidney stone, increased fluid intake was the one intervention that was clearly shown to reduce recurrent stone disease. This patient's urine volume is already at goal (>2.5 L/24 h) and increasing his fluids is unlikely to further reduce stone risk. In patients with multiple stone episodes and hypercalciuria, thiazide diuretics (Answer B) are effective in reducing urinary calcium and the incidence of future stones. The hydrochlorothiazide dosage shown to reduce stone frequency is 50 mg daily. However, starting with 25 mg daily is reasonable until documenting that serum potassium remains normal on this dosage. Hydrochlorothiazide dosages lower than 25 mg have not been studied.

Although potassium citrate supplementation may also be effective in reducing stones in this patient, sodium increases urinary calcium excretion, so sodium citrate (Answer E) would not be a good choice for him. Hydrochlorothiazide acts to enhance renal calcium reabsorption to reduce urinary calcium excretion. As noted above, increased sodium intake leads to increased sodium excretion and an obligatory loss of calcium in the urine; however, this patient's normal urinary sodium excretion indicates that is not the case here. Thus, reducing his dietary sodium (Answer D) is incorrect.

His urinary oxalate level is not elevated, so there would be no benefit in reducing his dietary intake of oxalate (Answer C).

Allopurinol (Answer A) can be used for patients with hyperuricosuria who continue to have active disease despite attempted dietary modification. However, this patient's urinary uric acid is not elevated.

EDUCATIONAL OBJECTIVE

Recommend hydrochlorothiazide to reduce hypercalciuria as a means to reduce the risk of additional kidney stones.

REFERENCE(S)

Voskaki I, al Qadreh A, Mengreli C, Sbyrakis S. Effect of hydrochlorothiazide on renal hypercalciuria. *Child Nephrol Urol.* 1992;12(1):6-9. PMID: 1606587

Yendt ER, Cohanim M. Prevention of calcium stones with thiazides. *Kidney Int.* 1978;13(5):397-409. PMID: 351268

Fink HA, Wilt TJ, Eidman KE, et al. Medical management to prevent recurrent nephrolithiasis in adults: a systematic review for an American College of Physicians Clinical Guideline [published correction appears in *Ann Intern Med.* 2013;159(3):230-232]. *Ann Intern Med.* 2013;158(7):535-543. PMID: 23546565

Reilly RF, Peixoto AJ, Desir GV. The evidence-based use of thiazide diuretics in hypertension and nephrolithiasis. *Clin J Am Soc Nephrol.* 2010;5(10):1893-1903. PMID: 20798254

20 ANSWER C) HYPOMAGNESEMIA

Hypomagnesemia (Answer C) impairs PTH release in response to low calcium and causes skeletal resistance to PTH. PTH resistance can occur with magnesium levels below 0.8 mg/dL (<0.3 mmol/L), with a decrease in PTH secretion occurring with more profound hypomagnesemia. Hypomagnesemia is most commonly due to malabsorption; chronic alcoholism; and medications such as proton-pump inhibitors, diuretics, and cisplatin. Despite relative hypoparathyroidism and PTH resistance, phosphate levels in these patients are usually normal or low, most likely due to poor intake. Magnesium disorders are the only reversible cause of hypoparathyroidism, and parenteral magnesium repletion resulted in a significant rise in this patient's PTH concentration. Calcium supplementation alone cannot correct hypocalcemia in the setting of magnesium deficiency.

While profound vitamin D deficiency (Answer E) can result in hypocalcemia and most likely contributed to this patient's low serum calcium, hypomagnesemia is the primary etiology in this case as evidenced by the low, not elevated, PTH concentration.

Chronic hypoparathyroidism (Answer B) is a rare disorder usually occurring after parathyroid surgery or associated with autoimmune disease. This patient has no evidence of neck surgery or other autoimmune conditions on physical examination. Acute alcohol intoxication can cause transient hypoparathyroidism associated with hypocalcemia, hypercalciuria, and hypermagnesuria; however, alcohol withdrawal (Answer A) has not been associated with low calcium.

Pancreatitis (Answer D) can result in hypocalcemia associated with precipitation of calcium soaps in the abdominal cavity. However, her amylase and lipase levels are only borderline elevated, which can occur with chronic alcohol abuse.

EDUCATIONAL OBJECTIVE

Identify hypomagnesemia as a cause of hypocalcemia.

REFERENCE(S)

Chase LR, Slatopolsky E. Secretion and metabolic efficacy of parathyroid hormone in patients with severe hypomagnesemia. *J Clin Endocrinol Metab.* 1974;38(3):363-371. PMID: 4360918

Fatemi S, Ryzen E, Flores J, Endres DB, Rude RK. Effect of experimental human magnesium depletion on parathyroid hormone secretion and 1,25-dihydroxyvitamin D metabolism. *J Clin Endocrinol Metab.* 1991;73(5):1067-1072. PMID: 1939521

21 ANSWER: C) Formal hearing test

This patient has the mildest form of osteogenesis imperfecta, known as type 1. Inheritance is autosomal dominant, but many mutations occur de novo, so family history may be negative. Patients with osteogenesis imperfecta type 1 have normal stature and little or no skeletal deformity. Fractures occur in childhood or adolescence and decrease markedly after puberty. Affected patients may then present in middle age with "osteoporosis." In 50% of patients, there is early-onset hearing loss before age 40 years, so it is important to screen for this with a formal hearing test (Answer C).

On physical examination, affected patients may have blue sclerae and evidence of easy bruising. Joint laxity can be present, but dentinogenesis imperfecta is usually absent, so a complete dental examination (Answer A) is not necessary now.

Because there is no increased risk for cardiac or kidney disease, echocardiography (Answer B) or kidney ultrasonography (Answer D) are not indicated. Young women with osteogenesis imperfecta type 1 who become pregnant should be considered to have high-risk pregnancies and require a team approach, but pregnancy is not contraindicated. Finally, bisphosphonates may need to be restarted in the future, particularly at the time of menopause or perimenopause given the risk for bone loss and fractures. However, there is no need to restart bisphosphonates now (Answer E).

The main therapy for osteogenesis imperfecta remains bisphosphonates (intravenous pamidronate, zoledronic acid, and oral bisphosphonates). Current limited evidence demonstrates that oral or intravenous bisphosphonates increase bone mineral density in adults with osteogenesis imperfecta. It is unclear whether oral or intravenous bisphosphonate treatment consistently decreases fractures, although multiple studies report this independently and no studies report an increased fracture rate with treatment. A systematic Cochrane database review did not show that bisphosphonates conclusively improve clinical status (reduce pain or improve growth and functional mobility) in persons with osteogenesis imperfecta. Denosumab has been used in rare case reports. Teriparatide does not dramatically change clinical outcomes.

EDUCATIONAL OBJECTIVE

Screen for nonskeletal risks associated with osteogenesis imperfecta type 1 such as hearing loss.

REFERENCE(S)

Van Dijk FS, Sillence DO. Osteogenesis imperfecta: clinical diagnosis, nomenclature and severity assessment. *Am J Med Genet A*. 2014;164A(6):1470-1481. PMID: 24715559

Thomas IH, DiMeglio LA. Advances in the classification and treatment of osteogenesis imperfecta. *Curr Osteoporos Rep*. 2016;14(1):1-9. PMID: 26861807

Shapiro JR, Thompson CB, Wu Y, Nunes M, Gillen C. Bone mineral density and fracture rate in response to intravenous and oral bisphosphonates in adult osteogenesis imperfecta. *Calcif Tissue Int*. 2010;87(2):120-129. PMID: 20544187

Cozzolino M, Perelli F, Maggio L, et al. Management of osteogenesis imperfecta type 1 in pregnancy: a review of literature applied to clinical practice. *Arch Gynecol Obstet*. 2016;293(6):1153-1159. PMID: 26781260

Dwan K, Phillipi CA, Steiner RD, Basel D. Bisphosphonate therapy for osteogenesis imperfecta. *Cochrane Database Syst Rev*. 2016;10:CD005088. PMID: 27760454

22 ANSWER: C) Multiple endocrine neoplasia type 1

Multiple endocrine neoplasia (MEN) type 1 (Answer C) due to pathogenic variants in the *MEN1* gene is inherited as an autosomal dominant disorder, although occasionally de novo variants occur. MEN type 1 is classically characterized by a predisposition for tumors of the parathyroid glands, anterior pituitary, and pancreatic islet cells. It is critical to think about and recommend genetic testing for MEN type 1 in all patients younger than 30 years who present with primary hyperparathyroidism. Up to 10% of all patients with primary hyperparathyroidism have a familial (germline) pathogenic variant. Hereditary syndromes should be suspected in patients with a personal history of other endocrine tumors (especially pancreatic-duodenal or pituitary) or a history of parathyroid disease, kidney stones, or pancreatic-duodenal/pituitary tumors in first-degree relatives. These syndromes should also be suspected and screened for in patients presenting with atypical or multigland parathyroid adenomas at any age. Only 2% to 4% of all patients with primary hyperparathyroidism present with multigland adenomas.

In addition to MEN type 1, other rarer causes of multiorgan syndromic primary hyperparathyroidism include MEN type 2A (Answer D) and 2B (Answer E), MEN type 4, and hyperparathyroidism–jaw tumor syndrome. The latter is caused by pathogenic variants in the *CDC73* gene, and inheritance is autosomal dominant with variable penetrance. It should be considered in a young patient (<35 years) with at least 2 first- or second-degree relatives with primary hyperparathyroidism; other findings can include ossifying fibromas of the maxilla or mandible in a patient or family member and uterine tumors.

This patient's family history includes his father with recurrent hyperparathyroidism and siblings with peptic ulcers (gastrinomas) suggesting a type of MEN. MEN type 2A is associated with primary hyperparathyroidism in about 30% of cases, but it is ruled out in this case by the absence of hypertension, spells, or medullary thyroid carcinoma in any of the affected individuals. In MEN type 2B, individuals may have multiple neuromas, distinctive facial features, and a "marfanoid" habitus; primary hyperparathyroidism is not a classic manifestation.

Hereditary activation of the calcium-sensing receptor (Answer B) would result in hypocalcemia, not hypercalcemia.

Autoimmune polyglandular syndrome type 1 (Answer A) is associated with hypoparathyroidism, not hyperparathyroidism, in addition to mucocutaneous candidiasis and autoimmune adrenal insufficiency.

EDUCATIONAL OBJECTIVE

Pursue the diagnosis of multiple endocrine neoplasia type 1 in young patients presenting with primary hyperparathyroidism.

REFERENCE(S)

Thakker RV, Newey PJ, Walls GV, et al; Endocrine Society. Clinical practice guidelines for multiple endocrine neoplasia 1 (MEN1). *J Clin Endocrinol Metab.* 2012;97(9):2990-3011. PMID: 22723327

Eastell R, Brandi ML, Costa AG, D'Amour P, Shoback DM, Thakker RV. Diagnosis of asymptomatic primary hyperparathyroidism: proceedings of the Fourth International Workshop. *J Clin Endocrinol Metab.* 2014;99(10):3570-3579. PMID: 25162666

Lassen T, Friis-Hansen L, Rasmussen AK, Knigge U, Feldt-Rasmussen U. Primary hyperparathyroidism in young people. When should we perform genetic testing for multiple endocrine neoplasia 1 (MEN-1)? *J Clin Endocrinol Metab.* 2014;99(11):3983-3987. PMID: 24731012

23 ANSWER: C) Nonadherence to treatment

When a patient on potent antiosteoporosis therapy has a poor response, such as a significant decline in bone mineral density, it is important to review the history, physical examination findings, medications, and laboratory results to look for secondary causes that may have been missed or developed in the interim. However, the most common cause for a poor outcome, particularly with self-administered medications, is treatment nonadherence (Answer C). Fifty percent of patients who start oral bisphosphonates are estimated to stop the drugs within 3 to 6 months. Many others take the drugs intermittently or improperly. Consequences of nonadherence include loss of bone mineral density, increased fracture risk, and higher health care costs. Other etiologies of nonresponse include calcium and/or vitamin D deficiencies, poor absorption of oral bisphosphonates, errors in DXA measurements, or underlying diseases that remain undiagnosed or untreated.

Malabsorption (Answer B) is unlikely given the adequate levels of calcium and vitamin D and the normal 24-hour urinary calcium excretion. Although patients who adhere to their treatment regimen may occasionally have inadequate absorption of bisphosphonates, this is much less common than nonadherence.

There is nothing in her laboratory findings to suggest an eating disorder (Answer E), and patients with an eating disorder should respond to oral bisphosphonate therapy if taken appropriately.

Positioning error by the DXA technician (Answer D) is unlikely to result in "bone loss" at both the spine and hip.

Finally, all oral bisphosphonates, when taken properly, have been shown to greatly reduce postmenopausal bone loss, although risedronate (Answer A) may be slightly less potent than alendronate.

EDUCATIONAL OBJECTIVE

Identify treatment nonadherence as the reason for poor response to osteoporosis therapy.

REFERENCE(S)

Modi A, Siris ES, Tang J, Sen S. Cost and consequences of noncompliance with osteoporosis treatment among women initiating therapy. *Curr Med Res Opin.* 2015;31(4):757-765. PMID: 25661017

Lewiecki EM, Watts NB. Assessing response to osteoporosis therapy. *Osteoporos Int.* 2008;19(10): 1363-1368. PMID: 18546030

24 ANSWER: A) Adynamic bone disease

The bone biopsy in this patient is most likely to show adynamic bone disease (Answer A), a variety of chronic kidney disease–mineral bone disorder (previously referred to as renal osteodystrophy). Adynamic bone disease is characterized by reduced osteoblasts and osteoclasts, markedly low bone turnover, and no accumulation of osteoid. It occurs in a high percentage of patients on dialysis (either peritoneal or hemodialysis) but also in patients with chronic kidney disease on conservative treatment. Serum PTH levels in patients with adynamic bone disease are relatively low; however, serum PTH levels in patients with chronic kidney disease without adynamic bone disease are generally higher than normal, so the PTH level in this patient is much lower than expected. In patients with end-stage kidney disease, there is resistance to PTH, due at least in part to increased N-terminal truncated PTH (7-84), which counteracts the effect of the 1-84 whole molecule on bone. This can be exacerbated by the use of cinacalcet, as well as overly aggressive treatment with calcitriol, both of which reduce PTH secretion. The low alkaline phosphatase is consistent with a low bone turnover state.

Osteomalacia (Answer C) would be characterized by a much lower 25-hydroxyvitamin D level and a higher alkaline phosphatase level.

Osteitis fibrosa cystica (Answer E) would be associated with very high PTH levels and secondary or tertiary hyperparathyroidism.

Mixed renal osteodystrophy (Answer B) would be associated with elements of both hyperparathyroidism and osteomalacia.

Osteoporosis (Answer D) may be present to some degree in patients with end-stage kidney disease, especially in those who have osteoporosis that predates the kidney disease. However, after 8 years of hemodialysis and suppression of PTH, the most likely cause of the bone fragility in this patient is adynamic bone disease, not osteoporosis.

EDUCATIONAL OBJECTIVE

Diagnose adynamic bone disease in a patient undergoing dialysis.

REFERENCE(S)

Kidney Disease: Improving Global Outcomes (KDIGO) CKD-MBD Update Work Group. KDIGO 2017 clinical practice guideline update for the diagnosis, evaluation, prevention, and treatment of chronic kidney disease-mineral and bone disorder (CKD-MBD). *Kidney Int Suppl (2011).* 2017;7(1):1-59. PMID: 30675420

Damasiewicz MJ, Nickolas TL. Rethinking bone disease in kidney disease. *JBMR Plus.* 2018;2(6): 309-322. PMID: 30460334

25 ANSWER: D) Severe hypocalcemia

Denosumab, a human monoclonal antibody against RANK ligand, is approved for treatment of osteoporosis, as well as metastatic solid tumors such as breast cancer. It is a very potent inhibitor of osteoclastic bone resorption. Unlike bisphosphonates, denosumab is not cleared via the kidneys and has no effect on kidney function (Answer E).

Although cases of osteonecrosis of the jaw (Answer B) have been reported with both bisphosphonates and denosumab, this is very unlikely after only a single dose of the drug.

Severe flulike syndromes (Answer C) (also known as "acute phase reactions") are much more common with intravenous bisphosphonates than with denosumab.

Potent antiresorptive agents such as denosumab have not been shown to impair fracture healing (Answer A).

The major adverse effect to be expected in this setting is profound, symptomatic hypocalcemia (Answer D) within 7 to 10 days following denosumab administration. Patients at greatest risk for this complication are those with significantly impaired kidney function and high bone turnover with elevated alkaline phosphatase, as demonstrated in this patient. The potent inhibition of osteoclastic bone resorption by denosumab stops the efflux of calcium from bone and can lower serum calcium dramatically. The usual physiologic responses to hypocalcemia, such as a rise in PTH and calcitriol production, that would normally lead to increased renal tubular reabsorption of calcium and increased gut absorption of calcium, will not work in the setting of kidney failure. This woman also has a very low vitamin D level. Therefore, even if kidney function were better, she would still be at risk for an inadequate homeostatic response due to very low vitamin D substrate.

EDUCATIONAL OBJECTIVE

Anticipate the risk of symptomatic hypocalcemia following denosumab in the setting of kidney failure.

REFERENCE(S)

Dave V, Chiang CY, Booth J, Mount PF. Hypocalcemia post denosumab in patients with chronic kidney disease stage 4-5. *Am J Nephrol.* 2015;41(2):129-137. PMID: 25790847

Body JJ, Bone HG, de Boer RH, et al. Hypocalcaemia in patients with metastatic bone disease treated with denosumab. *Eur J Cancer.* 2015;51(13):1812-1821. PMID: 26093811

Kinoshita Y, Arai M, Ito N, et al. High serum ALP level is associated with increased risk of denosumab-related hypocalcemia in patients with bone metastases from solid tumors. *Endocr J.* 2016; 63(5):479-484. PMID: 26860123

Stopeck AT, Lipton A, Body JJ, et al. Denosumab compared with zoledronic acid for the treatment of bone metastases in patients with advanced breast cancer: a randomized, double-blind study. *J Clin Oncol.* 2010;28(35):5132-5139. PMID: 21060033

26 ANSWER: B) 1000 IU (25 mcg) daily

Vitamin D deficiency is not uncommon among patients with primary hyperparathyroidism. In asymptomatic primary hyperparathyroidism, low levels of 25-hydroxyvitamin D are associated with higher bone turnover, lower bone density, and greater cardiovascular risk factors in some, but not all, studies. Several trials have shown that correction of 25-hydroxyvitamin D levels from less than 20 ng/mL (<49.9 nmol/L) to approximately 30 ng/mL (74.9 nmol/L) reduces serum PTH levels without significant increases in serum calcium or hypercalciuria. Guidelines from the Fifth International Workshop on the Management of Asymptomatic Primary Hyperparathyroidism recommend vitamin D supplementation in patient with a 25-hydroxyvitamin D level less than 30 ng/mL.

Given the possibility that some patients may be at risk for symptomatic worsening of hypercalcemia or hypercalciuria with vitamin D supplementation, it is recommended to start with cholecalciferol dosages of 600 to 1000 IU daily (Answer B) rather than much higher dosages, such as 4000 IU daily or 50,000 IU weekly (Answers C and D). A randomized controlled trial demonstrated that vitamin D supplementation up to 2800 IU (70 mcg) daily was safe in patients with primary hyperparathyroidism. In this older man with low bone mineral density, providing no supplementation (Answer E) would potentially worsen his bone loss over time and is therefore not recommended. A regimen of 400 IU daily (Answer A) is too modest to correct the vitamin D deficiency and help prevent bone loss.

The average serum 25-hydroxyvitamin D response to 1000 IU of vitamin D daily would be an increase of about 10 to 12 ng/mL (25.0-30.0 nmol/L) (in this vignette, the patient's level would be expected to increase from 22 ng/mL to 32 ng/mL [54.9 nmol/L to 79.9 nmol/L]). It takes 2 to 3 months of daily dosing to reach a steady state. The magnitude of increase varies widely, so it would be important to test him again.

EDUCATIONAL OBJECTIVE

Recommend appropriate vitamin D supplementation in patients with primary hyperparathyroidism.

REFERENCE(S)

Marcocci C, Bollerslev J, Khan AA, Shoback DM. Medical management of primary hyperparathyroidism: proceedings of the fourth International Workshop on the Management of Asymptomatic Primary Hyperparathyroidism. *J Clin Endocrinol Metab.* 2014;99(10):3607-3618. PMID: 25162668

Rolighed L, Rejnmark L, Sikjaer T, et al. Vitamin D treatment in primary hyperparathyroidism: a randomized placebo controlled trial. *J Clin Endocrinol Metab.* 2014;99(3):1072-1080. PMID: 24423366

Shah VN, Shah CS, Bhadada SK, Rao DS. Effect of 25 (OH) D replacements in patients with primary hyperparathyroidism (PHPT) and coexistent vitamin D deficiency on serum 25(OH) D, calcium and PTH levels: a meta-analysis and review of literature. *Clin Endocrinol (Oxf).* 2014;80(6):797-803. PMID: 24382124

Bilezikian JP, Khan AA, Silverberg SJ, et al; International Workshop on Primary Hyperparathyroidism. Evaluation and management of primary hyperparathyroidism: summary statement and guidelines from the Fifth International Workshop. *J Bone Miner Res.* 2022;37(11):2293-2314. PMID: 36245251

27 ANSWER: D) Low calcium, high PTH, high phosphate

This patient has Albright hereditary osteodystrophy with pseudohypoparathyroidism. Albright hereditary osteodystrophy is characterized by brachydactyly (classically described as shortening of the third, fourth, and fifth metacarpals), round facies, short stature, obesity, developmental delay, and subcutaneous calcifications. Albright hereditary osteodystrophy was described by Albright and colleagues in 1942 together with pseudohypoparathyroidism, historically the first reported hormone resistance syndrome. It is characterized by end-organ resistance to PTH associated with hypocalcemia, elevated PTH, and hyperphosphatemia (Answer D). Pseudohypoparathyroidism type 1A is the most common form of the disorder due to pathogenic variants in the *GNAS* gene, which encodes the α-subunit of G-protein coupled to the PTH receptor. Pathogenic variants prevent generation of adenyl cyclase when PTH binds to its receptor and, therefore, failure of signal transduction by PTH.

Interestingly, *GNAS* is imprinted in humans, so that expression of the allele for a specific tissue is dependent on whether the allele is inherited from the mother or father. Renal expression of *GNAS* is determined only by the maternal allele; a defect in the maternal allele results in pseudohypoparathyroidism. Patients with pseudohypoparathyroidism type 1A may have resistance to various other G-protein–coupled hormones, including TSH, LH, FSH, and GnRH. Paternally transmitted pathogenic variants in *GNAS* result in pseudopseudohypoparathyroidism, in which patients demonstrate the physical features of Albright hereditary osteodystrophy with no evidence of PTH resistance. As there is no renal tubular resistance to PTH, affected patients present with normal concentrations of calcium, phosphate, and PTH (Answer E); this answer is incorrect as this patient has symptoms of hypocalcemia (perioral and extremity numbness/tingling) and apparently inherited a *GNAS* pathogenic variant from his mother, who has a similar physical phenotype.

Low calcium, low PTH, and low phosphate (Answer A) can be seen with severe hypomagnesemia and nutritional deficiency. Low calcium, low PTH, and high phosphate (Answer B) can be seen with hypoparathyroidism. Low calcium, high PTH, and low phosphate (Answer C) can be seen with significant vitamin D deficiency or malabsorption. None of these disorders would present with evidence of Albright hereditary osteodystrophy.

EDUCATIONAL OBJECTIVE

Identify the physical and biochemical features of pseudohypoparathyroidism type 1A.

REFERENCE(S)

Linglart A, Levine MA, Jüppner H. Pseudohypoparathyroidism. *Endocrinol Metab Clin North Am.* 2018;47(4):865-888. PMID: 30390819

Mantovani G. Clinical review: pseudohypoparathyroidism: diagnosis and treatment. *J Clin Endocrinol Metab.* 2011;96(10):3020-3030. PMID: 21816789

28 ANSWER: E) Cholecalciferol, 50,000 IU (1250 mcg) weekly

The average serum 25-hydroxyvitamin D response to 1000 IU (25 mcg) of vitamin D daily for 8 to 12 weeks is an increase of 10 to 12 ng/mL (25.0-30.0 nmol/L). In this vignette, the patient's level would be expected to increase from 8 to 20 ng/mL (20.0 to 49.9 nmol/L) over a period of 2 to 3 months. Instead, due to class 3 obesity, his 25-hydroxyvitamin D level may only increase by a few nanograms per deciliter, a very blunted response. Therefore, cholecalciferol, 400 or 1000 IU daily (Answers B and C), would not normalize his 25-hydroxyvitamin D level.

Several studies have shown that patients who are overweight or obese require much higher dosages of vitamin D than normal-weight participants to achieve adequate levels. Patients with obesity are estimated to require 2 to 3 times the usual daily dose of cholecalciferol to achieve adequate levels. The mechanism is not well understood. The closest dosage to what would be needed to correct the vitamin D deficiency in this patient is cholecalciferol, 50,000 IU (1250 mcg) weekly (Answer E), which provides an average dosage of 7143 IU (179 mcg) daily. The dosage could be adjusted in 8 to 12 weeks after rechecking the 25-hydroxyvitamin D level. Giving 10,000 IU (250 mcg) cholecalciferol weekly (Answer D) would only provide about 1700 IU (42.5 mcg) daily and thus would not be adequate. Finally, there is no role for treating with activated vitamin D or calcitriol (Answer A) in this setting.

EDUCATIONAL OBJECTIVE

Recommend appropriate vitamin D supplementation for patients with obesity.

REFERENCE(S)

Heaney RP, Davies KM, Chen TC, Holick MF, Barger-Lux MJ. Human serum 25-hydroxycholecalciferol response to extended oral dosing with cholecalciferol. *Am J Clin Nutr.* 2003;77(1):204-210. PMID: 12499343

Ekwaru JP, Zwicker JD, Holick MF, Giovannucci E, Veugelers PJ. The importance of body weight for the dose response relationship of oral vitamin D supplementation and 25-hydroxyvitamin D in healthy volunteers. *PLoS One.* 2014;9(11):e111265. PMID: 25372709

Holick MF, Binkley NC, Bischoff-Ferrari HA, et al; Endocrine Society. Evaluation, treatment, and prevention of vitamin D deficiency: an Endocrine Society clinical practice guideline. *J Clin Endocrinol Metab.* 2011;96(7):1911-1930. PMID: 21646368

29 ANSWER: D) Potassium phosphate and calcitriol

This patient has tumor-induced osteomalacia caused by a benign mesenchymal tumor that is secreting FGF-23, which causes renal tubular loss of phosphorus and inhibits 1α-hydroxylase, resulting in low 1,25-dihydroxyvitamin D levels. Treatment should include both potassium phosphate and calcitriol (Answer D).

Potassium phosphate alone (Answer C) could result in secondary hyperparathyroidism since phosphate loading reduces serum calcium, thereby stimulating PTH release.

Treating with only cholecalciferol and calcitriol (Answer B) would not correct the hypophosphatemia. These tumors are typically located in the skin, bones, or connective tissue (eg, sinuses) and may be difficult to localize. Imaging to localize the tumor includes nuclear medicine imaging techniques such as bone scan, octreotide scan, or PET. In difficult cases, serum FGF-23 on selective venous sampling may be used to localize the extremity from which FGF-23 is being secreted. Tumor removal (if it can be located and removed) normalizes renal phosphate handling within hours to days. Burosumab has been approved for FGF-23–related hypophosphatemia in tumor-induced osteomalacia associated with mesenchymal tumors that cannot be localized or curatively resected in adults and children 2 years and older.

Neither alendronate (Answer A) nor zoledronic acid (Answer E) would improve his serum phosphate or osteomalacia.

EDUCATIONAL OBJECTIVE

Recommend appropriate treatment of hypophosphatemia due to tumor-induced osteomalacia.

REFERENCE(S)

Chong WH, Molinolo AA, Chen CC, Collins MT. Tumor-induced osteomalacia. *Endocr Relat Cancer.* 2011;18(3):R53-R77. PMID: 21490240

Hodgson SF, Clarke BL, Tebben PJ, Mullan BP, Cooney WP 3rd, Shives TC. Oncogenic osteomalacia: localization of underlying peripheral mesenchymal tumors with use of Tc 99m sestamibi scintigraphy. *Endocr Pract.* 2006;12(1):35-42. PMID: 16524861

Chong WH, Yavuz S, Patel SM, Chen CC, Collins MT. The importance of whole body imaging in tumor-induced osteomalacia. *J Clin Endocrinol Metab.* 2011;96(12):3599-3600. PMID: 22143830

Jan de Beur SM, Miller PD, Weber TJ, et al. Burosumab for the treatment of tumor-induced osteomalacia. *J Bone Miner Res.* 2021;36(4):627-635. PMID: 33338281

30 ANSWER: B) Measure calcium and PTH after stopping hydrochlorothiazide for 3 months

In this vignette, the dilemma is to decide whether the patient's laboratory values reflect true primary hyperparathyroidism or a drug effect from the thiazide diuretic. The best way to distinguish these possibilities is to stop hydrochlorothiazide for several weeks or months and repeat the calcium and PTH measurement (Answer B).

Starting cinacalcet (Answer E) is not indicated because her serum calcium is within 1 mg/dL of the upper normal limit and she is asymptomatic with regard to hypercalcemia.

Calculation of the calcium-to-creatinine clearance ratio (Answer A) to rule out familial hypocalciuric hypercalcemia (FHH) could be considered given the mild hypercalcemia and low urinary calcium excretion. However, the normal serum calcium value from 2 years ago, the patient's age, and the use of hydrochlorothiazide make this option a wrong choice. Patients with FHH usually have a positive family history, and the extremely high penetrance of FHH ensures that virtually all patients develop hypercalcemia by their third decade.

Measuring 1,25-dihydroxyvitamin D (Answer C) would not be informative or definitive.

Finally, an octreotide scan (Answer D) is used to diagnose neuroendocrine tumors but not parathyroid adenomas.

Thiazide diuretics reduce urinary calcium excretion and can cause mild hypercalcemia. In addition, some patients with latent or preexisting undiagnosed hyperparathyroidism may be prescribed thiazides, resulting in further elevations of serum calcium and an unmasking of the disorder. Following discontinuation of the thiazide, these individuals remain hypercalcemic, although perhaps less so, and are found to have surgically proven hyperparathyroidism. Thus, if a patient taking a thiazide becomes hypercalcemic, the drug should be withdrawn, if possible, and calcium and PTH should be assessed approximately 3 months later. Persistent hypercalcemia (with elevated or high-normal PTH) after drug withdrawal suggests that the thiazide has unmasked true primary hyperparathyroidism.

In a population-based study of residents of Olmsted County, Minnesota, thiazide-associated hypercalcemia was identified on average 5.2 years after initiating thiazides, and it persisted in 71% of patients who discontinued the thiazide. Among all patients with thiazide-associated hypercalcemia, 24% were subsequently diagnosed with primary hyperparathyroidism. The mean maximum serum calcium concentration in these patients was 10.85 mg/dL (2.7 mmol/L).

Although the optimal management strategy in patients with thiazide-related primary hyperparathyroidism is unclear, asymptomatic patients with unequivocal biochemical evidence of hyperparathyroidism weeks or months after stopping thiazides are best managed like patients with asymptomatic primary hyperparathyroidism. Interestingly, in patients with primary hyperparathyroidism who are not surgical candidates, introduction of thiazides may reduce hypercalciuria and PTH levels without significantly increasing serum calcium.

EDUCATIONAL OBJECTIVE

Evaluate hyperparathyroidism in patients taking thiazide diuretics.

REFERENCE(S)

Griebeler ML, Kearns AE, Ryu E, et al. Thiazide-associated hypercalcemia: incidence and association with primary hyperparathyroidism over two decades. *J Clin Endocrinol Metab.* 2016;101(3):1166-1172. PMID: 26751196

Tsvetov G, Hirsch D, Shimon I, et al. Thiazide treatment in primary hyperparathyroidism-a new indication for an old medication? *J Clin Endocrinol Metab.* 2017;102(4):1270-1276. PMID: 28388724

Riss P, Kammer M, Selberherr A, et al. The influence of thiazide intake on calcium and parathyroid hormone levels in patients with primary hyperparathyroidism. *Clin Endocrinol (Oxf).* 2016;85(2):196-201. PMID: PMID: 26921840

Wermers RA, Kearns AE, Jenkins GD, Melton LJ 3rd. Incidence and clinical spectrum of thiazide-associated hypercalcemia. *Am J Med.* 2007;120(10): 911.e9-e15. PMID: 17904464

31 ANSWER: B) Adjust FRAX score for trabecular bone score

Patients with type 1 and type 2 diabetes are at increased risk for fracture, above that predicted based on bone mineral density. The pathophysiology is most likely multifactorial and may be related to the accumulation of advanced glycosylation endpoints in the bone matrix resulting in more brittle bone and decreased bone formation due to interference with osteoblasts. No studies have directly assessed the performance of FRAX for predicting fractures in patients with type 1 diabetes. However, several have studied patients with type 2 diabetes. To account for the increased fracture risk in patients with type 2 diabetes, proposed adjustments include: (1) using trabecular bone score; (2) using rheumatoid arthritis in the FRAX calculator as a proxy; and (3) decreasing bone density downwards by 0.5 SD.

The trabecular bone score is a gray-level textural analysis that can be used to estimate trabecular microarchitecture, and it has been associated with fragility fractures in postmenopausal women and men, independent of bone density measurements. Trabecular bone score analysis is readily available from the lumbar spine DXA image without further imaging. The FRAX score can be adjusted for trabecular bone score on the website by clicking the box that appears after the fracture risk probabilities have been generated. By adjusting this patient's bone density for trabecular bone score (Answer B), her risk for hip fracture increases to 3.0%, above the treatment threshold, and pharmacologic osteoporosis therapy should be initiated.

Increasing her vitamin D supplementation further (Answer D) with a 25-hydroxyvitamin D concentration within the goal range would not be helpful.

Pioglitazone and canagliflozin have both been associated with increased fracture risk, and substitution of one for the other (Answer C) would not be of substantial benefit.

While adding dulaglutide (Answer A) should improve her hemoglobin A_{1c} and most likely decrease her fracture risk over time, it is not the best next step for her skeletal health.

This patient should receive pharmacologic therapy now for her bone health; waiting 2 years for interval bone density testing (Answer E) is not appropriate.

EDUCATIONAL OBJECTIVE

Manage bone health in patients with type 2 diabetes mellitus at increased fracture risk.

REFERENCE(S)

Camacho PM, Petak SM, Binkley N, et al. American Association of Clinical Endocrinologists/American College of Endocrinology clinical practice guidelines for the diagnosis and treatment of postmenopausal osteoporosis-2020 update. *Endocr Pract.* 2020;26(5):564-570. PMID: 32427503

Schacter GI, Leslie WD. DXA-based measurements in diabetes: can they predict fracture risk? *Calcif Tissue Int.* 2017;100(2):150-164. PMID: 27591864

World Health Organization Collaborating Centre for Metabolic Bone Diseases, University of Sheffield, UK. FRAX. Who Fracture Risk Assessment Tool. Available at: www.shef.ac.uk/FRAX. Accessed for verification May 2023.

32 ANSWER: E) Reduced calcium and calcitriol requirements during pregnancy

Alterations in calcium metabolism and requirements during pregnancy provide for adequate mineralization of the fetal skeleton. Calcitriol levels increase 2- to 5-fold in euparathyroid women in the first trimester of pregnancy to increase intestinal absorption of calcium. PTHrP levels increase by up to 3-fold by the third trimester, due to both placental and breast production. In women with hypoparathyroidism, these increased serum levels of calcitriol and PTHrP lead to a marked reduction in calcitriol and calcium requirements during pregnancy and nursing (Answer E). Serum calcium should be monitored closely, with a decrease in supplementation as needed.

The patient's increased 1,25-dihydroxyvitamin D level is due to increased production during pregnancy, as well as ingestion of calcitriol, and not due to granulomatous disease (Answer A).

The patient's increased PTHrP is due to production during pregnancy and not due to humoral hypercalcemia of malignancy (Answer B).

Recurrence of primary hyperparathyroidism (Answer D) has not been reported in a patient with chronic postoperative hypoparathyroidism.

A diagnosis of milk-alkali syndrome (Answer C) can be made in a patient with a history of hypercalcemia, alkalosis, and kidney impairment in the setting of a history of ingestion of calcium-rich products and exclusion of other causes of hypercalcemia. This patient has normal serum bicarbonate and kidney function, excluding this diagnosis.

EDUCATIONAL OBJECTIVE

Identify the reduction in calcitriol and calcium requirements during pregnancy and nursing in patients with hypoparathyroidism.

REFERENCE(S)

Khan AA, Clarke B, Rejnmark L, Brandi ML. Management of endocrine disease: hypoparathyroidism in pregnancy: review and evidence-based recommendations for management. *Eur J Endocrinol.* 2019;180(2):R37-R44. PMID: 30444723

Dobnig H, Kainer F, Stepan V, et al. Elevated parathyroid hormone related peptide levels after human gestation: relationship to changes in bone and mineral metabolism. *J Clin Endocrinol Metab.* 1995;80(12):3699-3707. PMID: 8530622

33 ANSWER: C) Fracture risk reduction = 50%, atypical femoral fracture risk = 5/10,000, osteonecrosis of the jaw risk = 1/100,000

This patient's calculated major osteoporotic fracture risk is 25% if untreated. Alendronate, risedronate, zoledronic acid, and denosumab have all been demonstrated to reduce the risk of vertebral and nonvertebral fractures, including hip fractures. While patients should be adequately counseled regarding risks of treatment, for patients with osteoporosis, the benefits of pharmacologic osteoporosis therapy far outweigh the risks. Her estimated fracture risk reduction with treatment is 50%, while her risk of atypical femoral fracture is approximately 5/10,000 person-years and her risk of osteonecrosis of the jaw is approximately 1/100,000 person-years (Answer C). The risks of atypical femoral fracture and osteonecrosis of the jaw increase with increasing duration of antiresorptive use, with higher risk generally beyond 5 years of use. The other answers overestimate or underestimate the benefits and risks. Of note, Asian individuals have a higher risk of atypical femoral fractures than nonAsian individuals.

EDUCATIONAL OBJECTIVE

Counsel a patient with osteoporosis regarding benefits and risks of antiresorptive therapy.

REFERENCE(S)

Camacho PM, Petak SM, Binkley N, et al. American Association of Clinical Endocrinologists/American College of Endocrinology clinical practice guidelines for the diagnosis and treatment of postmenopausal osteoporosis-2020 update. *Endocr Pract.* 2020;26(5):564-570. PMID: 32427503

Khosla S, Burr D, Cauley J, et al; American Society for Bone and Mineral Research. Bisphosphonate-associated osteonecrosis of the jaw: report of a task force of the American Society for Bone and Mineral Research. *J Bone Miner Res.* 2007;22(10): 1479-1491. PMID: 17663640

Shane E, Burr D, Ebeling PR, et al. Atypical subtrochanteric and diaphyseal femoral fractures: report of a task force of the American Society for Bone and Mineral Research. *J Bone Miner Res.* 2010;25(11):2267-2294. PMID: 20842676

Schilcher J, Koeppen V, Aspenberg P, Michaëlsson K. Risk of atypical femoral fracture during and after bisphosphonate use. *N Engl J Med.* 2014;371(10): 974-976. PMID: 25184886

Black DM, Geiger EJ, Eastell R, et al. Atypical femur fracture risk versus fragility fracture prevention with bisphosphonates. *N Engl J Med.* 2020;383(8): 743-753. PMID: 32813950

Diabetes Mellitus, Section 1 Board Review

Anne L. Peters, MD

1 ANSWER: A) *GCK*

GCK-related MODY (Answer A) is associated with relatively mild hyperglycemia that does not change over time. Specifically, it is not affected by sulfonylurea agents or any other oral medications and glucose levels do not change with insulin administration. It is an autosomal dominant condition, and in this patient's case, both of his children and more than 30 additional family members were found to have *GCK*-related MODY.

Pathogenic variants in the *KCNJ11* gene (Answer E) cause neonatal diabetes, which can be transient or recur later in life. *KCNJ11*-related MODY responds to sulfonylureas.

MODY due to pathogenic variants in the *HNF4A* (Answer D) or *HNF1A* (Answer B) genes is very responsive to treatment with sulfonylureas.

HNF1B-related MODY (Answer C) is associated with higher blood glucose levels, cystic kidneys, hypomagnesemia, genitourinary abnormalities, pancreatic atrophy, hyperuricemia, and gout.

EDUCATIONAL OBJECTIVE

Describe the different types of maturity-onset diabetes of the young (MODY) and associated clinical presentations.

REFERENCE(S)

Tosur M, Philipson LH. Precision diabetes: lessons learned from maturity-onset diabetes of the young (MODY). *J Diabetes Investig.* 2022;13(9):1465-1471. PMID: 35638342

Riddle MC, Philipson LH, Rich SS, *et al.* Monogenic diabetes: from genetic insights to population-based precision in care. Reflections from a *Diabetes Care* Editors' Expert Forum. *Diabetes Care.* 2020; 43(12):3117-3128. PMID: 33560999

Shields BM, McDonald TJ, Ellard S, Campbell MJ, Hyde C, Hattersley AT. The development and validation of a clinical prediction model to determine the probability of MODY in patients with young-onset diabetes. *Diabetologia.* 2012;55(5): 1265-1272. PMID: 22218698

2 ANSWER: B) Glutamic acid decarboxylase antibody assessment

In a relatively lean, younger individual with diabetes that does not respond to therapy for type 2 diabetes, it is important to rule out autoimmune type 1 diabetes, especially in the setting of possible autoimmune thyroid disease. Thus, guidelines from the American Diabetes Association/European Association for the Study of Diabetes recommend measuring glutamic acid decarboxylase antibodies (Answer B) to distinguish between adult-onset type 1 vs type 2 diabetes.

Genetic testing for MODY (Answer A) is not necessary because this patient lacks the sort of family history that would lead one to suspect MODY. Also, her glucose levels are very high, which is generally not associated with MODY.

Islet-cell antibodies (Answer C) are not useful for diagnosing type 1 diabetes.

Insulin levels (Answer D) could be normal or low in this individual. Therefore, measuring insulin would not be helpful in her diagnosis.

EDUCATIONAL OBJECTIVE

Determine the type of diabetes mellitus in a younger individual who could have type 1 or type 2 diabetes.

REFERENCE(S)

Holt RIG, DeVries JH, Hess-Fischl A, et al. The management of type 1 diabetes in adults. a consensus report by the American Diabetes Association (ADA) and the European Association for the Study of Diabetes (EASD). *Diabetes Care.* 2021;44(11): 2589-2625. PMID: 34593612

Merger SR, Leslie RD, Boehm BO. The broad clinical phenotype of type 1 diabetes at presentation. *Diabet Med.* 2013;30(2):170-178. PMID: 23075321

3 ANSWER: C) Add basal insulin and a GLP-1 receptor agonist

This patient wants to lower her glucose levels without weight gain. Adding a GLP-1 receptor agonist and basal insulin (Answer C) is the best approach to lower her glucose levels rapidly without excessive weight gain. Some literature suggests that persons with glutamic acid decarboxylase antibody–positive, adult-onset type 1 diabetes may retain the ability to respond to a GLP-1 receptor agonist.

Although a multiple daily injection insulin regimen (Answer D) could lower her glucose levels fairly quickly, it is likely to cause weight gain and is a complex approach to her diabetes management. She desires a simple regimen.

DPP-4 inhibitors (Answer A) only provide moderate hemoglobin A_{1c} reduction and do not work in persons with type 1 diabetes.

Adding an SGLT-2 inhibitor (Answer B) in the setting of evolving type 1 diabetes could lead to diabetic ketoacidosis.

EDUCATIONAL OBJECTIVE

Determine the best patient-centered treatment approach for an adult with newly diagnosed type 1 diabetes mellitus.

REFERENCE(S)

Buzzetti R, Tuomi T, Mauricio D, et al. Management of latent autoimmune diabetes in adults: a consensus statement from an international expert panel. *Diabetes.* 2020;69(10):2037-2047. PMID: 32847960

Pozzilli P, Leslie RD, Peters AL, et al. Dulaglutide treatment results in effective glycaemic control in latent autoimmune diabetes in adults (LADA): a post-hoc analysis of the AWARD-2, -4 and -5 Trials. *Diabetes Obes Metab.* 2018;20(6):1490-1498. PMID: 29377522

Davies MJ, Aroda VR, Collins BS, et al; Management of hyperglycemia in type 2 diabetes, 2022. A consensus report by the American Diabetes Association (ADA) and the European Association for the Study of Diabetes (EASD). *Diabetes Care.* 2022;45(11):2753-2786. PMID: 36148880

4 ANSWER: C) Obtain a family history

C-peptide should be measured in the nonfasting state (not fasting [Answer A]). Postprandial C-peptide measurement (Answer B) is recommended at diagnosis only if there are features of monogenic diabetes.

A family history should be obtained (Answer C) before ordering genetic testing for maturity-onset diabetes of the young (Answer D) (*see figure*).

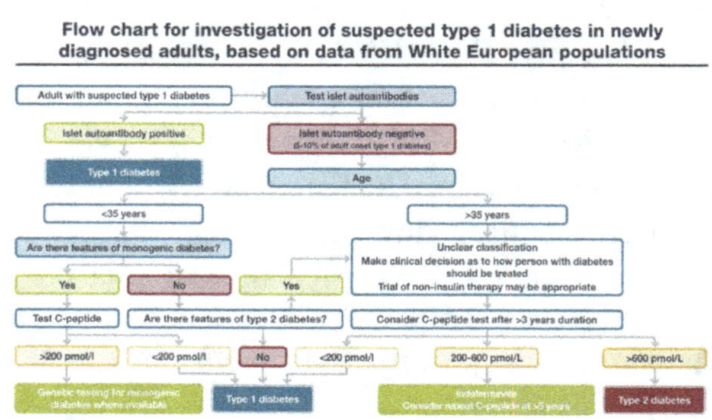

Reprinted from Holt Richard IG et al. *Diabetes Care* 1, 2021; 44(11): 2589–2625. © The American Diabetes Association.

EDUCATIONAL OBJECTIVE

Guide the process for diagnosing type 1 diabetes mellitus in an adult.

REFERENCE(S)

Holt RIG, DeVries JH, Hess-Fischl A, et al. The management of type 1 diabetes in adults. A consensus report by the American Diabetes Association (ADA) and the European Association for the Study of Diabetes (EASD). *Diabetes Care.* 2021;44(11):2589-2625. PMID: 34593612

Chung WK, Erion K, Florez JC, et al. Precision medicine in diabetes: a consensus report from the American Diabetes Association (ADA) and the European Association for the Study of Diabetes (EASD). *Diabetes Care.* 2020;43(7):1617-1635. PMID: 32561617

5 ANSWER: C) He will need to stay on multiple daily insulin injections or use an insulin pump

Immune checkpoint inhibitor–induced diabetes is generally permanent and requires treatment as insulin-deficient diabetes (thus, Answer C is correct and Answer A is incorrect). It is generally not associated with positive diabetes autoantibodies and occurs more commonly in people with a history of type 2 diabetes.

Oral medications (Answer B) are ineffective for treating this type of diabetes, which is caused by insulin deficiency.

Patients with immune checkpoint inhibitor–induced diabetes are very insulin deficient and require prandial insulin in addition to basal insulin (Answer D).

EDUCATIONAL OBJECTIVE

Manage immune checkpoint inhibitor–induced diabetes.

REFERENCE(S)

Chen X, Affinati AH, Lee Y, et al. Immune checkpoint inhibitors and risk of type 1 diabetes. *Diabetes Care.* 2022;45(5):1170-1176. PMID: 35238899

Shalit A, Sarantis P, Koustas E, Trifylli EM, Matthaios D, Karamouzis MV. Predictive biomarkers for immune-related endocrinopathies following immune checkpoint inhibitors treatment. *Cancers (Basel).* 2023;15(2):375. PMID: 36672324

Hattersley R, Nana M, Lansdown AJ. Endocrine complications of immunotherapies: a review. *Clin Med (Lond).* 2021;21(2):e212-e222. PMID: 33762389

6 ANSWER: D) Increase the insulin dosage

MT-TL1 pathogenic variants cause MIDD/mitochondrial encephalomyopathy, lactic acidosis, and strokelike episodes (MELAS). *MT-TL1* encodes the mitochondria tRNA for leucine, (tRNA-Leu). The same pathogenic variant causes several overlapping entities. Exactly which organs are affected is related to heteroplasmy, which refers to how mitochondria are distributed in various organs in embryogenesis, and there can be growing organ involvement over time.

The only treatment for MIDD/MELAS is insulin (Answer D). The patient's β cells are not working and nothing can fix these cells that are progressively impaired by sick mitochondria. Insulin secretion is impaired because the mitochondria are not metabolizing, but the (possible) effects in muscle cause long-term myopathy and muscle resistance to insulin, with some patients requiring hundreds of units of insulin per day.

Intensification of lifestyle efforts (Answer E) would not improve his glucose levels further. He is lean and very physically active. The defect in his mitochondria is not reversible by lifestyle alone.

Adding metformin (Answer C) is contraindicated because of a concern that its effect on mitochondrial function could cause metabolic acidosis.

A sulfonylurea (Answer B) would not work due to the mitochondrial dysfunction, although sulfonylureas can be effective in a variety of forms of maturity-onset diabetes of the young.

GLP-1 receptor agonists (Answer A) have not been shown to be effective in MIDD, and this individual is already quite lean and further weight loss is not recommended.

EDUCATIONAL OBJECTIVE

Guide treatment for maternally inherited diabetes and deafness.

REFERENCE(S)

Murphy R, Turnbull DM, Walker M, Hattersley AT. Clinical features, diagnosis and management of maternally inherited diabetes and deafness (MIDD) associated with the 3243A>G mitochondrial point mutation. *Diabet Med.* 2008;25(4):383-399. PMID: 18294221

Robinson KN, Terrazas S, Giordano-Mooga S, Xavier NA. The role of heteroplasmy in the diagnosis and management of maternally inherited diabetes and deafness. *Endocr Pract.* 2020;26(2):241-246. PMID: 31682520

Chung WK, Erion K, Florez JC, et al. Precision medicine in diabetes: a consensus report from the American Diabetes Association (ADA) and the European Association for the Study of Diabetes (EASD). *Diabetes Care.* 2020;43(7):1617-1635. PMID: 32561617

7 ANSWER: D) Reduce her correction dose at bedtime

Correcting hypoglycemia is always the first goal when evaluating a continuous glucose monitor tracing. This patient is experiencing low values at night, without symptoms. It is important to reduce the insulin dose that is causing the low glucose concentration; in this case, it appears to be a dose given at bedtime to correct a high glucose level. A discussion with the patient would be helpful to learn how she determines her bedtime correction dose. The correction dose at bedtime should be reduced (Answer D). Continuous glucose monitor alarms should be set to alert her to hypoglycemia, and her lower glucose target should be raised to 100 mg/dL (5.6 mmol/L) to restore her sensing of lows. Additionally, she needs to be certain she has unexpired glucagon at home, and her husband should be trained how to use it.

Increasing her daytime carbohydrate dose (Answer B) is not correct due to the presence of nocturnal lows. Although once her low nighttime values have been corrected, this strategy might be helpful.

Starting insulin pump therapy (Answer E) is not correct because the patient has been reluctant to use technology. First, hypoglycemia that has been occurring while on a multiple daily injection regimen should be corrected. Later, a conversation regarding additional technology, including use of an insulin pump (preferably with hybrid closed-loop technology), could be initiated.

Decreasing her long-acting insulin dosage (Answer A) is not correct because the hypoglycemia appears to be due to rapid-acting insulin administered later in the evening and her glucose values are high much of the day.

Although increasing her long-acting insulin dose (Answer C) may be necessary on further evaluation of her diabetes management, it is not her most immediate diabetes-related issue.

EDUCATIONAL OBJECTIVE

Make insulin dosage adjustments and treatment decisions in a person with type 1 diabetes on multiple daily insulin injections.

REFERENCE(S)

Rosenfeld C, Blevins T, Aleppo G, et al. Expert roundtable on continuous glucose monitoring. *Endocr Pract.* 2022;28(6):622-627. PMID: 35364329

Teo E, Hassan N, Tam W, Koh S. Effectiveness of continuous glucose monitoring in maintaining glycaemic control among people with type 1 diabetes mellitus: a systematic review of randomised controlled trials and meta-analysis. *Diabetologia.* 2022;65(4):604-619. PMID: 35141761

Battelino T, Danne T, Bergenstal RM, et al. Clinical targets for continuous glucose monitoring data interpretation: recommendations from the International Consensus on Time in Range. *Diabetes Care.* 2019;42(8):1593-1603. PMID: 31177185

Aleppo G, Webb K. Continuous glucose monitoring integration in clinical practice: a stepped guide to data review and interpretation. *J Diabetes Sci Technol.* 2019;(4):664-673. PMID: 30453772

Holt RIG, DeVries JH, Hess-Fischl A, et al. The management of type 1 diabetes in adults. A consensus report by the American Diabetes Association (ADA) and the European Association for the Study of Diabetes (EASD). *Diabetes Care.* 2021;44(11):2589-2625. PMID: 34593612

8 ANSWER: D) Teplizumab

Teplizumab (Answer D) slows but does not stop progression to type 1 diabetes. It is given as a once-daily infusion for 14 days. In a phase 2 clinical trial of individuals at high risk for developing type 1 diabetes, the median time to the diagnosis of type 1 diabetes was 48.4 months in the teplizumab group and 24.4 months in the placebo group; the disease was diagnosed in 19 (43%) of the participants who received teplizumab and in 23 (72%) of those who received placebo.

Neither insulin (Answer B) nor an intensive lifestyle regimen (Answer C) stops progression to type 1 diabetes. In one recent study, starting a tight degree of control with a hybrid closed-loop system immediately upon diagnosis did not modify progression of diabetes compared with that of a control group.

Golimumab (Answer A) is a human monoclonal antibody that has been approved for use in several autoimmune diseases. It has been studied in youth with new-onset type 1 diabetes and has shown some benefit in preserving endogenous insulin secretion. Golimumab is not currently indicated for treatment of type 1 diabetes at any stage.

EDUCATIONAL OBJECTIVE

Describe approaches for slowing the progression of stage 2 to stage 3 type 1 diabetes mellitus.

REFERENCE(S)

Herold KC, Bundy BN, Long SA et al. An Anti-CD3 antibody, teplizumab, in relatives at risk for type 1 diabetes. *N Engl J Med.* 2019;381(7):603-613. PMID: 31180194

LeFevre JD, Cyriac SL, Tokmic A, Pitlick JM. Anti-CD3 monoclonal antibodies for the prevention and treatment of type 1 diabetes: a literature review. *Am J Health Syst Pharm.* 2022;79(23):2099-2117. PMID: 36056809

Dayan CM, Korah M, Tatovic D, Bundy BN, Herold KC. Changing the landscape for type 1 diabetes: the first step to prevention. *Lancet.* 2019; 394(10205):1286-1296. PMID: 31533907

Sims EK, Besser REJ, Dayan C, et al; NIDDK Type 1 Diabetes TrialNet Study Group. Screening for type 1 diabetes in the general population: a status report and perspective. *Diabetes.* 2022;71(4):610-623. PMID: 35316839

9 ANSWER: A) Allow 15 minutes between the bolus and the meal

The most important variable that affects the risk of neonatal macrosomia is the postprandial glucose level. Women with diabetes who are pregnant or are planning pregnancy should try to normalize blood glucose levels to minimize congenital anomalies and other complications. The American Diabetes Association recommends that the hemoglobin A_{1c} level be less than 6.0% to 6.5% (<42-48 mmol/mol) during early pregnancy, with a lower target (<6.0% [<42 mmol/mol]) by the second and third trimesters. The American Diabetes Association also recommends maintaining fasting and preprandial glucose levels between 70 and 95 mg/dL (3.9-5.3 mmol/L) with either \ peak (1-hour) postprandial levels between 110 and 140 mg/dL (6.1 and 7.8 mmol/L) or 2-hour postprandial levels between 100 and 120 mg/dL (5.6 and 6.7 mmol/L). Although most of the patient's preprandial glucose levels are on target, there is clearly a pattern of elevated postprandial values that return to target at the completion of the rapid-acting insulin analogue's biologic activity (before the next check). It takes 10 to 15 minutes for a rapid-acting insulin analogue to enter the circulation from a subcutaneous depot, so allowing more time between the administration of aspart and the meal (Answer A) should correct the postprandial hyperglycemia.

Changing the sensitivity factor (Answer C) would only improve postprandial levels when preprandial levels are above target, which her log does not demonstrate.

Changing the insulin-to-carbohydrate ratio to 1:15 (Answer B) would give her *less* insulin before meals, not *more,* and would therefore worsen the postprandial hyperglycemia.

Increasing the detemir dosage (Answer E) would not be expected to affect postprandial glucose values specifically.

Continuing the same regimen (Answer D) is not correct, as changes to her regimen are needed because there is clearly a pattern of elevated postprandial values.

EDUCATIONAL OBJECTIVE

Develop a strategy, based on knowledge of insulin action, to improve postprandial glycemic control during pregnancy.

REFERENCE(S)

American Diabetes Association. 15. Management of diabetes in pregnancy: standards of medical care in diabetes-2023. *Diabetes Care.* 2023;46(Suppl 1): S254-S266. PMID: 36507645

McCance DR. Pregnancy and diabetes. *Best Pract Res Clin Endocrinol Metab.* 2011;25(6):945-958. PMID: 22115168

Kitzmiller JL, Block JM, Brown FM, et al. Managing preexisting diabetes for pregnancy: summary of evidence and consensus recommendations for care. *Diabetes Care.* 2008;31(5):1060-1079. PMID: 18445730

10 ANSWER: C) 6.0%

The risk of type 1 diabetes in children appears to be on the rise and can be affected by several factors, including geography, age, sex, family history, and environment. The risk of developing type 1 diabetes increases from 0.4% in individuals with no family history of the disease to 4% to 8% in offspring of an affected parent (thus, Answer C is correct). Having an affected father confers a higher risk than having an affected mother. The risk rises to as high as 30% when both parents have type 1 diabetes.

EDUCATIONAL OBJECTIVE

Counsel patients about the magnitude of risk of type 1 diabetes mellitus developing in the offspring of an affected parent.

REFERENCE(S)

Krischer JP, Liu X, Lernmark A, et al; TEDDY Study Group. The influence of type 1 diabetes genetic susceptibility regions, age, sex, and family history on the progression from multiple autoantibodies to type 1 diabetes: a TEDDY study report. *Diabetes.* 2017;66(12):3122-2129. PMID: 28903990

van Esch SC, Cornel MC, Snoek FJ. "I am pregnant and my husband has diabetes. Is there a risk for my child?" A qualitative study of questions asked by email about the role of genetic susceptibility to diabetes. *BMC Public Health.* 2010;10:688. PMID: 21067573

Mehers KL, Gillespie KM. The genetic basis for type 1 diabetes. *Br Med Bull.* 2008;88(1):115-129. PMID: 19088009

Aly TA, Ide A, Jahromi MM, et al. Extreme genetic risk for type 1A diabetes. *Proc Natl Acad Sci U S A.* 2006;103(38):4074-14079. PMID: 16966600

11 ANSWER: E) Recommend overnight basal testing

This patient has fasting hyperglycemia, which has multiple possible causes. Therefore, it is necessary to have the patient test 2 to 3 times at night for a few days (Answer E) to see what is truly happening before making dose adjustments. Ideally, he could be convinced to wear a blinded continuous glucose monitor to more fully ascertain what is happening at night.

Neither increasing the basal rate 1 or 2 hours before morning hyperglycemia is typically observed (Answer C) nor increasing the basal rate overnight (Answer D) is the best recommendation.

Changing the method of insulin delivery would not be expected to correct the fasting hyperglycemia, and including long-acting insulin, as one would find in a multiple daily injection regimen (Answer A), might increase the incidence of hypoglycemia.

Eliminating the bedtime snack (Answer B) would only help if the patient were hyperglycemic throughout the night, which is unknown.

EDUCATIONAL OBJECTIVE

Recommend overnight basal testing to assess fasting hyperglycemia.

REFERENCE(S)

Davies MJ, Aroda VR, Collins BS, et al. Management of hyperglycaemia in type 2 diabetes, 2022. A consensus report by the American Diabetes Association (ADA) and the European Association for the Study of Diabetes (EASD), *Diabetologia.* 2022;65(12):1925-1966. PMID: 36151309

Nimri R, Nir J, Phillip M. Insulin pump therapy. *Am J Ther.* 2020;27(1):e30-e41. PMID: 31833871

12 ANSWER: E) History of previous ulceration

The lifetime risk of developing a foot ulcer in persons with diabetes mellitus is about 25%. Multiple factors are associated with an increased risk of ulceration, including previous ulceration or amputation, the presence of peripheral neuropathy with loss of protective sensation, foot deformity, and suboptimally controlled diabetes. Options A, B, and E are all risk factors for the development of future ulcers, but the strongest predictive factor is a history of previous ulceration (Answer E), with an odds ratio of 56.8 and up to a 10-fold increased risk for amputation.

Other factors are absent ankle reflexes (Answer B) associated with neuropathy (odds ratio, 6.48), abnormal response to monofilament testing (Answer A) (odds ratio, 18.42), and male gender (odds ratio, 2.15).

Peripheral vascular disease (Answer C) is an important prognostic factor for delayed wound healing and amputations but not a strong independent predictor of foot ulceration.

Callus formation (Answer D) does not predispose to foot ulcers.

EDUCATIONAL OBJECTIVE

Identify predictors of increased risk of foot ulcers.

REFERENCE(S)

Van Netten JJ, Raspovic A, Lavery LA, et al; International Working Group on the Diabetic Foot. Prevention of foot ulcers in the at-risk patient with diabetes: a systematic review. *Diabetes Metab Res Rev.* 2020;36(Suppl 1):e3270213. PMID: 26340966

Hicks CW, Canner JK, Mathiousdakis N, Lippincott C, Sherman RL, Abularrage CJ. Incidence and risk factors associated with ulcer recurrence among patients with diabetic foot ulcers treated in a multidisciplinary setting. *J Surg Res.* 2020;246:243-250. PMID: 31610352

Ahmad J. The diabetic foot. *Diabetes Metab Syndr.* 2016;10(1):48-60. PMID: 26072202

Noor S, Zubair M, Ahmad J. Diabetic foot ulcer--a review on pathophysiology, classification and microbial etiology. *Diabetes Metab Syndr.* 2015;9(3):192-199. PMID: 25982677

Moura Neto A, Zantut-Wittmann DE, Fernandes TD, Nery M, Parisi MCR. Risk factors for ulceration and amputation in diabetic foot: study in a cohort of 496 patients. *Endocrine.* 2013;44(1):119-124. PMID: 23124278

Boulton AJ, Armstrong DG, Albert SF, et al; American Diabetes Association; American Association of Clinical Endocrinologists. Comprehensive foot examination and risk assessment: a report of the task force of the foot care interest group of the American Diabetes Association, with endorsement by the American Association of Clinical Endocrinologists. *Diabetes Care.* 2008;31(8):1679-1685. PMID: 18663232

13 ANSWER: E) Temporarily relax his tight glucose targets

Up to 30% of patients with type 1 or longstanding type 2 diabetes mellitus have impaired or absent awareness of hypoglycemia. As plasma glucose levels fall, compromised physiologic counterregulatory defenses include failure of an increase in glucagon secretion and attenuated epinephrine secretion. This, together with inability to reduce circulating insulin levels, results in the clinical syndrome of defective counterregulation, which markedly increases the risk of recurrent severe hypoglycemia. Hypoglycemia-attenuating defense against subsequent hypoglycemia is a concept referred to as hypoglycemia-associated autonomic failure (HAAF). The mainstay therapy for HAAF is the scrupulous avoidance of hypoglycemia. Patients with hypoglycemia unawareness and/or severe hypoglycemia and tight control should be advised to relax their glucose targets for a period to allow awareness to potentially return with adrenergic symptoms (Answer E).

A glucagon emergency kit (Answer B) should be available, but it would not help if he were alone. Additionally, it is used only as a last resort and does not address the hypoglycemia unawareness.

Although a hybrid closed-loop system (Answer A) may help reduce hypoglycemia, it would not address the underlying cause of the hypoglycemia unawareness or guarantee its avoidance. There would also be a delay in initiating pump therapy and a learning curve regarding its use. Finally, hybrid closed-loop therapy has not been shown to reduce the number of episodes of severe hypoglycemia, although it can help reduce overt hypoglycemia in certain populations.

While a number of educational programs focusing on hypoglycemia detection and avoidance (Answer C) (Dose Adjustment for Normal Eating [DAFNE], Blood Glucose Awareness Training [BGAT], Hypoglycemia Awareness and Avoidance [HAAT]) have demonstrated effectiveness in reducing the occurrence of hypoglycemia, such an education program is not the most immediate fix for the patient, but it would be an important part of his subsequent follow-up.

Lastly, although exercise in people with type 1 diabetes can cause hypoglycemia, the timing and type of exercise impact its effect. Therefore, discussing how to exercise without causing hypoglycemia is important and can generally be accomplished without stopping it completely (Answer D).

EDUCATIONAL OBJECTIVE

Recommend management of severe hypoglycemia and hypoglycemia unawareness in type 1 diabetes mellitus.

REFERENCE(S)

Rickels MR. Hypoglycemia-associated autonomic failure, counterregulatory responses, and therapeutic options in type 1 diabetes. *Ann N Y Acad Sci.* 2019;1454(1):68-79. PMID: 31389033

Cryer PE. Mechanisms of hypoglycemia-associated autonomic failure in diabetes. *N Engl J Med.* 2013;69(4):362-372. PMID: 23883381

Teo E, Hassan N, Tam W, Koh S. Effectiveness of continuous glucose monitoring in maintaining glycaemic control among people with type 1 diabetes mellitus: a systematic review of randomised controlled trials and meta-analysis. *Diabetologia.* 2022;65(4):604-619. PMID: 35141761

Reddy M, Jugnee N, Anantharaja S, Oliver N. Switching from flash glucose monitoring to continuous glucose monitoring on hypoglycemia in adults with type 1 diabetes at high hypoglycemia risk: the Extension Phase of the I HART CGM Study. *Diabetes Technol Ther.* 2018;20(11):751-757. PMID: 30265562

De Valk HW, Lablanche S, Bosi E, et al. Study of MiniMed 640G Insulin Pump with SmartGuard in prevention of low glucose events in adults with type 1 diabetes (SMILE): design of a hypoglycemia prevention trial with continuous glucose monitoring data as outcomes. *Diabetes Technol Ther.* 2018;20(11):758-766. PMID: 30325656

14 ANSWER: D) Nonadherence to insulin therapy

Hospitalizations for diabetic ketoacidosis are increasing in the United States. Diabetic ketoacidosis is a common, life-threatening complication of diabetes, accounting for as many as 4% to 9% of all hospital admissions in patients with diabetes. Diabetic ketoacidosis is the leading cause of mortality among children and young adults with type 1 diabetes, accounting for 50% of all deaths in this population. Most cases of diabetic ketoacidosis are associated with type 1 diabetes, but 1 in 5 cases of diabetic ketoacidosis are associated with type 2 diabetes.

Diabetic ketoacidosis has many precipitating causes, with one of the most common being undertreatment or omission of insulin doses (Answer D). There are higher prevalence rates of eating disorders among persons with type 1 diabetes, as compared with rates in their peers without diabetes. Given the detailed meal planning, precision in food portions, and constant monitoring of food intake (carbohydrates in particular) related to insulin doses recommended for diabetes management, persons with diabetes may be inherently more prone to issues revolving around food. Eating disorders and disordered eating behaviors—especially insulin omission—are associated with suboptimal glycemic control and serious risk for increased morbidity, including diabetic ketoacidosis and mortality. Insulin omission is sometimes viewed as a weight-control strategy.

Although this patient's serum creatinine concentration is elevated, there is clear evidence of volume depletion, and this is a more likely reason for her azotemia than acute kidney injury (Answer A).

Infection (Answer C) can cause insulin resistance and diabetic ketoacidosis, but this young woman has no signs or symptoms of injection. Evidence of infection, such as a urinary tract infection, should be ruled out.

Unrecognized pregnancy (Answer B) is also a precipitating factor for diabetic ketoacidosis, but this patient is taking an oral contraceptive pill. Nonetheless, a pregnancy test is needed to rule out this possibility.

EDUCATIONAL OBJECTIVE

Identify eating disorders and omission of insulin doses as a cause of diabetic ketoacidosis in type 1 diabetes.

REFERENCE(S)

Self WH, Evans CS, Jenkins CA, et al; Pragmatic Critical Care Research Group. Clinical effects of balanced crystalloids vs saline in adults with diabetic ketoacidosis: a subgroup analysis of cluster randomized clinical trials. *JAMA Netw Open.* 2020;3(11):e2024596. PMID: 33196806

Vellanki P, Umpierrez GE. Increasing hospitalizations for DKA: a need for prevention programs. *Diabetes Care.* 2018;41(9):1839-1841. PMID: 30135197

Hanlan ME, Griffith J, Patel N, Jaser SS. Eating disorders and disordered eating in type 1 diabetes: prevalence, screening, and treatment options. *Curr Diab Rep.* 2013. PMID: 24022608

Steenkamp DW, Alexanian SM, McDonnell ME. Adult hyperglycemic crisis: a review and perspective. *Curr Diab Rep.* 2013;13(1):130-137. PMID: 23115048

Guenette MD, Hahn M, Cohn TA, Teo C, Remington GJ. Atypical antipsychotics and diabetic ketoacidosis: a review. *Psychopharmacology (Berl).* 2013;226(1):1-12. PMID: 23344556

Kitabchi AE, Umpierrez GE, Miles JM, Fisher JN. Hyperglycemic crises in adult patients with diabetes. *Diabetes Care.* 2009;32(7):1335-1343. PMID: 19564476

15 ANSWER: B) Plan to do anerobic exercise prior to aerobic exercise

Management of type 1 diabetes before, during, and after exercise can be challenging but is very important to do correctly. Multiple guidelines and review articles have recently been published. A key concept to exercising without hypoglycemia is the idea of insulin on-board, which may need to be reduced 30 to 120 minutes before aerobic exercise. Usually, it is considered optimal for patients to begin aerobic exercise at a blood glucose concentration above 150 mg/dL (>8.3 mmol/L). Additionally, trend arrows on continuous glucose monitoring can be helpful in guiding glucose management during exercise. At the end of aerobic exercise, glucose levels may increase, which is generally associated with an increase in lactate levels.

In general, anerobic or resistance exercise (Answer B) does not lower glucose levels, and if done before aerobic exercise it can reduce the risk for hypoglycemia during the aerobic exercise. Thus, this is the best recommendation.

The basal insulin dose usually needs to be reduced 30 or more minutes before exercise to reduce insulin on-board. Thus, reducing the basal rate immediately before exercise (Answer C) is incorrect.

Aerobic exercise is safe to start if the glucose concentration is above 150 mg/dL (>8.3 mmol/L), not above 100 mg/dL (>5.6 mmol/L) (Answer D).

Most people with type 1 diabetes need 15 to 30 g of simple carbohydrates for every 30 minutes of aerobic exercise, not 30 to 45 g (Answer A).

EDUCATIONAL OBJECTIVE

Advise patients with type 1 diabetes mellitus about the effects of exercise on the risk of hypoglycemia.

REFERENCE(S)

Riddell MC, Peters AL. Exercise in adults with type 1 diabetes mellitus. *Nat Rev Endocrinol.* 2023;19(2): 98-111. PMID: 36316391

Scott SN, Fontana FY, Cocks M, et al; Study of Integrative Biology of Exercise in Diabetes. Post-exercise recovery for the endurance athlete with type 1 diabetes: a consensus statement. *Lancet Diabetes Endocrinol.* 2021;9(5):304-317. PMID: 33864810

Riddell MC, Scott SN, Fournier PA, et al. The competitive athlete with type 1 diabetes. *Diabetologia.* 2020;63(8):1475-1490. PMID: 32533229

Yardley JE, Kenny GP, Perkins BA, et al. Resistance versus aerobic exercise: acute effects on glycemia in type 1 diabetes. *Diabetes Care.* 2013;36(3):537-542. PMID: 23172972

16 ANSWER: E) >90%

The annual incidence of diabetic retinopathy ranges from 2.2% to 12.7%, and the incidence of progression ranges from 3.4% to 12.3%. Progression to proliferative diabetic retinopathy is higher in individuals with mild disease than in those with no disease at baseline. Understanding the available treatment options for persons with diabetic retinopathy is key because targeted glycemic control, blood pressure, and lipid control has been shown to reduce both the incidence and progression of retinopathy.

The American Diabetes Association recommends retinopathy screening by an eye specialist within 5 years of the diagnosis of type 1 diabetes in adults. Patients with type 2 diabetes should have an initial dilated and comprehensive eye examination by an ophthalmologist or optometrist at the time of the diabetes diagnosis, because microvascular changes can begin before diagnosis if prediabetes has been present. Female patients should be advised to have a dilated eye exam before conception or during the first trimester of pregnancy, and then every trimester and for 1 year postpartum. If any level of diabetic retinopathy is present, subsequent dilated retinal examinations for patients with type 1 (or type 2) diabetes should be repeated at least annually by an ophthalmologist or optometrist. If retinopathy is progressive or sight-threatening, examinations are required more frequently.

Management recommendations call for optimizing glycemic control, blood pressure, and lipids to reduce the risk or slow the progression of retinopathy. It is important to emphasize to the patient that attention to lifestyle and pharmacotherapeutic measures to optimize blood glucose, blood pressure, and lipids can be highly effective and would indeed reduce risk of vision loss due to retinopathy by more than 90% (Answer E). Effective metabolic control would significantly reduce her risk of progression to proliferative retinopathy, macular edema, and the need for laser or alternative treatments, thus protecting sight.

If retinopathy does advance, current therapeutic options can be remarkably effective at preventing severe vision loss when administered in an appropriate and timely manner.

EDUCATIONAL OBJECTIVE

Counsel patients regarding the effect of appropriate medical care on the risk of vision loss in type 1 diabetes mellitus.

REFERENCE(S)

American Diabetes Association. 11. Microvascular complications and foot care: standards of medical care in diabetes-2020. *Diabetes Care.* 2020;43(Suppl 1):S135-S151. PMID: 31862754

Sabanayagam C, Banu R, Chee ML, et al. Incidence and progression of diabetic retinopathy: a systematic review. *Lancet Diabetes Endocrinol.* 2019;7(2): 140-149. PMID: 30005958

Bloomgarden ZT. Screening for and managing diabetic retinopathy: current approaches. *Am J Health Syst Pharm.* 2007;64(17 Suppl 12):S8-S14. PMID: 17720893

17 ANSWER: A) Assessment for ketones

In patients with type 1 diabetes, the urine should be tested for ketones (Answer A) if the blood glucose concentration is above 300 mg/dL (>16.7 mmol/L) for unexplained reasons, especially if the person feels unwell at the time. Testing for ketonuria should also be performed during periods of illness or stress or if there are symptoms compatible with ketoacidosis such as nausea, vomiting, and abdominal pain. If ketonuria is present in the setting of hyperglycemia, diabetic ketoacidosis should be suspected and the patient should be ideally sent to the emergency department for more testing (serum ketones, electrolytes, bicarbonate, pH, etc) and treated accordingly with intravenous fluids and insulin drip if diabetic ketoacidosis is indeed present.

While basal rate testing (Answer B), diabetes education (Answer C), and a continuous glucose sensor (Answer D) are all needed to help this patient achieve a lower hemoglobin A_{1c}, none of these options is the best immediate step now. These steps can be done over weeks to months. Therapy for stress management (Answer E) is appropriate if she is willing to explore it, but again, this is not immediately necessary.

EDUCATIONAL OBJECTIVE

Determine when urine ketones should be measured in a patient with type 1 diabetes mellitus.

REFERENCE(S)

Albanese-O'Neill A, Wu M, Miller KM, et al; T1D Exchange Clinic Network. *Diabetes Care.* 2017;40(4):e38-e39. PMID: 28100607

Marks BE, Wolfsdorf JI. Monitoring of pediatric type 1 diabetes. *Front Endocrinol (Lausanne).* 2020;11:128. PMID: 32256447

Cao X, Zhang X, Xian Y, Wu J, et al. The diagnosis of diabetic acute complications using the glucose-ketone meter in outpatients at endocrinology department. *Int J Clin Exp Med.* 2014;7(12):5701-5705. PMID: 25664094

Weber C, Kocher S, Neeser K, Joshi SR. Prevention of diabetic ketoacidosis and self-monitoring of ketone bodies: an overview. *Curr Med Res Opin.* 2009;25(5):1197-1207. PMID: 19327102

Goldstein DE, Little RR, Lorenz RA, et al. Tests of glycemia in diabetes. *Diabetes Care.* 2004;27(7): 1761-1773. PMID: 15220264

18 ANSWER: B) Measurement of tissue transglutaminase antibodies

The incidence of celiac disease in individuals with type 1 diabetes is 5% to 7%. Affected patients may report typical symptoms of celiac sprue (bloating, diarrhea, abdominal pain, weight loss) or be relatively asymptomatic. Sometimes a chronic inflammatory rash (dermatitis herpetiformis) develops suddenly, lasts for weeks to months, and may also be associated with other gastrointestinal diseases. The best initial test is measurement of tissue transglutaminase antibodies (Answer B).

Colonoscopy (Answer A) would not be diagnostic.

An upper gastrointestinal series with small-bowel follow-through (Answer E) would probably show nonspecific small-bowel findings but would also not be diagnostic.

TPO antibody measurement (Answer C) is irrelevant to this case.

A skin biopsy (Answer D) should diagnose the rash as dermatitis herpetiformis, but it would not identify the specific associated gastrointestinal condition—in this case, celiac disease.

EDUCATIONAL OBJECTIVE

Recognize the signs and symptoms of celiac disease and initiate appropriate evaluation.

REFERENCE(S)

Vermeersch P, Geboes K, Marien G, Hoffman I, Hiele M, Bossuyt X. Serological diagnosis of celiac disease: comparative analysis of different strategies. *Clin Chim Acta.* 2012;413(21-22):1761-1767. PMID: 22771970

Elwenspoek MM, Thom H, Sheppard AL, et al. Defining the optimum strategy for identifying adults and children with coeliac disease: systematic review and economic modelling. *Health Technol Assess.* 2022;26(44):1-310. PMID: 36321689

Eland I, Klieverik L, Mansour AA, Al-Toma A. Gluten-free diet in co-existent celiac disease and type 1 diabetes mellitus: is it detrimental or beneficial to glycemic control, vascular complications, and quality of life? *Nutrients.* 2022;15(1):199. PMID: 36615856

Salmi T, Hervonen K. Current concepts of dermatitis herpetiformis. *Acta Derm Venereol.* 2020;100(5): adv00056. PMID: 32039457

19 ANSWER: E) Weight loss and exercise to prevent type 2 diabetes

The diagnostic abnormalities documented by oral glucose tolerance testing in this patient are impaired fasting glucose and impaired glucose tolerance, both signifying prediabetes. Therefore, weight loss and exercise should be recommended to prevent type 2 diabetes (Answer E). He does not have diabetes because the fasting glucose level is less than 126 mg/dL (<7.0 mmol/L), and the 2-hour value from the oral glucose tolerance test is less than 200 mg/dL (<11.1 mmol/L). The 1-hour value is elevated, but this can occur in persons with prediabetes, and it is not a standard parameter for the diagnosis of diabetes. Diagnosis of diabetes on the basis of fasting glucose requires 2 separate abnormal values but repeating this measurement (Answer A) in a patient such as this one who has a nondiagnostic level is not indicated. Thus, initiating metformin (Answer D) is incorrect because the patient does not have diabetes.

Common forms of maturity-onset diabetes of the young (MODY) are associated with autosomal dominant inheritance, and the presented family history (with neither parent being affected) is not consistent with this diagnosis. MODY is also rare. Thus, genetic screening (Answer C) is incorrect.

Although insulin resistance can be inferred from measurement of insulin during an oral glucose tolerance test (Answer B), this is not likely to affect this patient's management.

The American Diabetes Association criteria for the diagnosis of diabetes are as follows:

1. Hemoglobin A_{1c} ≥6.5% (≥48 mmol/mol). The test should be performed in a laboratory using a method that is certified by the National Glycohemoglobin Standardization Program and standardized to the Diabetes Control and Complications Trial assay.*

   OR

2. Fasting plasma glucose ≥126 mg/dL (≥7.0 mmol/L). Fasting is defined as no caloric intake for at least 8 hours.*

   OR

3. Two-hour plasma glucose value ≥200 mg/dL (≥11.1 mmol/L) during an oral glucose tolerance test. The test should be performed as described by the World Health Organization, using a glucose load containing the equivalent of 75-g anhydrous glucose dissolved in water.*

   OR

4. In a patient with classic symptoms of hyperglycemia or hyperglycemic crisis, a random plasma glucose value ≥200 mg/dL (≥11.1 mmol/L).

*In the absence of unequivocal hyperglycemia, criteria 1 to 3 should be confirmed by repeated testing.

EDUCATIONAL OBJECTIVE

Diagnose prediabetes on the basis of results from oral glucose tolerance testing.

REFERENCE(S)

American Diabetes Association. 2. Classification and diagnosis of diabetes: standards of medical care in diabetes-2020. *Diabetes Care.* 2020;43(Suppl 1): S14-S31. PMID: 31862745

Kumar R, Nandhini LP, Kamalanathan S, Sahoo J, Vivekanadan M. Evidence for current diagnostic criteria of diabetes mellitus. *World J Diabetes.* 2016;7(17):396-405. PMID: 27660696

Inzucchi SE. Clinical practice. Diagnosis of type 2 diabetes. *N Engl J Med.* 2012;367(6):542-550. PMID: 22873534

Chivese T, Hirst J, Matizanadzo JT, et al. The diagnostic accuracy of HbA_{1c}, compared to the oral glucose tolerance test, for screening for type 2 diabetes mellitus in Africa-A systematic review and meta-analysis. *Diabet Med.* 2022;39(4):e14754. PMID: 34854127

Gordon DK, Hussain M, Kumar P, Khan S, Khan S. The sickle effect: the silent titan affecting glycated hemoglobin reliability. *Cureus.* 2020;12(8):e9685. PMID: 32923278

20 ANSWER: A) Insulin degludec; take it at his convenience once daily

The duration of action of insulin degludec (Answer A) is longer than 42 hours; the half-life is approximately 25 hours and it reaches steady state in 2 to 3 days. It may be given safely and effectively with a minimum of 8 hours and maximum of 40 hours between doses. This makes it well suited to use during travel, as long as the patient takes it once daily.

NPH insulin at bedtime, given at the same time when traveling (Answer C), is an impractical regimen as it is difficult to give it at the same time when crossing multiple time zones.

Insulin detemir may be given once daily at bedtime but reducing the dose by 50% when traveling (Answer B) would lead to hyperglycemia.

The half-life of U300 insulin glargine (Answer D) is about 23 hours. It reaches a steady state in 4 days, and the duration of action is 36 hours or less. Data regarding U300 insulin support its safety and efficacy up to a ± 3-hour window for administration, so this also may not be ideal for dosing when traveling.

EDUCATIONAL OBJECTIVE

Optimize basal insulin therapy for travel across time zones.

REFERENCE(S)

Ritzel R, Rouseel R, Bolli GB, et al. Patient-level meta-analysis of the EDITION 1, 2 and 3 studies: glycaemic control and hypoglycaemia with new insulin glargine 300 U/ml versus glargine 100 U/mL in people with type 2 diabetes. *Diabetes Obes Metab.* 2015;17(9):859-867. PMID: 25929311

Matheiu C, Hollander P, Miranda-Palma B, et al. Efficacy and safety of insulin degludec in a flexible dosing regimen vs insulin glargine in patients with type 1 diabetes (BEGIN: Flex T1): a 26-week randomized, treat-to-target trial with a 26-week extension. *J Clin Endocrinol Metab.* 2013;98(3):1154-1162. PMID: 23393185

21 ANSWER: D) Referral for retinal examination

In a 2-year trial (SUSTAIN-6) of patients with type 2 diabetes and high cardiovascular risk, more events of diabetic retinopathy complications occurred in patients treated with semaglutide (3.0%) compared with placebo (1.8%). The difference was seen very early in the trial (in the first 2 to 8 weeks). The absolute risk increase for diabetic retinopathy complications was higher among patients with a history of diabetic retinopathy at baseline (semaglutide, 8.2%; placebo, 5.2%) than among patients without a known history of diabetic retinopathy (semaglutide, 0.7%; placebo, 0.4%). Rapid improvement in glucose control has been associated with a temporary worsening of diabetic retinopathy. The applicability of such an association to semaglutide and retinopathy is unclear, and a direct effect of semaglutide cannot be ruled out. The effect of long-term glycemic control with semaglutide on diabetic retinopathy complications has not been studied. Patients with a history of diabetic retinopathy should be monitored for progression. Thus, this patient should be referred for a retinal examination (Answer D) at his follow-up visit.

GLP-1 receptor agonists have a boxed warning regarding the risk of C-cell tumors observed in rodents and a warning regarding acute pancreatitis. However, measuring calcitonin (Answer B) is not recommended unless there is a suspicion for medullary thyroid carcinoma based on thyroid biopsy, family history, or presence of multiple endocrine neoplasia type 2.

Similarly, it is not recommended to measure serum amylase and lipase (Answer A) unless the patient has gastrointestinal symptoms suggestive of acute pancreatitis.

GLP-1 receptor agonists have a warning regarding renal impairment/acute kidney injury, but this is in the setting of a patient with baseline kidney dysfunction and severe gastrointestinal symptoms (diarrhea, vomiting) leading to dehydration with subsequent worsening of the renal impairment. Thus, creatinine measurement (Answer C) is not necessary now.

Routine thyroid ultrasonography (Answer E) is not recommended for patients taking on GLP-1 receptor agonists any more than it is recommended for any other patient. However, if a thyroid nodule is found on clinical examination, standard evaluation and follow-up with thyroid ultrasonography is recommended.

EDUCATIONAL OBJECTIVE

Monitor for progression of diabetic retinopathy in a patient with diabetes mellitus taking a GLP-1 receptor agonist.

REFERENCE(S)

Marso SP, Bain SC, Consoli A, et al; SUSTAIN-6 Investigators. Semaglutide and cardiovascular outcomes in patients with type 2 diabetes. *N Engl J Med.* 2016;375(19):1834-1844. PMID: 27633186

Drab SR. Glucagon-like peptide-1 receptor agonists for type 2 diabetes: a clinical update of safety and efficacy. *Curr Diabetes Rev.* 2016;12(4):403-413. PMID: 26694823

22 ANSWER: C) Empagliflozin

Empagliflozin (Answer C) has been proven to reduce progression to chronic kidney disease and has proven cardiovascular disease benefit.

In one of the clinicals trials with canagliflozin (Answer B), there was an unexpected increase in lower-extremity amputation. This concern is noted as a warning in the package insert. Given that there is an alternative agent in this class (empagliflozin), it seems reasonable to use it preferentially. An approximately 2-fold increased risk of lower limb amputations associated with canagliflozin use was observed in CANVAS and CANVAS-R, 2 large, randomized, placebo-controlled trials evaluating patients with type 2 diabetes who had either established cardiovascular disease or were at risk for cardiovascular disease. In CANVAS, canagliflozin-treated patients and placebo-treated patients had 5.9 and 2.8 amputations per 1000 patients per year, respectively. In CANVAS-R, canagliflozin-treated patients and placebo-treated patients had 7.5 and 4.2 amputations per 1000 patients per year, respectively. The risk of lower-limb amputations was observed at both the 100 mg and 300 mg once-daily regimens. Lower-limb infections, gangrene, and diabetic foot ulcers were the most common precipitating medical events leading to the need for amputation. The risk of amputation was highest in patients with a baseline history of amputation, peripheral vascular disease, and neuropathy.

DPP-4 inhibitors (Answer E) have no proven benefit on chronic kidney disease and are not recommended as the next step in therapy in this patient with chronic kidney disease and cardiovascular disease. In the cardiovascular outcome trial SAVOR-TIMI, 3.5% of patients who received saxagliptin were hospitalized for heart failure vs 2.8% of patients who received placebo. This is the same as 35 of every 1000 patients compared with 28 of every 1000 patients. Risk factors included history of heart failure or kidney impairment, as in the current case.

Neither bexagliflozin (Answer A) nor ertugliflozin (Answer D) has primary evidence of reducing chronic kidney disease progression.

EDUCATIONAL OBJECTIVE

List contraindications of various oral agents used to treat type 2 diabetes mellitus.

REFERENCE(S)

Neal B, Perkovic V, Mahaffey KW, et al; CANVAS Program Collaborative Group. Canagliflozin and cardiovascular and renal events in type 2 diabetes. *N Engl J Med.* 2017;377(7):644-657. PMID: 28605608

Scirica BM, Bhatt DL, Braunwald E, et al; SAVOR-TIMI 53 Steering Committee and Investigators. Saxagliptin and cardiovascular outcomes in patients with type 2 diabetes mellitus. *N Engl J Med.* 2013;369(14):1317-1326. PMID: 23992601

ElSayed NA, Aleppo G, Aroda VR, et al; American Diabetes Association. 9. Pharmacologic approaches to glycemic treatment: standards of care in diabetes-2023. *Diabetes Care.* 2023;46(Suppl 1): S140-S157. PMID: 36507650

23 ANSWER: C) Cannabis

Cannabis use (Answer C) has been shown to cause an unusual form of diabetic ketoacidosis, with a more alkalotic pH. These individuals tend to have vomiting before they are ketotic, and symptoms may be due to hyperemesis caused by the cannabis. This causes ketosis followed by hyperglycemia.

He is not hypotensive or hypoglycemic, so he does not likely have adrenal insufficiency (Answer A).

He has no evidence of infection (Answer D).

While alcohol intoxication (Answer B) is also an important consideration, typically in this setting the glucose level is low due to suppression of gluconeogenesis.

Insulin rationing (Answer E) can occur if patients lack access to medical care/health insurance, but this patient seems to be continuing to administer insulin and take care of his diabetes, even though he has moved away from home.

EDUCATIONAL OBJECTIVE

Identify features of cannabis-mediated diabetic ketoacidosis.

REFERENCE(S)

Kinney GL, Akturk HK, Taylor DD, Foster NC, Shah VN. Cannabis use is associated with increased risk for diabetic ketoacidosis in adults with type 1 diabetes: findings from the T1D Exchange Clinic Registry. *Diabetes Care.* 2020;43(1):247-249. PMID: 3168116

Akturk HK, Snell-Bergeon J, Kinney GL, Champakanath A, Monte A, Shah VN. Differentiating diabetic ketoacidosis and hyperglycemic ketosis due to cannabis hyperemesis syndrome in adults with type 1 diabetes. *Diabetes Care.* 2022;45(2():481-483. PMID: 34880067

24 ANSWER: A) Chronic autoimmune urticaria

Chronic autoimmune urticaria (Answer A) is a syndrome that occurs at an increased frequency in patients with autoimmune disorders. Type 1 diabetes and Hashimoto thyroiditis are commonly associated with this condition. In general, chronic autoimmune urticaria is treated symptomatically, but in severe cases omalizumab has been used. The etiology is thought to be due to autoantibodies to the IgE receptors.

Flea bites (Answer B) are unlikely given the rash's location and appearance. Flea bites are a consideration in the differential diagnosis of scattered pruritic lesions, but this would not specifically be associated with diabetes.

Necrobiosis lipoidica diabeticorum (Answer D) is a rare, chronic, granulomatous skin disorder that affects 0.3% of patients with diabetes. The skin lesions are characterized by thinning of the skin, dilated capillaries, and lipid deposits. This appearance is quite different from the lesions seen in this case. While the etiology and pathogenesis of necrobiosis lipoidica diabeticorum is still controversial, it is thought that microangiopathy has an important role. The legs are the most common site for necrobiosis lipoidica diabeticorum, but involvement of other areas such as the abdomen, upper extremities, and scalp has been described. Benefit has been reported from different treatment regimens such as corticosteroid therapy (topical, intralesional and systemic), enhancers of wound healing, surgery, and immunomodulating therapies (including photochemotherapy).

Perforating collagenosis (Answer E) is not correct, although it is more common in persons with diabetes. It is not a diffuse process as is seen in the photograph in this vignette. Perforating collagenosis presents as hyperkeratotic papules with transepidermal elimination of degenerated material, including collagen or elastic fibers. It is generally diagnosed with a biopsy. This condition may be difficult to treat, but it often responds to light therapy.

Insulin allergy (Answer C) is unlikely due to the location of the lesions and the timing of the reaction. If it were an insulin allergy, the lesions would start as a localized reaction at the injection site. Before the introduction of recombinant human insulin to the market in the early 1980s, insulin allergy was a common occurrence. Allergy to human insulin preparations, although rare, still occurs. When insulin allergy is suspected, it is important to rule out causes such as allergies to inactive ingredients in the insulin formulation (eg, protamine sulfate, zinc, and metacresol) and allergies to latex or alcohol swabs that are used in the insulin preparation and injection process. Allergies to inactive ingredients in the insulin formulation can often be resolved by switching to a different type of insulin that does not contain the responsible inactive ingredient. In rare cases, an individual can be allergic to the insulin molecule itself. Insulin allergy may present as a localized reaction at the injection site or a more severe, generalized reaction that can range from urticaria to anaphylaxis.

EDUCATIONAL OBJECTIVE

Differentiate among specific skin disorders associated with diabetes mellitus.

REFERENCE(S)

Murdaca G, Paladin F, Borro M, Ricciardi L, Gangemi S. Prevalence of autoimmune and autoinflammatory diseases in chronic urticaria: pathogenetic, diagnostic and therapeutic implications. *Biomedicines.* 2023;11(2):410. PMID: 36830946

Müller CSL, Bourg C, Schweitzer LF, Friesenhahn-Ochs B, Pföhler C. Injection site reaction to various insulins as type III allergy with urticarial vasculitis in a patient with type I diabetes mellitus. *Am J Dermatopathol.* 2023;45(2):86-89. PMID: 36669070

25 ANSWER: C) At least every 3 years

In asymptomatic adults, diabetes screening should be considered in patients who are overweight or obese and have 1 or more of the following risk factors: first-degree relative with diabetes, high-risk race/ethnicity, history of cardiovascular disease, hypertension, HDL-cholesterol concentration less than 35 mg/dL (<0.91 mmol/L), and/or triglyceride level greater than 250 mg/dL (>2.83 mmol/L), polycystic ovary syndrome (in women), and physical inactivity.

Patients with prediabetes should have annual testing, and women diagnosed with gestational diabetes should have lifelong testing at least every 3 years (Answer C).

According to the American Diabetes Association guidelines, screening for diabetes should begin at age 35 years regardless of other factors such as ethnicity, family history, BMI, blood pressure, and dyslipidemia.

EDUCATIONAL OBJECTIVE

Select the appropriate screening frequency for type 2 diabetes/prediabetes in a woman with a history of gestational diabetes mellitus.

REFERENCE(S)

ElSayed NA, Aleppo G, Aroda VR, et al; American Diabetes Association. 2. Classification and diagnosis of diabetes: standards of medical care in diabetes-2023. *Diabetes Care.* 2023;46(Suppl 1):S14-S40. PMID: 36507649

US Preventive Services Task Force. Final Recommendation Statement. Abnormal Blood Glucose and Type 2 Diabetes Mellitus: Screening. April 2018. https://www.uspreventiveservicestaskforce.org/Page/Document/RecommendationStatementFinal/screening-for-abnormal-blood-glucose-and-type-2-diabetes

Pottie K, Jaramillo A, Lewin G, et al; Canadian Task Force on Preventive Health Care. Recommendations on screening for type 2 diabetes in adults. *CMAJ.* 2012;184(15):1687-1696. PMID: 23073674

26 ANSWER: B) Hydralazine

Cardiovascular autonomic neuropathy is associated with mortality independent of other cardiovascular risk factors. This woman has supine hypertension and a marked orthostatic drop in blood pressure, both systolic and diastolic upon arising. This presentation is consistent with orthostatic hypotension due to autonomic neuropathy. She does not, however, have a fixed tachycardia that often accompanies autonomic neuropathy. About one-half of persons with neurogenic orthostatic hypotension are hypertensive in the supine position. Supine hypertension promotes nocturnal sodium excretion, and orthostatic hypotension and may predispose to cardiovascular and renal disease. These reasons provide a rationale for treating supine hypertension. Given the lack of evidence from clinical trials on which to base therapy, recommendations are necessarily based on expert opinion and observations in small case series.

Pharmacologic treatment must be individualized. Persons with autonomic failure are highly sensitive to vasodilators, and hydralazine (Answer B) often effectively lowers nocturnal blood pressure without exacerbating orthostatic symptoms the next morning.

Due to $\alpha 2$ adrenoreceptor-mediated vasoconstriction, clonidine (Answer A) may paradoxically raise blood pressure in patients with pure autonomic failure.

β-Adrenoreceptor blockade alone (Answer E) may not lower supine blood pressure unless a drug with additional vasodilator properties is used. However, nebivolol, which is a vasodilating β-adrenergic blocker, can effectively lower nighttime hypertension.

Patients with neurogenic orthostatic hypotension and supine hypertension are highly sensitive to pressor drugs. Medications such as nonsteroidal anti-inflammatory drugs (Answer C) in commonly prescribed dosages can elicit a substantial pressor response and should be avoided. Midodrine (Answer D) is a vasopressor agent that is used to treat refractory orthostatic hypotension.

Relative to nonpharmacologic treatments for neurogenic orthostatic hypotension and supine hypertension, modest orthostatic stress can substantially lower blood pressure. Therefore, raising the head of the bed by 10 to 20 degrees has been applied to ameliorate supine blood pressure. The intervention also attenuates pressure-induced natriuresis, nocturnal volume loss, and orthostatic symptoms the next day. Water drinking may elicit a profound pressor response. This "osmopressor response" has a rapid onset within minutes, reaches a maximum after approximately 30 minutes, and is sustained for 60 to 90 minutes. Therefore, patients should limit drinking water 60 to 90 minutes before bedtime depending on their sensitivity to the osmopressor response. Finally, patients with orthostatic hypotension can also exhibit postprandial hypotension. A snack before bedtime may lower supine blood pressure in such cases. Compared with other macronutrients, carbohydrates result in larger blood pressure drops. Limitations to trying this approach clearly exist for a patient with obesity and uncontrolled diabetes.

Table. Management of supine hypertension[a]

Management of supine hypertension
Avoid offending agents
Avoid lying down during the day
Avoid rest in the seated position
Beware of "hidden" pressor agents
Ibuprofen
Indomethacin
Atomoxetine
Limit water ingestion near bedtime
Avoid fludrocortisone in favor of short-acting pressor agents when possible
Nonpharmacologic treatments
Tilt the whole bed head up by approximately 10 degrees; in patients who do not tolerate this measure, tilt only the head of the bed up 30 degrees
Carbohydrate-rich snack at bedtime
If alcohol is consumed, small amount at bedtime
Pharmacologic treatments
Consider individualized antihypertensive treatment taken at bedtime
Monitor nighttime blood pressure with 24-hour ambulatory blood pressure monitors
Monitor before starting treatment to see if patient "dips" to a normal pressure later in the night
Monitor to evaluate treatment efficacy
[a]These recommendations are based on expert opinion and results from small-scale studies. Larger-scale trials with hard clinical endpoints do not exist.

Table adapted from Jordan J, Fanciulli A, Tank J, et al. Management of supine hypertension in patients with neurogenic orthostatic hypotension: scientific statement of the American Autonomic Society, European Federation of Autonomic Societies, and the European Society of Hypertension. *J Hypertens.* 2019;37(8):1541-1546.

This patient is off the multiple antihypertensive agents she was taking before hospital admission. While proximally due to dehydration secondary to her intercurrent viral illness, her hypertension was most likely driven by high sodium intake, which masked her orthostatic hypotension, and blood pressure–lowering agents were added sequentially even though it is not clear that she was taking any of them regularly. Her orthostasis improved with hydration during the hospital stay. Her blood pressure should be monitored closely following discharge. Once she has equilibrated and is taking hydralazine, 24-hour ambulatory blood pressure monitoring would be useful to ensure her blood pressure management is optimized. Medical nutrition therapy as an outpatient should be recommended.

EDUCATIONAL OBJECTIVE

Recommend treatment options for diabetes-related cardiovascular autonomic neuropathy with supine hypertension.

REFERENCE(S)

ElSayed Na, Aleppo G, Aroda VR, et al; American Diabetes Association. 12. Retinopathy, neuropathy, and foot care: standards of care in diabetes-2023. *Diabetes Care.* 2023;46(Suppl 1): S203-S215. PMID: 36507636

Jordan J, Fanciulli A, Tank J, et al. Management of supine hypertension in patients with neurogenic orthostatic hypotension: scientific statement of the American Autonomic Society, European Federation of Autonomic Societies, and the European Society of Hypertension. *J Hypertens.* 2019;37(8):1541-1546. PMID: 30882602

Diabetes Mellitus, Section 2 Board Review

Marie E. McDonnell, MD

27 ANSWER: B) Endoscopic ultrasonography

The combination of hypophosphatemic hypercalcemia and insulin-dependent fasting hypoglycemia in a young person strongly indicates the diagnosis of multiple endocrine neoplasia (MEN) type 1. Imaging of the pancreas (Answer B) is the best next step to guide surgical management. MEN type 1, or Wermer syndrome, is a rare autosomal dominant disorder caused by germline pathogenic variants in the tumor suppressor gene *MEN1*, which encodes the menin protein. While nearly 100% of individuals with MEN type 1 have clinical manifestations by age 50 years, the prevalence is only 50% by age 20. Many individuals remain undiagnosed in young adulthood, especially if they are adopted and have no knowledge of their family history.

While genetic testing (Answer C) for germline *MEN1* pathogenic variants is important for the diagnosis, available guidelines indicate that the presence of two MEN type 1–associated conditions is adequate to make the diagnosis. Imaging will not only confirm diagnosis, but measurements of size and presence of metastatic disease are key elements in the management of patients with MEN type 1 to determine appropriate therapeutic strategies. Since this patient has had a severe hypoglycemic event and appears mildly volume depleted based on serum urea nitrogen and creatinine concentrations, potentially due to hypercalcemia, there is some urgency to address management, which will likely involve surgery for both multifocal parathyroid and insulin-producing tumors.

Among all available diagnostic imaging modalities, endoscopic ultrasonography is considered by expert consensus to be the most sensitive for the diagnosis of duodenopancreatic neuroendocrine neoplasia and should be used as the first imaging test whenever a specialized endosonographer is available. MRI is a good alternative, while CT is considered the last choice because of low sensitivity and radiation exposure (with the expectation that future surveillance imaging is likely to follow over the course of the patient's life). Lastly, in some cases where detection is difficult by imaging, selective arterial calcium stimulation (Answer E) is used to detect regional increases in pancreatic insulin secretion to guide surgical approach. This is not, however, a reasonable first step.

Despite this short, nonobserved fast, the laboratory test results obtained are adequate for the diagnosis of insulin-dependent hypoglycemia, and neither a formal mixed-meal test (Answer D) nor formal observed fasting (Answer A) would add substantial value to the evaluation. Because the episode was documented while fasting, postbariatric hypoglycemia can be ruled out.

Both primary hyperparathyroidism and insulinoma due to MEN type 1 are known to have delayed diagnosis due to subclinical presentations or their symptoms being attributed to other conditions. After the diagnosis of MEN type 1 was confirmed in this patient, her care team concluded that because both bariatric surgery and pregnancy are known to cause fluctuations in weight and blood glucose/insulin sensitivity, these recent conditions likely temporarily obscured her condition. Moreover, since calcium is normally lower during the second and third trimesters of pregnancy due to hemodilution, hypercalcemia would most likely have been missed.

EDUCATIONAL OBJECTIVE

Determine when to formally evaluate postbariatric hypoglycemia for alternative causes.

REFERENCE(S)

Brandi ML, Agarwal SK, Perrier ND, Lines KE, Valk GD, Thakker RV. Multiple endocrine neoplasia type 1: latest insights. *Endocr Rev.* 2021;42(2):133-170. PMID: 33249439

Niederle B, Selberherr A, Bartsch DK, et al. Multiple endocrine neoplasia type 1 and the pancreas: diagnosis and treatment of functioning and non-functioning pancreatic and duodenal neuro-endocrine neoplasia within the MEN1 syndrome - an International Consensus Statement. *Neuroendocrinology.* 2021;111(7):609-630. PMID: 32971521

28 ANSWER: D) Increase the losartan dosage to 50 mg daily

This patient is at high risk of advanced chronic kidney disease given her multiple risk factors (suboptimal glycemic control, cigarette smoking, A3 level albuminuria, reduced estimated glomerular filtration rate) and her relatively young age. Importantly, this patient has prioritized reducing her treatment burden specifically by stopping some of her medications; the benefit of adding a new medication needs to be weighed carefully with the risk of her becoming frustrated and nonadherent.

With her current medication regimen including a GLP-1 receptor agonist, HMG CoA reductase inhibitor, and an angiotensin receptor blocker, she is on a reasonable path for organ protection, a clear overall strategy to prolong survival and quality of life. However, the cardiorenal benefit of the angiotensin receptor blocker depends heavily on dosage and the degree of blood pressure control achieved, with the greatest risk reduction seen at the highest dosage. In addition, considering data from large randomized controlled trials of persons with and without diabetes, blood pressure less than 130/80 mm Hg is recommended to reduce cardiovascular mortality and slow progression of chronic kidney disease among patients with diabetes. Lower targets (eg, <120 mm Hg systolic) should be considered in patients with severe albuminuria (≥300 mg/g creat). As this patient is only on 25% of the highest losartan dosage and remains far from target, the best next step is to titrate the medication to arrive at the maximum tolerated dosage (Answer D) before considering the addition of another medication.

While it is true that empagliflozin (Answer A) and finerenone (Answer B) reduce progression of chronic kidney disease, both of these agents lower blood pressure modestly. Thus, the best initial step is to optimize the angiotensin receptor blocker. There is no expected secondary benefit from empagliflozin on glycemic control, as her hemoglobin A_{1c} is already excellent.

Increasing the dulaglutide dosage (Answer C) may modestly accelerate weight loss, but it would not appreciably affect the progression of chronic kidney disease.

Switching to semaglutide (Answer E) might be considered in this case for 2 indications: (1) to promote less weight regain after bariatric surgery given known differences in weight-loss potency and/or (2) to potentially have a better effect on slowing progression of chronic kidney disease than dulaglutide. However, because these 2 agents have not been compared in a head-to-head randomized clinical trial to answer either of these specific questions, a switch is not clearly indicated. Moreover, she continues to lose weight successfully (no indication of weight regain).

EDUCATIONAL OBJECTIVE

Maximize evidence-based strategies for slowing the progression of chronic kidney disease in patients with diabetes mellitus.

REFERENCE(S)

de Boer IH, Khunti K, Sadusky T, et al Diabetes management in chronic kidney disease: a consensus report by the American Diabetes Association (ADA) and Kidney Disease: improving global outcomes (KDIGO). *Diabetes Care.* 2022;45(12): 3075-3090. PMID: 36189689

Weir MR. Angiotensin II receptor blockers: the importance of dose in cardiovascular and renal risk reduction. *J Clin Hypertens (Greenwich)*. 2004;6(6): 315-323. PMID: 15187494

Sloan LA. Review of glucagon-like peptide-1 receptor agonists for the treatment of type 2 diabetes mellitus in patients with chronic kidney disease and their renal effects. *J Diabetes*. 2019;11(12):938-948. PMID: 31318152

29 ANSWER: C) Stop metformin

Regardless of how estimated glomerular filtration rate is determined, landmark randomized controlled trials have demonstrated that a decline in glomerular filtration rate after starting an SGTL-2 inhibitor is common. It is reversible in most cases and is generally not an indicator of risk of acute kidney injury. Independent of the initial glomerular filtration rate decline, SGLT-2 inhibitors are associated with overall kidney protection with improved albuminuria, decreased progression to severe albuminuria, and reduction of risk from worsening kidney impairment, kidney replacement therapy, or death of kidney-related causes. Pooled results of the 4 large randomized controlled trials that published results on kidney outcomes also demonstrated that risk of acute kidney injury is significantly lower with SGLT-2 inhibitor treatment. However, given the reduced clearance of metformin with a lower estimated glomerular filtration rate and the low but potential risk of lactic acidosis, the prevailing guidance from professional kidney and diabetes societies is to discontinue metformin (Answer C) whenever the glomerular filtration rate falls below 30 mL/min per 1.73 m^2.

Based on current guidance derived from reported patterns from prospective trials, if the creatinine concentration declines by 30% or more within 4 weeks of starting an SGLT-2 inhibitor, the medication could reasonably be held and the patient could be carefully assessed for volume depletion. Otherwise, the drug can be continued. The increase in creatinine observed in this case after starting empagliflozin is approximately 23%, and the glomerular filtration rate reduction is 6 mL—both of which are considered to be within a range that can be observed without discontinuation of the SGLT-2 inhibitor. Therefore, stopping empagliflozin (Answers D and E) is incorrect.

This patient likely has multifactorial chronic kidney disease, but assuming he had been screened for diabetes over time, diabetes may not be a major contributor. Individuals with HIV are at increased risk for chronic kidney disease through multiple comorbidities for which they are at increased risk, including diabetes, obesity, hypertension, and coinfection with hepatitis C. Recent data from several large randomized controlled trials, including EMPA-KIDNEY (empagliflozin) and DAPA-CKD (dapagliflozin), enrolled more than 4000 participants with or without diabetes and a glomerular filtration rate of 20 and 25 mL/min per 1.73 m^2, respectively, to an SGLT-2 inhibitor compared with standard of care. In both trials, the SGLT-2 inhibitor significantly reduced a composite kidney outcome, defined in EMPA-KIDNEY as end-stage kidney disease, a sustained decrease in glomerular filtration rate to less than 10 mL/min per 1.73 m^2, a sustained decrease in glomerular filtration rate 40% or greater from baseline, or death of kidney-related causes. Considering the compendium of available data, regardless of the etiology of kidney disease, an SGLT-2 inhibitor such as empagliflozin is indicated to reduce progression of chronic kidney disease.

While assessing overall hydration is reasonable, the blood pressure lowering observed is the average seen across clinical trials (≥4 mm Hg systolic blood pressure), suggesting that there has not been significant volume depletion to explain the glomerular filtration rate decline. Thus, advising increased hydration (Answer A) is incorrect.

As the cause of his baseline kidney disease is already established, and the increased creatinine is explained by the addition of the SGLT-2 inhibitor, there is no role for a diagnostic kidney biopsy (Answer B).

EDUCATIONAL OBJECTIVE

Describe expected changes in estimated glomerular filtration rate within a month following initiation of SGLT-2 inhibitor.

REFERENCE(S)

Kidney Disease: Improving Global Outcomes (KDIGO) Diabetes Work Group. KDIGO 2022 clinical practice guideline for diabetes management in chronic kidney disease. *Kidney Int.* 2022;102(5S):S1-S127. PMID: 36272764

Meraz-Muñoz AY, Weinstein J, Wald R. eGFR decline after SGLT2 inhibitor initiation: the tortoise and the hare reimagined. *Kidney360.* 2021;2(6):1042-1047. PMID: 35373074

Neuen BL, Young T, Heerspink HJL, et al. SGLT2 inhibitors for the prevention of kidney failure in patients with type 2 diabetes: a systematic review and meta-analysis. *Lancet Diabetes Endocrinol.* 2019;7(11):845-854. PMID: 31495651

Kraus BJ, Weir MR, Bakris GL, et al. Characterization and implications of the initial estimated glomerular filtration rate 'dip' upon sodium-glucose cotransporter-2 inhibition with empagliflozin in the EMPA-REG OUTCOME trial. *Kidney Int.* 2021;99(3):750-762. PMID: 33181154

30 ANSWER: A) Add semaglutide and discontinue insulin aspart

The scenario described in this vignette is increasingly common because individuals with type 2 diabetes are living longer (due to reduced cardiovascular death rates) and developing progressive insulin deficiency with age. The goals of care are multimodal in older adults and include the recognition of common syndromes that should be used to determine care strategies. These include, but are not limited to, frailty, mild cognitive impairment, hypoglycemia, and marked glucose variability. The GLP-1 receptor agonist drug class has been identified in type 2 diabetes to be as potent as basal insulin, but in insulin-deficient individuals, it can be used to minimize insulin requirements, reduce regimen complexity, and improve glycemic variability. The combination of a GLP-1 receptor agonist and basal insulin reduces overall insulin requirements while lowering both weight and hemoglobin A_{1c}. This was recently demonstrated in a "real-world" observational study where among those who added a GLP-1 receptor agonist to basal-bolus insulin regimens, 81% were able to discontinue prandial insulin. This deintensification approach (Answer A) would be expected to reduce hypoglycemia risk without sacrificing glycemic control.

Most guidelines agree that a reasonable hemoglobin A_{1c} target for adults is below 8.0% (<64 mmol/mol), or below 8.5% (<69 mmol/mol) in the presence of poor overall health. Importantly, hemoglobin A_{1c} must be evaluated for accuracy given common interfering problems, including anemia. Based on this patient's mean glucose from the continuous glucose monitoring data and the ADAG study (A1C-Derived Average Glucose), there is good correlation in this case. Thus, there is no need to measure hemoglobin A_{1c} and hemoglobin and perform iron studies (Answer C).

As for time-in-range using continuous glucose monitoring, the American Diabetes Association 2023 Standards of Care address the interpretation of the ambulatory glucose profile in patients who are either at high risk of hypoglycemia or are frail. While there are many definitions of frailty, this patient's reduced functional status at minimum indicates the prefrail state, and her cognitive impairment suggests high risk of hypoglycemia. For these individuals, the recommended time-in-range is 50% or more (vs ≥70% in nonfrail patients/those at lower risk) and less than 1% below range (vs <4% in nonfrail/lower risk). Based on this guidance, the only concern here is the 4% of time spent below 70 mg/dL (<3.9 mmol/L) and the high risk of hypoglycemia.

The best next step for this patient is to reconsider her treatment regimen to reduce hypoglycemia risk and optimize quality of life, which would include elective hip replacement with optimal postoperative outcomes. In light of a reasonable mean fasting glucose value, postmeal glycemic control—as is commonly the case in older adults—explains her hyperglycemia and elevated hemoglobin A_{1c}. Increasing her basal insulin dosage would not address postmeal glycemic control (Answer E). Increasing mealtime insulin (Answer B) may be an effective approach, but it would increase her risk of hypoglycemia. Given the present clinical need to undergo surgery, achieving overall better glycemic control and a lower preoperative hemoglobin A_{1c} and/or average glucose is consistent with current guidelines.

Suggesting no change to her regimen (Answer D) would dismiss the surgical team's concern for perioperative risk.

EDUCATIONAL OBJECTIVE

Appropriately use potent noninsulin agents to deintensify insulin regimens.

REFERENCE(S)

LeRoith D, Biessels GJ, Braithwaite SS, et al. Treatment of diabetes in older adults: an Endocrine Society clinical practice guideline. *J Clin Endocrinol Metab.* 2019;104(5):1520-1574. PMID: 30903688

Falcetta P, Nicolì F, Citro F, et al. De-intensification of basal-bolus insulin regimen after initiation of a GLP-1 RA improves glycaemic control and promotes weight loss in subjects with type 2 diabetes. *Acta Diabetol.* 2023;60(1):53-60. PMID: 36166172

Nathan DM, Kuenen J, Borg R, Zheng H, Schoenfeld D, Heine RJ; A1c-Derived Average Glucose (ADAG) Study Group. Translating the A1C assay into estimated average glucose values. *Diabetes Care.* 2008;31(8):1473-1478. PMID: 18540046

Korytkowski MT, Muniyappa R, Antinori-Lent K, et al. Management of hyperglycemia in hospitalized adult patients in non-critical care settings: an Endocrine Society clinical practice guideline. *J Clin Endocrinol Metab.* 2022;107(8):2101-2128. PMID: 35690958

31 ANSWER: D) Platelet count

The generic report of "fatty infiltration of the liver" is a common incidental finding on CT, ultrasonography, or MRI imaging in persons at high risk of nonalcoholic fatty liver disease (NAFLD) and is often dismissed as benign. NAFLD is the term used to identify the broad spectrum of the disease ranging from nonalcoholic fatty liver with macrovesicular hepatic steatosis only (or with mild inflammation) to steatohepatitis (nonalcoholic steatohepatitis [NASH]) to cirrhosis in the absence of ongoing or recent consumption of significant amounts of alcohol (defined as ingestion of >21 standard drinks per week in men and >14 standard drinks per week in women over a 2-year period preceding evaluation) or the presence of other secondary causes of fatty liver disease. Recent studies in adults estimate that NAFLD is prevalent in more than 70% of people with type 2 diabetes, half of whom have NASH, a precursor of cirrhosis. NASH also adds significantly to the already increased risk of cancer seen among those with diabetes and/or obesity.

In recognition of the global problem of underestimated risk by clinicians and evidence showing that early diagnosis can prevent future cirrhosis, recent guidance documents have called for routine screening for NASH in individuals at high risk. This is largely in response to data showing that between 12% and 20% of persons with type 2 diabetes have clinically significant fibrosis in developed countries around the world.

The FIB-4 tool has recently been recommended by several professional societies to be the most cost-effective first discriminatory test to determine risk of cirrhosis. The tool estimates the risk of hepatic cirrhosis and is calculated from the computation of age, plasma aminotransferase concentrations (AST and ALT), and platelet count (mdcalc.com/calc/2200/fibrosis-4-fib-4-index-liver-fibrosis). A value less than 1.3 is considered lower risk, while a value greater than 2.67 is considered to be high probability of advanced fibrosis. FIB-4 has an area under the receiver–operating characteristic curve of only 0.78 to 0.80; for this reason, for those of intermediate risk, a confirmatory test is suggested. This includes a simple outpatient test to measure hepatic stiffness, namely vibration-controlled transient elastography. It would be premature to order the elastography (Answer E) without first assessing this patient's platelet count (Answer D).

Liver biopsy (Answer C) would not be considered if the FIB-4 score were lower than 1.3.

Hemoglobin (Answer B) does not factor into predicting NASH.

This patient had an unexpected platelet count of $100 \times 10^3/\mu L$ (normal $>150 \times 10^3/\mu L$), and his FIB-4 score was in the high-risk range (>3). He was referred to a hepatologist.

The FIB-4 score was initially developed to predict the risk of clinically significant scarring, a precursor to clinical cirrhosis, in people with coinfection of HIV and hepatitis C. FIB-4 has since been used broadly in high-risk populations including those with obesity and type 2 diabetes. Many studies have illustrated that other tests are either not sensitive or specific enough. Specifically, relying on transaminitis as an indicator is not sensitive, yet relying on abdominal imaging alone indicates the presence of intrahepatic fat and does not indicate its clinical relevance. While whole-body densitometry (Answer A) could indicate the percentage of body fat, which could predict the risk of fatty liver, it has not been studied to predict risk of cirrhosis.

EDUCATIONAL OBJECTIVE

Screen and diagnose nonalcoholic steatohepatitis in individuals with diabetes mellitus.

REFERENCE(S)

Sterling RK, Lissen E, Clumeck N, et al. Development of a simple noninvasive index to predict significant fibrosis patients with HIV/HCV co-infection. *Hepatology*. 2006;43(6):1317-1325. PMID: 16729309

Kanwal F, Shubrook JH, Younossi Z, et al. Preparing for the NASH epidemic: a call to action. *Obesity (Silver Spring)*. 2021;29(9):1401-1412. PMID: 34365735

ElSayed NA, Aleppo G, Aroda VR, et al, American Diabetes Association. 4. Comprehensive medical evaluation and assessment of comorbidities: standards of care in diabetes-2023. *Diabetes Care*. PMID: 36507651

32 ANSWER: E) Simultaneous kidney and pancreas transplant from the same deceased donor

Individuals with end-stage kidney disease (ESKD) and type 1 diabetes should be considered for dual kidney and pancreas transplant due to increased survival and improved quality of life. While many factors play into candidacy for transplant, including functional status, cardiovascular health, and personal support system, the choice of transplant type is relevant.

There are 2 main transplant options for this patient. Simultaneous pancreas-kidney (SPK) transplant is a transplant of the 2 organs from the same deceased donor, while pancreas after kidney (PAK) transplant is a sequential transplant whereby the kidney is transplanted before the pancreas. The advantage of the SPK is that preoperative preparation and postoperative risk are addressed for a single operation, and that normalization of glucose due to the pancreas graft promotes long-term survival of the kidney graft. However, the advantage of a preselected and matched live kidney donor for optimal graft survival is sacrificed with the SPK.

Following the first world consensus conference on pancreas transplant, the authors concluded that SPK offers better survival in most cases over PAK, even in the presence of a live kidney donor option. However, for older patients approaching 60 years, given that wait times for SPK are substantially longer than 2 years, reducing time living with ESKD by providing a transplant with a high-quality live kidney donor is likely to offer a survival advantage over waiting several years for SPK from the same deceased donor. The patient in this vignette is relatively young, has been living with ESKD for a short time, and her center reports short-to-average wait times. Thus, SPK (Answer E) is the best option for her. PAK (Answer C) is a second-line option.

Pancreas transplant before kidney (Answer D) is not performed mainly because the survival advantage for this patient in all scenarios is primarily through kidney transplant, and it should be prioritized over pancreas transplant in ESKD.

Although islet transplant (Answers A and B) holds much promise, especially stem cell–derived cells, cadaveric islet transplant currently has limited benefit duration and is still reserved in research settings only for individuals with severe, recurrent hypoglycemia. One phase 3 study of human cadaveric islet-after-kidney transplant in patients with type 1 diabetes did show short-term benefit, but less than half of patients maintained initial improvements after 3 years.

EDUCATIONAL OBJECTIVE

Balance risks and benefits of different options for pancreas transplant in individuals with end-stage kidney disease.

REFERENCE(S)

Boggi U, Vistoli F, Andres A, et al. First World Consensus Conference on pancreas transplantation: part II – recommendations. *Am J Transplant.* 2021;21(Suppl 3):17-59. PMID: 34245223

Markmann JF, Rickels MR, Eggerman TL, et al. Phase 3 trial of human islet-after-kidney transplantation in type 1 diabetes. *Am J Transplant.* 2020;21(4):1477-1492. PMID: 32627352

33 ANSWER: A) Add basal insulin

Advancing β-cell failure is a reality for most people after 20 or more years with classic type 2 diabetes. Although maintaining optimal or reduced body weight and use of insulin-sensitizing antidiabetes agents are likely to delay the onset of symptomatic insulin deficiency or the need for insulin replacement for glycemic control, there is currently no validated approach to preserve β-cell function in type 2 diabetes. As advised by the American Diabetes Association, individuals with type 2 diabetes who report symptoms of insulin deficiency, including excess urination (also increased or new nocturia as in this case), who are managed on sufficiency potent combination noninsulin therapy should start insulin therapy. In most cases, insulin should be started by the addition of intermediate- or long-acting basal insulin (Answer A).

Stopping other agents (Answer E) is not necessary and would likely result in rapid decline in glucose control during insulin titration.

The DPP-4 inhibitor linagliptin (Answer B) would not only duplicate the mechanism of action of the dulaglutide, it lacks adequate potency and would not address the insulin-deficient state.

Pioglitazone (Answer C), a thiazolidinedione, has good potency but increases fracture risk in postmenopausal women and risk for new-onset congestive heart failure. Pioglitazone is not the best choice in the absence of a unique indication (eg, fatty liver disease or inability to take/tolerate alternatives).

EDUCATIONAL OBJECTIVE

Identify the appropriate time to start basal insulin in patients with type 2 diabetes mellitus.

REFERENCE(S)

ElSayed NA, Aleppo G, Aroda VR, et al; American Diabetes Association. 9. Pharmacologic approaches to glycemic treatment: standards of care in diabetes-2023. *Diabetes Care.* 2023;46(Suppl 1): S140-S157. PMID: 36507650

34 ANSWER: D) Metformin therapy

In neonatology, small-for-gestational-age (SGA) is usually defined as a birth weight below the 10th percentile for gestational age, but it can also be defined as a birth weight and/or length of at least 2 SDs below the mean for gestational age, based on data derived from an appropriate reference population. Infants born SGA are at increased risk of perinatal morbidity, persistent short stature, and metabolic alterations in later life. SGA followed by rapid weight gain during early postnatal life has been associated with increased long-term risks for central obesity, insulin resistance, impaired glucose tolerance, type 2 diabetes, hypertension, increased fat mass, and cardiovascular disease.

In the MiTy trial (Metformin in Women With Type 2 Diabetes in Pregnancy), 502 women with type 2 diabetes during pregnancy from 25 centers in Canada and 4 in Australia were randomly assigned to receive either metformin, 1000 mg twice daily, or placebo, added to insulin. Compared with women in the placebo group, metformin-treated women achieved better glycemic control, required less insulin, gained less weight, and had fewer cesarean deliveries, but the prevalence of SGA was nearly double in the metformin arm vs the placebo group (relative risk, 1.96 [1.10-3.64]; *P* = .026). The importance of this finding remains uncertain because it was not clear that the observed SGA represented a pathological outcome due to intrauterine growth retardation. Moreover, in a recently published follow-up study, these differences were not significant after infancy. Therefore, in addition to counseling this patient about metformin, it is important to discuss that some of the strongest predictors of SGA include having had a prior SGA baby and either the mother or father's birth weight being low, a common scenario that likely reflects constitutive SGA due to genetic and epigenetic factors, and is less likely to reflect an underlying pathology.

Maternal age (Answer A) has been shown to positively correlate with higher birth weights, likely due in part to insulin resistance.

Low-normal blood pressure (Answer B) in the second trimester does not predict birth size, per se, but it does indicate a much lower risk of preeclampsia, which is a major risk factor for SGA.

Glycemic control below recommended targets may increase the risk of SGA, although this is unclear and may be related more to dietary restriction, which can increase the risk. This patient's glycemic control (Answer C) is normal for pregnancy, and her 15 lb (6.8 kg) weight gain indicates that her diet is not restricted (Answer E).

EDUCATIONAL OBJECTIVE

Identify factors affecting fetal growth in the setting of pregestational type 2 diabetes mellitus.

REFERENCE(S)

Feig DS, Donovan LE, Zinman B, et al; MiTy Collaborative Group. Metformin in women with type 2 diabetes in pregnancy (MiTy): a multicentre, international, randomised, placebo-controlled trial. *Lancet Diabetes Endocrinol*. 2020;8(10):834-844. PMID: 32946820

Finken MJJ, van der Steen M, Smeets CCJ, et al. Children born small for gestational age: differential diagnosis, molecular genetic evaluation, and implications. *Endocr Rev.* 2018;39(6):851-894. PMID: 29982551

35 ANSWER: C) Advise the surgeon that the patient's current hemoglobin A_{1c} is acceptable for the planned surgical procedure

In the recent update of the Endocrine Society's clinical practice guideline on the management of hyperglycemia in the hospital, the panel of experts addressed the question of acceptable glycemic control leading up to elective surgery. They performed a meta-analysis of available studies and found that, overall, better glycemic control led to lower postoperative complications, including infection, respiratory complications, and reduced length of hospital stay. Even though most of the studies compared outcomes associated with preoperative hemoglobin A_{1c} values less than 7.0% or ≥7.0% (<53 mmol/mol or ≥53 mmol/mol), none of the available investigations were randomized controlled trials. Due to overall uncertainty and concerns for both equity, feasibility, and the consequences of delaying surgery in persons with diabetes, the panel suggested a target hemoglobin A_{1c} value less than 8.0% (<64 mmol/mol) as a feasible goal for identifying patients who are not at higher risk for postoperative complications (Answer C). In addition, despite very limited data regarding the effect of preoperative blood glucose levels on postoperative outcomes, the panel suggested a blood glucose target 100 to 180 mg/dL (5.6-10 mmol/L) 1 to 4 hours preoperatively, which this patient appears to be achieving most of the time based on his reported fasting blood glucose readings. Importantly, the recommendation applies only to patients scheduled for elective surgical procedures. In addition, when choosing to delay an operation due to hemoglobin A_{1c}, factors that may affect hemoglobin A_{1c} levels must be considered, such as anemia, hemoglobinopathies, chronic kidney failure, and alcoholism.

Given this patient's age and the variability in his glucose readings, his hemoglobin A_{1c} elevation is likely due to postmeal glycemic control, which could be addressed by adding a premeal rapid-acting insulin dose (Answer B). However, given some postmeal values in the reference range (ie, <140 mg/dL [<7.8 mmol/L]), doing this now would increase his risk of hypoglycemia.

Similarly, increasing the basal insulin dosage (Answer D) will likely lower his hemoglobin A_{1c} by reducing fasting glucose and overall average glycemia, but since some of his fasting glucose values are in the usual target range, this is not the best choice.

Lastly, adding a long-acting sulfonylurea (Answer A) is likely to increase the risk of unexpected hypoglycemia, which he appears to already be having based on his symptoms with mild physical activity.

EDUCATIONAL OBJECTIVE

Recommend acceptable preoperative glycemic control.

REFERENCE(S)

Korytkowski MT, Muniyappa R, Antinori-Lent K, et al. Management of hyperglycemia in hospitalized adult patients in non-critical care settings: an Endocrine Society clinical practice guideline. *J Clin Endocrinol Metab.* 2022;107(8):2101-2128. PMID: 35690958

36 ANSWER: A) Dapagliflozin

There are 3 priorities to address in this patient: organ protection given new-onset ischemic congestive heart failure and albuminuric chronic kidney disease, potency to achieve necessary glycemic control, and obesity management/weight loss. Since the SGLT-2 inhibitor dapagliflozin (Answer A) can address all 3 of these priorities, it is an optimal choice at this time.

While the GLP-1 receptor agonist semaglutide (Answer D) can address glycemic control and weight management, the presence of ischemic cardiomyopathy with reduced ejection fraction and albuminuric nephropathy take management precedence given the combined potential of reduced morbidity and mortality.

Pioglitazone (Answer C) is contraindicated in the setting of congestive heart failure, and even without a formal diagnosis his ejection fraction is reduced and this drug should be avoided.

Insulin glargine (Answer B) may be an effective glucose-lowering agent, but it does not address the additional priorities in his diabetes care and it supports weight gain.

While sitagliptin (Answer E) is weight-neutral, it does not offer organ-protection qualities independently of (modest) glycemic control.

EDUCATIONAL OBJECTIVE

Select an appropriate second-line agent to manage hyperglycemia in a patient with type 2 diabetes mellitus.

REFERENCE(S)

Kato ET, Silverman MG, Mosenzon O, et al. Effect of dapagliflozin on heart failure and mortality in type 2 diabetes mellitus. *Circulation.* 2019;139(22):2528-2536. PMID: 30882238

ElSayed NA, Aleppo G, Aroda VR, et al; American Diabetes Association. 11. Chronic kidney disease and risk management: standards of care in diabetes-2023. *Diabetes Care.* 2023;46(Suppl 1):S191-S202. PMID: 36507634

ElSayed NA, Aleppo G, Aroda VR, et al, American Diabetes Association. 9. Pharmacologic approaches to glycemic treatment: standards of care in diabetes-2023. *Diabetes Care.* 2023;46(Suppl 1): S140-S157. PMID: 36507650

37 ANSWER: E) Insulin glargine, 30 units once daily, plus a scheduled regular insulin dose plus correction scale administered every 6 hours

When selecting a subcutaneous insulin regimen for this man with diabetes mellitus, an effort should be made to prescribe a physiologic basal-bolus regimen that will meet both his basal insulin requirements and nutritional insulin needs.

Based on his weight and extrapolating from randomized controlled trials in noncritically ill patients, this patient requires at least 0.5 units/kg per day of insulin, or approximately 50 units, with at least half of this requirement as basal insulin. However, because his recent overnight insulin rate is 1.5 units/h, his basal insulin requirement can be safely estimated at 80% of 1.5 × 24 hours = 36 units, or 30 units (Answer E). Therefore, Answer A would be too low and Answer D would be too high. His nutritional insulin requirement needs to be considered separately as he begins enteral feeding. Based on current guidelines, this is accomplished with scheduled regular insulin every 6 hours or scheduled rapid-acting insulin every 4 hours. Answer B suggests use of basal insulin plus correction scale alone, rather than scheduled nutritional insulin in addition to correction as needed, and is therefore incorrect.

Only 1 published randomized controlled trial has examined specific subcutaneous insulin regimens in patients with diabetes who are receiving enteral nutrition. Fifty patients were randomly assigned to sliding-scale regular insulin alone or sliding-scale regular insulin plus glargine. By the end of the insulin titration period, 48% of the patients randomly assigned to sliding-scale regular insulin alone required the addition of NPH insulin to the regimen for persistent hyperglycemia (blood glucose >180 mg/dL [>10 mmol/L]). Even if scheduled, regular insulin without basal insulin (Answer C) is not recommended.

In the 2022 update of the Endocrine Society's clinical practice guideline on the management of hyperglycemia in the hospital, the question was addressed of whether an NPH-based or long-acting basal-based regimen was superior for achieving glycemic control. After careful review of 2 systematic reviews, 1 randomized controlled trial, and 3 nonrandomized controlled trials, the guideline development panel concluded that there were no important differences in benefits or harms in the outcomes with regimens based either on NPH or once-daily basal insulin. However, because this patient is unknown to the hospital, he could have type 1 diabetes. Thus, a regimen that includes a once-daily long-acting insulin is likely to be a safer, more reliable approach to provide consistent basal insulin replacement.

EDUCATIONAL OBJECTIVE

Recommend a physiologic basal-bolus insulin regimen for patients receiving enteral nutrition.

REFERENCE(S)

Korytkowski MT, Muniyappa R, Antinori-Lent K, et al. Management of hyperglycemia in hospitalized adult patients in non-critical care settings: an Endocrine Society clinical practice guideline. *J Clin Endocrinol Metab.* 2022;107(8):2101-2128. PMID: 35690958

Low Wang CC, Hawkins M, Gianchandani R, Dungan K. Glycemic control in the setting or parenteral nutrition or enteral nutrition via tube-feeding. In: Draznin B, ed. Managing Diabetes and Hyperglycemia in the Hospital Setting. American Diabetes Association; 2016.

38 ANSWER: B) Insulin degludec/liraglutide combination injectable

This patient has macrovascular disease as illustrated by the recent transient ischemic attack and nearly absent peripheral pulses. Her ongoing cigarette smoking compounds her high risk for a cardiovascular event. The GLP-1 receptor agonists semaglutide and dulaglutide reduce the risk of major adverse cardiovascular events when used in combination with metformin, and semaglutide specifically has shown a reduction in stroke, albeit in secondary post hoc outcomes analyses. Additionally, her degree of hyperglycemia places her at increased risk of stroke based on large epidemiologic studies and warrants an approach with high-potency glucose-lowering agents.

This patient requires an agent that she can tolerate that ideally would address her hyperglycemia and risk for major adverse cardiovascular events. The basal insulin/GLP-1 receptor agonist fixed-ratio coformulations (Answer B) have a lower risk of nausea than GLP-1 receptor agonists given alone. The combined formulation makes it possible to titrate both the basal insulin and the GLP-1 receptor agonist, starting at a low dosage and titrating upwards at a slow and steady rate, which is hypothesized to be the reason that nausea rates are lower than when the GLP-1 receptor agonists are given as single agents. Nausea rates for both fixed-ratio coformulations are relatively low. In the DUAL studies, the rate was 8% to 9% for the combination insulin degludec/liraglutide injection, and in the pooled clinical trials for the combination insulin glargine/lixisenatide combination, the rate was 10%.

When administered as single agents, nausea rates for dulaglutide (Answer A) are higher than for the fixed-ratio coformulations and are reported to be in the range of 20% to 30%.

The dual GLP-1/GIP drug tirzepatide (Answer E) has the same adverse effect profile as the GLP-1 receptor agonist drug class and has not yet shown evidence of reduced major adverse cardiovascular events.

Insulin glargine alone (Answer C) should be considered once it is clear that the patient is unable to tolerate GLP-1 receptor agonist therapy given the potential vascular benefit.

While pioglitazone (Answer D) reduces risk of stroke after transient ischemic attack, it takes several weeks to have an effect and is not potent enough to achieve necessary hemoglobin A_{1c} lowering by at least 2% to achieve the target of less than 7.0% (<53 mmol/mol).

EDUCATIONAL OBJECTIVE

Explain the potential for gastrointestinal adverse effects of GLP-1 receptor agonists alone compared with that of new fixed-ratio combination basal insulin plus GLP-1 receptor agonist formulations.

REFERENCE(S)

ElSayed NA, Aleppo G, Aroda VR, et al; American Diabetes Association. 9. Pharmacologic approaches to glycemic treatment: standards of care in diabetes-2023. *Diabetes Care.* 2023;46(Suppl 1):S140-S157. PMID: 36507650

Rosenstock J, Aronson R, Grunberger G, et al; LixiLan-O Trial Investigators. Benefits of LixiLan, a titratable fixed-ratio combination of insulin glargine plus lixisenatide, versus insulin glargine and lixisenatide monocomponents in type 2 diabetes inadequately controlled on oral agents: the LixiLan-O randomized trial. *Diabetes Care.* 2016;39(11):2026-2035. PMID: 27527848

Freemantle N, Mamdani M, Visboll T, Kongso JH, Kvist K, Bain SC. IDegLira versus alternative intensification strategies in patients with type 2 diabetes inadequately controlled on basal insulin therapy. *Diabetes Ther.* 2015;6(4):573-591. PMID: 26582052

39 ANSWER: B) She has a 50% chance of having a hemoglobin A_{1c} level <7.0% (<53 mmol/mol) on no medications in 3 years

This patient has an excellent chance for ideal outcomes following bariatric surgery in the setting of diabetes and obesity. The STAMPEDE trial (Surgical Therapy and Medications Potentially Eradicate Diabetes Efficiently) is one of the first prospective randomized controlled trials to compare traditional medical therapy for type 2 diabetes with either gastric bypass surgery or sleeve gastrectomy. Diabetes remission was defined as a hemoglobin A_{1c} level less than 6.0% (<42 mmol/mol) while on no glucose-lowering medications, but the trial also looked at a higher yet clinically relevant cutoff of less than 7.0% (<53 mmol/mol). At the 3-year time point, 58% of patients had a hemoglobin A_{1c} level less than 7.0% (<53 mmol/mol) while on no medications. Factors that increased the chances of achieving this target included duration of diabetes less than 8 years and good weight loss within the first year, as in this patient's case. These findings are supported by a more recent study published by this group comparing Roux-en-Y gastric bypass with other bariatric procedures, showing that the probability of remission at 3 years after Roux-en-Y gastric bypass was 48% unadjusted and 42% adjusted for baseline hemoglobin A_{1c}, diabetes duration, insulin use, and sex. Since this patient was not on insulin and had a 5-year history of diabetes, her chances are evening higher. Based on available data, 50% (Answer B) is a reasonable expectation.

In a more recent study, Mingrone et al showed the diabetes remission rate (defined here as a hemoglobin A_{1c} value less than 6.5% [<48 mmol/mol] on no treatment) was 37.5% with Roux-en-Y gastric bypass at 5 years and 25% at 10 years. This is much higher than 10% (thus, Answer C is incorrect). This is consistent with the 3-year interim analysis of the Alliance of Randomized Trials of Medicine vs Metabolic Surgery in Type 2 Diabetes (ARMMS-T2D) study, the 5-year results of which will be published in 2023.

While her risk of microvascular complications is reduced, this reduction was found to be 19% per year of diabetes remission (hemoglobin A_{1c} <6.5% [<48 mmol/mol]), not 40% in the less than 1 year after surgery that she is currently (thus, Answer A is incorrect).

In the STAMPEDE trial, investigators also found that quality of life after surgery was superior to the changes observed after medical therapy alone, which also depended on the duration of diabetes (thus, Answer D is incorrect).

EDUCATIONAL OBJECTIVE

Explain predictors based on data from randomized controlled trials that predict remission of diabetes mellitus after gastric bypass surgery.

REFERENCE(S)

Schauer PR, Bhatt DL, Kirwan JP, et al; STAMPEDE Investigators. Bariatric surgery versus intensive medical therapy for diabetes - 5-year outcomes. *N Engl J Med.* 2017;376(7):641-651. PMID: 28199805

Schauer PR, Bhatt DL, Kirwan JP, et al; STAMPEDE Investigators. Bariatric surgery versus intensive medical therapy for diabetes--3-year outcomes. *N Engl J Med.* 2014;370(21):2002-2013. PMID: 24679060

Kirwan JP, Courcoulas AP, Cummings DE, et al. Diabetes remission in the Alliance of Randomized Trials of Medicine Versus Metabolic Surgery in Type 2 Diabetes (ARMMS-T2D). *Diabetes Care.* 2022;45(7):1574-1583. PMID: 35320365

Mingrone G, Panunzi S, De Gaetano A, et al. Metabolic surgery versus conventional medical therapy in patients with type 2 diabetes: 10-year follow-up of an open-label, single-centre randomised controlled trial. *Lancet.* 2021;397(10271): 293-304. PMID: 33485454

40 ANSWER: B) Diabetic radiculopathy

Diabetic neuropathy has myriad manifestations and is generally more common in patients with long disease duration and suboptimal glycemic control. Classification is subdivided into somatosensory, motor, and autonomic. The most common presentation involves damage to sensory nerve fibers and typically affects the distal extremities in a "stocking-glove" distribution. Affected patients describe numbness, paresthesias, and occasionally sharp, lancinating pains. Less common manifestations are acute sensory neuropathies characterized by sudden pain and dysesthesias in the distribution of one or more individual peripheral nerves or nerve roots. The patient in this vignette has left flank and left upper quadrant discomfort in the distribution of left nerve root T10. This may be seen in acute diabetic mononeuropathy or radiculitis (Answer B).

Autonomic dysfunction (Answer A) may affect one or several organ systems, including the vasculature (orthostatic hypotension), the heart (silent ischemia, abnormal cardiac rhythms), the gastrointestinal tract (gastroparesis, constipation, diarrhea from bacterial overgrowth), and the urinary bladder (atonic bladder, chronic urinary tract infections, overflow incontinence). It does not cause pain syndromes. Herpes zoster (Answer C) can cause localized pain in a pattern similar to the one described here, but it does not cause dramatic tenderness. However, the pain can precede the typical rash but not usually for 1 week.

Pancreatitis (Answer D) is unlikely without more nausea and pain in relation to eating. In this patient, the normal amylase and lipase values and normal findings on CT also make this unlikely.

Lastly, a small amount of blood in the urine is not uncommon in persons who have had diabetes for more than 10 years, especially if they have chronic kidney disease (as evidenced by proteinuria). While nephrolithiasis (Answer E) can produce flank pain and hematuria, it should be apparent on CT and passing the stone would relieve most of the pain.

EDUCATIONAL OBJECTIVE

Diagnose rare syndromes of diabetic neuropathy.

REFERENCE(S)

Tesfaye S, Boulton AJ, Dyck PJ, et al; Toronto Diabetic Neuropathy Expert Group. Diabetic neuropathies: update on definitions, diagnostic criteria, estimation of severity, and treatments. *Diabetes Care.* 2010;33(10):2285-2293. PMID: 20876709

Casellini CM, Vinik AI. Clinical manifestations and current treatment options for diabetic neuropathies. *Endocr Pract.* 2007;13(5):550-566. PMID: 17872358

41 ANSWER: E) Switch to U500 insulin, 300 units in divided doses

This patient has severe insulin resistance and uncontrolled diabetes, probably related to long-term use of high-dosage steroids. She is taking 300 to 350 units of insulin daily (3.5 to 4.0 units/kg), reflecting severe insulin resistance. Although there is evidence that the addition of insulin sensitizers can improve glycemic control in patients with type 2 diabetes treated with insulin, this patient is too severely affected to get much benefit from a thiazolidinedione (Answer C) or metformin. And while the SGLT-2 inhibitor canagliflozin (Answer A) can improve glycemia and cause modest weight loss that could improve insulin sensitivity, this is unlikely to have the desired potency to impact glycemic control. In addition, the risk of a complex vulvovaginal candida infection while taking this drug class is high given her treatment with high-dosage steroids. Addition of another dose of insulin glargine (Answer B), even at a dose of 100 units, is unlikely to get her to target and would require her taking more than 5 injections per day.

The most effective approach is to switch her regimen to the highly concentrated form of U500 insulin (Answer E). While she is already taking more than 300 units of insulin per day, concentrated insulin has been observed to have better absorption characteristics, and it is wise to start with a dose similar to what the patient is currently on if control is suboptimal, or reducing the dose by 20% to 30% if control is adequate. Lastly, U500 has the advantage of having a duration of action of up to 13 to 24 hours, permitting adequate delivery with 2 or 3 injections per day. This may be helpful in this case as the patient is expressing concerning diabetes distress related to injections. To further address this in the future, U500 via insulin pump (Answer D) may also be considered.

EDUCATIONAL OBJECTIVE

Treat severe insulin resistance.

REFERENCE(S)

Lane WS, Cochran EK, Jackson JA, et al. High-dose insulin therapy: is it time for U-500 insulin? *Endocr Pract.* 2009;15(1):71-79. PMID: 19211405

Hood RC, Arakaki RF, Wysham C, Li YG, Settles JA, Jackson JA. Two treatment approaches for human regular U-500 insulin in patients with type 2 diabetes not achieving adequate glycemic control on high-dose U-100 insulin therapy with or without oral agents: a randomized, titration-to-target clinical trial. *Endocr Pract.* 2015;21(7):782-793. PMID: 25813411

Ma X, Benson CT, Prescilla R, et al. Pharmacokinetics and pharmacodynamics of human regular U-500 insulin administered via continuous subcutaneous insulin infusion versus subcutaneous injection in adults with type 2 diabetes and high-dose insulin requirements. *J Diabetes Sci Technol.* 2022;16(2):401-407. PMID: 33242998

42 ANSWER: B) Diagnostic continuous glucose monitoring

This patient's hemoglobin A_{1c} level is higher than would be expected based on the reported home blood glucose readings. A hemoglobin A_{1c} value of 8.4% (68 mmol/mol) corresponds with an estimated average glucose value of 194 mg/dL (10.8 mmol/L). There is evidence that he is having nocturnal hypoglycemia. Continuous glucose monitoring (CGM) technology (Answer B) has been used as a tool to document the incidence and magnitude of both hypoglycemia and hyperglycemia in adults with diabetes. In adults with type 2 diabetes, even in those with apparently well-controlled diabetes, CGM has shown that hypoglycemia and excessive postprandial glycemic excursions are common. In older patients, CGM has demonstrated that hypoglycemia is extremely common and often asymptomatic, and even when the hemoglobin A_{1c} level is 8.0% or greater (≥64 mmol/mol), CGM has documented hypoglycemia rates to be as high as 65%. Ninety-five percent of these low values were not detected by traditional fingerstick blood glucose testing, nor by symptoms, which increases risk of harm to the patient. This patient does not monitor his blood glucose frequently, so it would be helpful to start diagnostic CGM, which will determine the time(s) of day and to what degree hypoglycemia is present, if he has rebound hyperglycemia after such episodes, and his postprandial blood glucose trends. This will facilitate optimal adjustment of his insulin doses and provide insight into how his diet and physical activity are affecting his glycemic control.

Glycosylated albumin (Answer C) is similar to fructosamine, a measure of glycosylation of serum proteins, and it is a reasonable alternative to hemoglobin A_{1c} for assessing long-term glucose control with an advantage in cases where red blood cell turnover is altered. However, there is no reason to doubt the hemoglobin A_{1c} in this man, and measuring glycosylated albumin is only likely to validate that his overall glycemic control is suboptimal.

Measuring C-peptide (Answer A) may detect residual β-cell function, but this man with longstanding diabetes who is taking 65 units of insulin daily will not be able to stop insulin therapy, so this information would not be clinically important now.

Finally, insulin antibodies (Answer D), which were relatively common when patients were treated with insulins extracted from bovine and porcine pancreas, caused both hyperglycemia and hypoglycemia by binding injected insulin and releasing it intermittently. However, antibodies in response to human insulins or analogues such as insulin glargine are rare and there is not much evidence that this patient's blood glucose values are erratic, which is a hallmark of the clinical presentation when antibodies are present.

EDUCATIONAL OBJECTIVE

Interpret measures of glycemic control in the setting of type 2 diabetes mellitus.

REFERENCE(S)

ElSayed NA, Aleppo G, Aroda VR, et al, American Diabetes Association. 7. Diabetes technology: standards of care in diabetes-2023. *Diabetes Care.* 2023;46(Suppl 1):S111-S127. PMID: 36507635

Beck RW, Connor CG, Mullen DM, Wesley DM, Bergenstal RM. The fallacy of average: how using HbA1c alone to assess glycemic control can be misleading. *Diabetes Care.* 2017;40(8):994-999. PMID: 28733374

American Diabetes Association. eAG/A1C Conversion Calculator. Available at: https://professional.diabetes.org/diapro/glucose_calc. Accessed for verification June 2023.

43 ANSWER: A) Adrenal insufficiency

This patient with type 1 diabetes and possibly hypothyroidism (as evidenced by her elevated TSH) most likely has adrenal insufficiency (Answer A) with an autoimmune basis. In a patient with type 1 diabetes who experiences progressive decline in total daily insulin requirements with no obvious precipitating factors, it is important to consider a diagnosis of adrenal insufficiency. This woman has a classic presentation, namely persistent hypoglycemia and a falling insulin requirement. She also has orthostatic hypotension, defined as a decrease in systolic blood pressure greater than 20 mm Hg and a reflex increase in heart rate upon standing, which may or may not occur at the time the diagnosis is considered. Biochemical features of adrenal insufficiency such as mild hyperkalemia or hyponatremia, which are seen with acute adrenal insufficiency, are often not present in these patients.

Orthostatic hypotension can also result from cardiovascular autonomic neuropathy (Answer B), but one would not expect a reflex increase in heart rate if this were the case.

In the setting of cardiovascular autonomic neuropathy, signs of advanced peripheral neuropathy (Answer E) are often present (they are mild this case).

Although this patient with longstanding type 1 diabetes may also have hypothyroidism (Answer C), it would not cause orthostatic hypotension.

Gitelman syndrome (Answer D) is a renal tubulopathy caused by inactivating pathogenic variants in the *SLC12A3* gene encoding the thiazide-sensitive chloride cotransporter in the distal convoluted tubule. It is characterized by salt-wasting in addition to hypokalemic metabolic acidosis due to compensatory hyperaldosteronism. Affected individuals are typically normotensive. Given the normal potassium and orthostasis in this patient, Gitelman syndrome is incorrect.

EDUCATIONAL OBJECTIVE

Identify the clinical signs and symptoms suggestive of adrenal insufficiency in the setting of type 1 diabetes mellitus.

REFERENCE(S)

Chantzichristos D, Eliasson B, Johannsson G. Disease burden and treatment challenges in patients with both Addison's disease and type 1 diabetes mellitus. *Eur J Endocrinol.* 2020;183(1):R1-R11. PMID: 32299062

Cutolo M. Autoimmune polyendocrine syndromes. *Autoimmun Rev.* 2014;13(2):85-89. PMID: 24055063

Vinik AI, Ziegler D. Diabetic cardiovascular autonomic neuropathy. *Circulation.* 2007;115(3):387-397. PMID: 17242296

44 ANSWER: C) Decrease the evening dose of NPH insulin to 20 units and give it at bedtime

Human NPH insulin remains the least expensive basal insulin available; therefore, it is important to understand its pharmacokinetics and how to appropriately adjust dosages. This patient has suboptimal glycemic control. Her fasting blood glucose values vary widely, which is a pattern that often indicates nocturnal low glucose values. She clearly has overnight hypoglycemia periodically. These findings are due to the pharmacokinetics of NPH as a basal insulin. When given with the evening meal, the peak effect is in the early morning, and if only a small evening meal is consumed, hypoglycemia overnight can occur. However, because the effect of NPH insulin does not last 12 hours in all patients, glucose control is lost in some by the time of waking. She is experiencing both these effects. A good solution is to move her insulin to bedtime administration and to lower the dose. Importantly, shifting her evening NPH dose to bedtime will lower her risk for nocturnal hypoglycemia because the insulin effect will be most marked at breakfast. Thus, decreasing the evening dose of NPH insulin to 20 units and giving it at bedtime (Answer C) is the best course of action. While a bedtime snack (Answer B) may be protective against low glucose overnight and could be used as needed, this is a less reliable approach because the snack may be forgotten/missed on occasion, placing her at risk of hypoglycemia after taking her usual NPH dose.

Despite her high hemoglobin A_{1c} level, increasing her NPH insulin dose to 28 units (Answers D and E) would exacerbate the tendency for overnight lows.

No data in the vignette indicate whether she needs prandial insulin, so adding 6 units of regular insulin before meals and stopping glipizide (Answer A) is also incorrect. Further fingerstick blood glucose testing after meals would be required to determine whether she needs mealtime insulin.

EDUCATIONAL OBJECTIVE

Manage insulin dosing using NPH insulin in a patient with type 2 diabetes mellitus.

REFERENCE(S)

Malkani S. Are newer insulins always the better option? *Curr Opin Endocrinol Diabetes Obes.* 2019;26(2):77-83. PMID: 30694828

Leahy JL. Insulin treatment in type 2 diabetes mellitus. *Endocrinol Metab Clin North Am.* 2012;41(1): 119-144. PMID: 22575410

45 ANSWER: A) Add empagliflozin, 10 mg daily

Heart failure is highly prevalent in patients with diabetes, occurring in more than 1 in 5 patients with diabetes who are older than 65 years. Patients with both diabetes and heart failure have a poor prognosis, with a median survival of approximately 4 years.

This patient has American Heart Association Class II Congestive Heart Failure, which is characterized by slight limitation in physical activity. Recommending no change in her regimen (Answer E) would be inadequate. Cardiovascular outcome trials of SGLT-2 inhibitors (Answer A) among persons with type 2 diabetes have demonstrated significant effect on cardiovascular outcomes, including risk for hospitalizations for heart failure, as shown in the table.

Trial	Outcomes	
EMPA-REG (n = 7020 with established cardiovascular disease) - empagliflozin		
	Study drug	**Placebo**
Risk for heart failure admissions	2.7% (hazard ratio, 0.65; CI, 0.50-0.85)	4.1%
CANVAS (n = 10,142 with high cardiovascular risk) - canagliflozin		
	Study drug	**Placebo**
Risk for heart failure hospitalization	5.5/1000 patient-years (hazard ratio, 0.67; CI, 0.52-0.87)	8.7/1000 patient-years
CVD-REAL (n = 309,045) observational comparison SGLT-2 inhibitors vs other antihyperglycemic drugs		
Risk for heart failure hospitalization	39% lower risk of heart failure with SGLT-2 inhibitors	
DECLARE-TIMI 58 (n = 17,160 with or at risk for cardiovascular disease) - dapagliflozin		
Hospitalization rate for heart failure	Hazard ratio, 0.73 for study drug; 95% CI, (0.61-0.88)	

Empagliflozin reduced the primary major adverse cardiovascular event (MACE) endpoint compared with placebo treatment (10.5% vs 12.5%; hazard ratio, 0.86; 95% CI, 0.74-0.99). This reflects a reduced rate of hospitalizations for heart failure as shown in the table. This was an effect shown independent of glycemic control, and it has been subsequently found in persons without diabetes who have heart failure. Therefore, while this patient has achieved excellent glycemic control, management of her heart failure should be considered an independent indication for the empagliflozin.

The GLP-1 receptor agonist semaglutide (Answer D) in oral formulation did not show significant reduction in MACE, and no GLP-1 receptor agonists have been shown to significantly reduce risk for hospitalization due to heart failure.

No prospective randomized controlled trial has evaluated whether metformin (Answer C) is the optimal first-line agent in patients with diabetes and heart failure, but the EmpaREG trial did maintain metformin as background therapy and hence there is no reason to withhold it.

Finally, the new agent tirzepatide (Answer B) is a highly potent dual GLP-1/GIP agonist that would be ideal in the setting of obesity and/or suboptimal glycemic control. However, cardiovascular benefit has not been established. The SURPASS Cardiovascular Outcome Trial is expected to be completed in October 2024.

EDUCATIONAL OBJECTIVE

Manage antihyperglycemic agents in a patient with type 2 diabetes mellitus and congestive heart failure.

REFERENCE(S)

ElSayed NA, Aleppo G, Aroda VR, et al, American Diabetes Association. 10. Cardiovascular disease and risk management: standards of care in diabetes-2023. *Diabetes Care.* 2023;46(Suppl 1): S158-S190. PMID: 36507632

Zinman B, Wanner C, Lachin JM, et al; EMPA-REG OUTCOME Investigators. Empagliflozin, cardiovascular otucomes, and mortality in type 2 diabetes. *N Engl J Med.* 2015;373(22):2117-2128. PMID: 26378978

46 ANSWER: C) Insulin autoantibody assessment

Hypoglycemia in patients without diabetes mellitus has a broad differential. In unprovoked hypoglycemia in patients with preexisting autoimmune disease (such as Graves disease), the possibility of insulin autoantibody syndrome (Hirata disease) should be strongly considered. In this condition, first described by Hirata et al in 1970, autoantibodies (IgG) are produced that bind insulin with variable affinity, which may result in glucose intolerance. Sudden dissociation of prebound insulin from the antibody results in unpredictable episodes of hypoglycemia. This can be seen as a rare adverse reaction to methimazole, and almost all cases of methimazole-induced insulin autoimmune syndrome are reported in East Asia, especially in Japan. This association is due to the DRB1*0406 genotype, which is relatively common in persons of East Asian descent, and it is exclusively associated with an elevated risk of developing methimazole-induced insulin autoimmune syndrome. Additionally, the specific allelic combination of HLA-Bw62/Cw4/DR4 carrying DRB1*0406 is a major genetic risk factor. Thus, the best next step in this vignette is an insulin autoantibody assessment (Answer C).

All the other answer choices are unlikely to reveal the precise cause of the hypoglycemia. A sulfonylurea screen (Answer E) is appropriate in all cases in which endogenous insulin and C-peptide hypersecretion are demonstrated. It is an unlikely culprit here, however, given the strong history of autoimmunity and the lack of apparent access to antihyperglycemic drugs.

Both C-peptide and insulin levels should be measured. In Hirata disease, increased insulin levels are usually demonstrated, particularly if the insulin assay cannot distinguish between bound and unbound insulin. C-peptide levels are variable, but usually detectable.

There is nothing in the history to suggest hypoadrenalism. Although cortisol (Answer A) should be measured routinely in the evaluation of hypoglycemia, it is most likely to be normal (or high if obtained when the patient has hypoglycemia).

Elevated circulating IGF-2 (Answer B) is a rare, paraneoplastic cause of hypoglycemia that occurs in the setting of large, solid malignant masses. Individuals with this condition are generally unwell (unlike this patient).

Metanephrines (Answer D) secreted by a pheochromocytoma can increase, rather than decrease, blood glucose levels.

EDUCATIONAL OBJECTIVE

Investigate causes of hypoglycemia unrelated to treatment of diabetes mellitus.

REFERENCE(S)

Cappellani D, Macchia E, Falorni A, Marchetti P. Insulin autoimmune syndrome (Hirata disease): a comprehensive review fifty years after its first description. *Diabetes Metab Syndr Obes.* 2020;13: 963-978. PMID: 32308449

Uchigata Y, Kuwata S, Tsushima T, et al. Patients with Graves' disease who developed insulin autoimmune syndrome (Hirata disease) possess HLA-Bw62/Cw4/DR4 carrying DRB1*0406. *J Clin Endocrinol Metab.* 1993;77(1):249-254. PMID: 8325948

47 ANSWER: C) Fructosamine measurement

Hemoglobin A_{1c} measurement is the criterion standard test to assess the quality of glycemic control in patients with diabetes. Unfortunately, hemoglobin A_{1c} (Answer D) cannot be used as a metric of glycemic control in all patients. Of greatest importance is its unreliability in the setting of hemoglobinopathies, such as sickle-cell disease, or other causes of increased red blood cell turnover. Because glycation of hemoglobin A increases over the life of a red cell, conditions that shorten red blood cell lifespan cause an artificially reduced hemoglobin A_{1c} level, whether measurement is point of care or done in the laboratory. In this setting, other markers of long-term glucose control should be considered. Fructosamine (Answer C), a measure of glycosylated plasma proteins, is proportional to the mean blood glucose over the previous 2 weeks and may be used in place of hemoglobin A_{1c} in this patient because it is not dependent on red blood cell turnover.

Measuring postprandial glucose levels (Answer A) is not likely to add much in this case, as they are generally proportional to fasting values.

Urinary glucose testing (Answer E) is imprecise and only estimates recent levels of circulating glucose concentrations.

C-peptide (Answer B) only gives a rough estimate of β-cell function and not glycemic control.

EDUCATIONAL OBJECTIVE

Explain the relationship between hemoglobinopathies and hemoglobin A_{1c}.

REFERENCE(S)

National Glycohemoglobin Standardization Program (NGSP) website. NGSP: HbA1c Assay Interferences. www.ngsp.org/interf.asp. Accessed for verification March 2023.

Lorenzo-Medina M, De-La-Iglesia S, Ropero P, Nogueria-Salgueriro P, Santana-Benitez J. Effects of hemoglobin variants on hemoglobin A1c values measured using a high-performance liquid chromatography method. *J Diabetes Sci Technol.* 2014;8(6):1168-1176. PMID: 25355712

Sacks DB, Arnold M, Bakris GL, et al; National Academy of Clinical Biochemistry; Evidence-Based Laboratory Medicine Committee of the American Association for Clinical Chemistry. Guidelines and recommendations for laboratory analysis in the diagnosis and management of diabetes mellitus. *Diabetes Care.* 2011;34(6):e61-e99. PMID: 21617108

48 ANSWER: B) Fasting glucose

A higher risk of insulin resistance and diabetes has been described in patients with HIV infection who are on antiretroviral therapy compared with risk in uninfected patients. According to the American Diabetes Association guidelines, patients with HIV should be screened for diabetes and prediabetes with a fasting glucose measurement (Answer B) before starting antiretroviral therapy, at the time of switching antiretroviral therapy, and 3 to 6 months after starting or switching antiretroviral therapy. If initial screening results are normal, measuring fasting glucose every year is advised.

In several studies, hemoglobin A_{1c} measurement (Answer E) has been found to underestimate glycemic levels in HIV-infected patients when compared with other diagnostic methods. Explanations for the lower-than-expected hemoglobin A_{1c} values in these patients have been hypothesized. For example, higher mean cell volume and hemolysis are more prevalent in HIV-infected patients. High mean cell volume, as a marker of a greater proportion of younger erythrocytes that have a shorter time to become glycated, suggests greater red blood cell turnover in HIV-infected patients.

Fructosamine (Answer C) and C-peptide (Answer A) are not used to diagnose diabetes. Glutamic acid decarboxylase 65 antibodies (Answer D) can distinguish type 1 from type 2 diabetes once diabetes has been diagnosed.

EDUCATIONAL OBJECTIVE

Appropriately screen for diabetes mellitus in persons with HIV infection.

REFERENCE(S)

Coelho AR, Moreira FA, Santos AC, et al. Diabetes mellitus in HIV-infected patients: fasting glucose, A1c, or oral glucose tolerance test – which method to choose for the diagnosis? *BMC Infect Dis.* 2018;18(309):1-13. PMID: 29980190

Kim PS, Woods C, Georgoff P, et al. A1C underestimates glycemia in HIV infection. *Diabetes Care.* 2009;32(9):1591-1593. PMID: 19502538

ElSayed NA, Aleppo G, Aroda VR, et al; American Diabetes Association. 2. Classification and diagnosis of diabetes: standards of care in diabetes-2023. *Diabetes Care.* 2023;46(Suppl 1):S19-S40. PMID: 36507649

49 ANSWER: C) Serum vitamin B_{12}

This patient has recent onset of peripheral neuropathy and ataxia. She has been on high-dosage metformin for a long time, making vitamin B_{12} deficiency (Answer C) the most likely diagnosis. Metformin reduces intestinal absorption of vitamin B_{12} in up to 30% of patients and lowers serum vitamin B_{12} concentrations in 5% to 10%. The dosage and duration of metformin use correlate with the risk of vitamin B_{12} deficiency. While the mechanism is not entirely clear, most evidence points to interference with food-derived B_{12} absorption, primarily in the ileum. The most common neurologic findings in vitamin B_{12} deficiency are symmetric paresthesias or numbness and gait problems. Neuropsychiatric symptoms can be present even in the absence of anemia or macrocytosis, and the lack of these hematologic changes cannot be used to exclude vitamin B_{12} deficiency as a cause of neuropsychiatric symptoms. The current American Diabetes Association standards of care recommend periodic measurement of vitamin B_{12} levels in metformin-treated patients, especially in those with anemia or peripheral neuropathy.

Cortisol measurement (Answer A) is incorrect because there is no evidence of adrenal insufficiency: the patient has no weight loss, hypotension, or electrolyte abnormalities.

Taking proton-pump inhibitors can lead to magnesium deficiency (Answer B), which would present as hypocalcemia, hypokalemia, and neuromuscular hyperexcitability, none of which are present in this patient.

Biotin can affect TSH levels (Answer E) in certain assays, mimicking hyperthyroidism, unlike in this patient who has a high TSH concentration. In addition, abnormalities in TSH would not explain this patient's ataxia and peripheral neuropathy.

Time-below-range (Answer D) would indicate whether she is having hypoglycemia, but specific episodes would then have to be correlated with her symptoms. Moreover, gate imbalance is not an expected symptom of recurrent hypoglycemia.

EDUCATIONAL OBJECTIVE

Identify vitamin B_{12} deficiency as an adverse effect of metformin therapy.

REFERENCE(S)

Yang W, Cai X, Ji L, et al. Associations between metformin use and vitamin B_{12} levels, anemia, and neuropathy in patients with diabetes: a meta-analysis. *J Diabetes.* 2019;11(9):729-743. PMID: 30615306

Bell DSH. Metformin-induced vitamin B12 deficiency can cause or worsen distal symmetrical, autonomic and cardiac neuropathy in the patient with diabetes. *Diabetes Obes Metab.* 2022;24(8):1423-1428. PMID: 35491956

ElSayed NA, Aleppo G, Aroda VR, et al; American Diabetes Association. 9. Pharmacologic approaches to glycemic treatment: standards of care in diabetes-2023. *Diabetes Care.* 2023;46(Suppl 1):S140-S157. PMID: 36507650

50 ANSWER: B) Glipizide

This patient has severe hypoglycemia due to intake of glipizide (sulfonylurea) (Answer B), which stimulates β cells to release insulin, C-peptide, and proinsulin.

A plasma insulin concentration of 3 µIU/mL or higher (≥20.8 pmol/L) by immunochemiluminometric assay when the plasma glucose concentration is below 55 mg/dL (<3.1 mmol/L) indicates insulin excess and is consistent with hyperinsulinemia (either from insulinoma, exogenous insulin, or sulfonylurea).

Plasma C-peptide distinguishes endogenous from exogenous hyperinsulinemia (Answer E) at a cutoff of 0.6 ng/mL (0.20 nmol/L). In patients with insulinoma or sulfonylurea intake, the C-peptide concentration is at least 0.6 ng/mL or higher (≥0.20 nmol/L) as opposed to the setting of exogenous insulin intake where the C-peptide concentration is less than 0.6 ng/mL (<0.20 nmol/L). A plasma proinsulin concentration of 44.1 pg/mL or greater (≥5 pmol/L) is seen in the setting of insulinoma or sulfonylurea intake. Because of the antiketogenic effect of insulin, plasma β-hydroxybutyrate concentrations are lower in patients with an insulinoma than in patients without. All patients with hyperinsulinemia or IGF-mediated hypoglycemia have plasma β-hydroxybutyrate values of 28 mg/dL or less (≤2700 µmol/L). Obviously, a plasma sulfonylurea screen will reveal the sulfonylurea agent causing the hypoglycemia.

In adrenal insufficiency (Answer A) and hepatic failure (Answer C), plasma insulin is less than 3 µIU/mL (<20.8 pmol/L), plasma C-peptide is less than 0.6 ng/mL (<0.2 nmol/L), plasma proinsulin is less than 44.1 pg/mL (<5 pmol/L), and plasma β-hydroxybutyrate is greater than 28 mg/dL (>2700 µmol/L).

In IGF-2–secreting tumors (Answer D), plasma insulin is less than 3 µIU/mL (<20.8 pmol/L), plasma C-peptide is less than 0.6 ng/mL (<0.2 nmol/L), plasma proinsulin is less than 44.1 pg/mL (<5 pmol/L), *but* plasma β-hydroxybutyrate is 28 mg/dL or less (≤2700 µmol/L).

EDUCATIONAL OBJECTIVE

Interpret laboratory test results associated with hypoglycemia.

REFERENCE(S)

Cryer PE, Axelrod L, Grossman AB, et al; Endocrine Society. Evaluation and management of adult hypoglycemic disorders: an Endocrine Society clinical practice guideline. *J Clin Endocrinol Metab.* 2009;94(3):709-728. PMID: 19088155

Service FJ, O'Brien PC. Increasing serum betahydroxybutyrate concentrations during the 72-hour fast: evidence against hyperinsulinemic hypoglycemia. *J Clin Endocrinol Metab.* 2005;90(8):4555-4558. PMID: 15886243

51 ANSWER: B) Decrease insulin degludec to 20 units at bedtime; discontinue nateglinide; continue alogliptin

Individuals with recurrent treatment-associated hypoglycemia can experience hypoglycemia unawareness or hypoglycemia-associated autonomic failure. Hypoglycemia unawareness is characterized by a reduction in the sympathoadrenal and autonomic responses and is more common in those with longer duration of type 2 diabetes and in older adults. This syndrome can lead to a prolonged exposure to hypoglycemia, resulting in loss of consciousness, seizures, or brain damage. However, it is possible to improve glycemic control and reduce the frequency of hypoglycemia with short-term relaxation of glycemic targets. This hypoglycemia avoidance includes reducing insulin therapy for several weeks to allow the patient's blood glucose levels to run a little higher, thereby increasing sensitivity to symptoms. In addition, the glycemic targets in older patients are more relaxed, with a hemoglobin A_{1c} goal between 7.0% and 8.0% (53-64 mmol/mol). Accordingly, this patient's insulin dosage should be decreased by 20% to 30% given recurrent clinically important hypoglycemia (<55 mg/dL [<3.1 mmol/L]), and insulin secretagogues (eg, nateglinide, which is a meglitinide) should be discontinued (Answer B).

Although approaches that discontinue the insulin secretagogue are preferred, replacing degludec with the same dose of insulin detemir (Answer C) or NPH (Answer D) would not resolve the issue. An approach that continues the use of an insulin secretagogue (Answer A) should be avoided. Alogliptin is a DPP-4 inhibitor that enhances glucose-dependent insulin secretion (as opposed to meglitinides and sulfonylureas) and it does not increase the risk of hypoglycemia.

EDUCATIONAL OBJECTIVE

Manage hypoglycemia in patients with type 2 diabetes mellitus.

REFERENCE(S)

LeRoith D, Biessels GJ, Braithwaite SS, et al. Treatment of diabetes in older adults: an Endocrine Society* clinical practice guideline. *J Clin Endocrinol Metab.* 2019;104(5):1520-1574. PMID: 30903688

Neumiller JJ, Munshi MN. Geriatric syndromes in older adults with diabetes. *Endocrinol Metab Clin North Am.* 2023;52(2):341-353. PMID: 36948783

Sircar M, Bhatia A, Munshi M. Review of hypoglycemia in the older adult: clinical implications and management. *Can J Diabetes.* 2016;40(1):66-72. PMID: 26752195

Cryer PE. Diverse causes of hypoglycemia-associated autonomic failure in diabetes. *N Engl J Med.* 2004;350(22):2272-2279. PMID: 15163777

52 ANSWER: B) Atorvastatin

This patient has relatively longstanding type 1 diabetes with minimal evidence of microvascular complications. With 2 discrepant and borderline urinary albumin-to-creatinine ratios and with a preserved estimated glomerular filtration rate, he does not meet criteria for chronic kidney disease. However, he is at increased cardiovascular risk; statin therapy (Answer B) should be considered to lower his elevated LDL cholesterol and to reduce his risk of death from cardiovascular causes.

While most prospective studies showing the benefit of statin therapy in diabetes have exclusively enrolled those with type 2 diabetes, meta-analyses that have included type 1 diabetes studies indicate that the benefit extends to this group. The Heart Protection Study tested the effect of statin therapy to lower cardiovascular events and set out to recruit patients who would not have been recruited the earlier cardiology trials and included a cohort with type 1 diabetes. Investigators found that the reductions in cardiovascular events due to statin therapy were not different from those in patients with type 2 diabetes, but the confidence intervals were wide. The Cholesterol Treatment Trialists' Collaborators performed a meta-analysis of cholesterol-lowering therapy in 14 trials of statins, including the Heart Protection Study. Among the included participants, 1466 had type 1 diabetes, and 17,220 had type 2 diabetes; the analysis showed a 21% relative risk reduction in major cardiovascular events in persons with type 1 diabetes.

As all participants in the Cholesterol Treatment Trialists' study were older than 40 years, the American Diabetes Association recommends starting statin therapy in patients with type 1 diabetes at this age, but notes that starting therapy earlier should be considered for patients with either increased cardiovascular risk or established kidney disease. This patient has a strong family history of cardiovascular disease, so statin therapy is indicated.

Although an SGLT-2 inhibitor (Answer C) would be indicated in the case of type 2 diabetes and chronic kidney disease (for which he does not yet meet criteria), it is not recommended for use in type 1 diabetes given the increased risk of euglycemic ketoacidosis.

Based on the findings of several prospective studies, the American Diabetes Association standards of care and Kidney Disease: Improving Global Outcomes guidelines do not recommend blockade of the angiotensin-renin axis using an ACE inhibitor (Answer A) or an angiotensin-receptor blocker (Answer D) for the primary prevention of chronic kidney disease in persons with diabetes who have normal blood pressure, normal urinary albumin-to-creatinine ratio (<30 mg/g creat), and normal estimated glomerular filtration rate.

Lastly, there is no evidence for vitamin B_{12} supplementation (Answer E) as a preventive measure to reduce complications in type 1 diabetes.

EDUCATIONAL OBJECTIVE

Prescribe statin therapy for patients with type 1 diabetes mellitus.

REFERENCE(S)

Collins R, Armitage J, Parish S, Sleigh P, Peto R; Heart Protection Study Collaborative Group. MRC/BHF Heart Protection Study of cholesterol-lowering with simvastatin in 5963 people with diabetes: a randomised placebo-controlled trial. *Lancet.* 2003;361(9374):2005-2016. PMID: 12814710

Cholesterol Treatment Trialists' (CTT) Collaborators. Efficacy of cholesterol-lowering therapy in 18,686 people with diabetes in 14 randomised trials of statins: a meta-analysis. *Lancet.* 2008;371(9607):117-125. PMID: 18191683

ElSayed NA, Aleppo G, Aroda VR, et al; American Diabetes Association. 10. Cardiovascular disease and risk management: standards of care in diabetes-2023. *Diabetes Care.* 2023;46(Suppl 1): S158-S190. PMID: 36507632

Female Reproduction Board Review

Margaret Flynn Lippincott, MD

1 ANSWER: E) Selective serotonin reuptake inhibitor

This patient has premenstrual dysphoric disorder (PMDD) or premenstrual disorder (PMD). Women with PMD/PMDD experience a wide variety of cyclic and recurrent physical, emotional, behavioral, and cognitive symptoms that start in the luteal phase and diminish and stop after the onset of menses. Major symptoms include affective symptoms such as depression, angry outbursts, irritability, and anxiety, and somatic symptoms such as breast pain, bloating, swelling, and headache. In this case, the patient's symptoms are interfering with her daily life.

While exercise (Answer C) can help with symptoms, the first-line treatment is a selective serotonin reuptake inhibitor (Answer E). Selective serotonin reuptake inhibitors can be given continuously or cyclically limited to the luteal phase of the cycle.

GnRH agonists, such as leuprolide (Answer D), can be used to suppress ovulation in treatment-resistant, moderately severe cases of PMDD cases. However, she would require hormone therapy, including progesterone, which could trigger PMDD.

A continuous low-dose oral contraceptive pill (Answer B), specifically one containing drospirenone, is considered second-line treatment for mild to moderate PMDD and could be considered if the patient desires contraception.

There is no high-quality evidence that acupuncture (Answer A) improves PMDD symptoms.

EDUCATIONAL OBJECTIVE

Recommend treatment options for women with premenstrual dysphoric disorder.

REFERENCE(S)

Ismaili E, Walsh S, O'Brien PMS, et al; Consensus Group of the International Society for Premenstrual Disorders. Fourth consensus of the International Society for Premenstrual Disorders (ISPMD): auditable standards for diagnosis and management of premenstrual disorder. *Arch Womens Ment Health.* 2016;19(6):953-958. PMID: 27378473

Marjoribanks J, Brown J, O'Brien PMS, Wyatt K. Selective serotonin reuptake inhibitors for pre-menstrual syndrome. *Cochrane Database Syst Rev.* 2013;2013(6):CD001396. PMID: 23744611

Carlini SV, Lanza di Scalea T, McNally ST, Lester J, Deligiannidis KM. Management of premenstrual dysphoric disorder: a scoping review. *Int J Womens Health.* 2022;14:1783-1801. PMID: 36575726

2 ANSWER: A) Continuous low-dose oral contraceptive pill

This woman has primary ovarian insufficiency and is perimenopausal. Once she achieves menopause, she should be treated with hormone therapy until the average age of menopause (50 or 51 years). She is currently symptomatic and is a good candidate for hormonal therapy for her vasomotor symptoms. She does not have any contraindications to therapy (eg, personal or family history of breast cancer or venous thromboembolism). The patient is not yet menopausal and requires contraceptive management. The contraceptive pill should be provided continuously (Answer A) to prevent bothersome vasomotor symptoms that would occur during the placebo week of the pill pack.

Gabapentin (Answer B) could be used as adjuvant treatment if she continues to experience symptoms on hormone therapy.

A low-dose transdermal estradiol patch (Answer E) could be used to treat her symptoms if she had a cycle every 3 months and did not require contraception. Providing hormone therapy (Answer D) can increase irregular bleeding in perimenopausal women and is not the best answer due to the need for contraceptive management.

EDUCATIONAL OBJECTIVE

Select the best treatment options for women with premature ovarian insufficiency who require contraception.

REFERENCE(S)

Panay N, Anderson RA, Nappi RE, et al. Premature ovarian insufficiency: an International Menopause Society White Paper. *Climacteric.* 2020;23(5):426-446. PMID: 32896176

Christin-Maitre S, Givony M, Albarel F, et al. Position statement on the diagnosis and management of premature/primary ovarian insufficiency (except Turner Syndrome). *Ann Endocrinol (Paris).* 2021;82(6):555-571. PMID: 34508691

3 ANSWER: D) Sleep study

Polycystic ovary syndrome is a common disorder that occurs in 6% to 8% of women. Affected patients usually present with hirsutism, acne, and irregular menses. Sixty percent of affected women develop obesity. In addition to being at increased risk for impaired glucose tolerance and type 2 diabetes mellitus (5 to 10 times that of age-matched control women), women with polycystic ovary syndrome are also at high risk for sleep apnea. Given this patient's history of daytime sleepiness, the most likely diagnosis is sleep apnea, and a sleep study (Answer D) should be ordered.

While women with polycystic ovary syndrome are at increased risk for nonalcoholic fatty liver disease and nonalcoholic steatohepatitis, the Endocrine Society recommends against routine screening with liver function tests (Answer A). In addition, AST and ALT were already measured in this patient, as these values are used along with platelet count and patient age to generate a FIB-4 score, which rules out hepatic fibrosis.

Although she has gained weight and reports fatigue, she has no other features that strongly suggest hypercortisolism (white striae are common with weight gain). Thus, late-night salivary cortisol measurement is not necessary.

Metformin (Answer C) is not first-line therapy for obesity. Metformin could be considered as a part of the treatment for metabolic syndrome; however, this patient does not have metabolic syndrome.

She does have mild acne, and although initiation of spironolactone (Answer E) could be considered, it is more important to assess for sleep apnea given her symptoms.

EDUCATIONAL OBJECTIVE

Counsel patients about the increased risk of sleep apnea associated with polycystic ovary syndrome.

REFERENCE(S)

Legro RS, Arslanian SA, Ehrmann DA, et al; Endocrine Society. Diagnosis and treatment of polycystic ovary syndrome: an Endocrine Society clinical practice guideline. *J Clin Endocrinol Metab.* 2013;98(12):4565-4592. PMID: 24151290

Rosenzweig JL, Bakris GL, Berglund LF, et al. Primary prevention of ASCVD and T2DM in patients at metabolic risk: an Endocrine Society clinical practice guideline. *J Clin Endocrinol Metab.* 2019;104(9):3939-3985. PMID: 31365087

Sterling RK, Lissen E, Clumeck N, et al. Development of a simple noninvasive index to predict significant fibrosis patients with HIV/HCV co-infection. *Hepatology.* 2006;43(6):1317-1325. PMID: 16729309

4 ANSWER: B) GnRH agonist, continuous estradiol patch, and continuous micronized progesterone

Women with premenstrual disorder (PMD)/premenstrual dysphoric disorder (PMDD) experience a wide variety of cyclic and recurrent physical, emotional, behavioral, and cognitive symptoms that start in the luteal phase and diminish and stop after the onset of menses. Major symptoms include affective symptoms such as depression, angry outbursts, irritability, and anxiety and somatic symptoms such as breast pain, bloating and swelling, and headache. In this case, first- and second-line therapies have failed. GnRH agonists (Answers A, B, and C), such as leuprolide, can be used to suppress ovulation in patients with treatment-resistant, moderately severe PMDD. GnRH agonists should be paired with hormone therapy to prevent hypoestrogenemia. Hormone replacement with a continuous estradiol patch and continuous micronized progesterone (Answer B) minimizes the risk of triggering PMDD while providing appropriate hormone therapy.

Unopposed estrogen (Answer A) is not recommended for this patient who has a uterus because of the risk for endometrial hyperplasia and cancer.

Cyclic progesterone (Answer C) can trigger PMDD and is not recommended.

GnRH agonist therapy should be trialed prior to a woman pursuing surgical oophorectomy and hysterectomy (Answers D and E).

EDUCATIONAL OBJECTIVE

Recommend treatment options for women with treatment-resistant premenstrual dysphoric disorder.

REFERENCE(S)

Ismaili E, Walsh S, O'Brien PMS, et al; Consensus Group of the International Society for Premenstrual Disorders. Fourth consensus of the International Society for Premenstrual Disorders (ISPMD): auditable standards for diagnosis and management of premenstrual disorder. *Arch Womens Ment Health.* 2016;19(6):953-958. PMID: 27378473

Carlini SV, Lanza di Scalea T, McNally ST, Lester J, Deligiannidis KM. Management of premenstrual dysphoric disorder: a scoping review. *Int J Womens Health.* 2022;14:1783-1801. PMID: 36575726

5 ANSWER: B) Estradiol patch (50 mcg) and progesterone (100 mg) daily

The Study of Women's Health Across the Nation (SWAN), a multisite longitudinal, epidemiologic study, found that menopausal vasomotor symptoms last on average 7 years (4.5 years after final menstrual period). Black women have persistent vasomotor symptoms that can last for up to 10 years. For some women, vasomotor symptoms last for a lifetime. Hormone therapy is the most effective treatment for vasomotor symptoms and other symptoms of the climacteric. Benefits may exceed risks for most symptomatic postmenopausal women who are younger than 60 years or for whom it has been less than 10 years since the onset of menopause. Hormone therapy should be used for the shortest duration needed to effectively treat the patient's symptoms. Endocrine Society clinical practice guidelines encourage shared decision-making. Risk stratification for cardiovascular disease and breast cancer risk is recommended to assess the risk of hormone therapy and method of administration. This patient is at intermediate cardiovascular disease risk; therefore, she should be offered transdermal menopausal hormone therapy accompanied by continuous or cyclical progesterone therapy (Answer B).

She should not be offered oral estradiol therapy (Answer E) based on her intermediate cardiovascular risk, but this could be an option if her breast cancer and cardiovascular risk were both low.

Gabapentin (Answer D) could be used for vasomotor symptoms if hormone therapy is contraindicated or if the patient does not want to use hormone therapy. Gabapentin does not address her genitourinary symptoms.

Selective serotonin reuptake inhibitors can also be used if hormone therapy is contraindicated or as adjunctive therapy.

Vaginal estradiol (Answer C) is an effective therapy for her genitourinary symptoms, but not for her hot flushes.

She has a uterus, so estradiol therapy alone (Answer A) is contraindicated.

EDUCATIONAL OBJECTIVE

Recommend appropriate hormone therapy for symptomatic postmenopausal women based on cardiovascular disease and breast cancer risk.

REFERENCE(S)

Avis NE, Crawford SL, Greendale G, et al; Study of Women's Health Across the Nation. Duration of menopausal vasomotor symptoms over the menopause transition. *JAMA Intern Med.* 2015;175(4):531–539. PMID: 25686030

Stuenkel CA, Davis SR, Gompel, et al. Treatment of symptoms of the menopause: an Endocrine Society clinical practice guideline. *J Clin Endocrinol Metab.* 2015;100(11):3975-4011. PMID: 26444994

Bassuk SS, Manson JE. Menopausal hormone therapy and cardiovascular disease risk: utility of biomarkers and clinical factors for risk stratification. *Clin Chem.* 2014;60(1):68-77. PMID: 24379312

6 **ANSWER: A) Anxiety and depression**

Sleep disturbances are common in perimenopausal and postmenopausal women. A bothersome feature of hot flushes is that they are more common at night than during the day and are typically associated with arousal from sleep. However, some women experience insomnia even in the absence of hot flushes. Anxiety and depression symptoms (Answer A) also contribute to sleep disturbances, particularly during perimenopause, when there is a high rate of new-onset or recurrent mood disorders. Primary sleep disorders such as restless legs syndrome are also common in this population.

Normal aging (Answer D) is associated with sleep disturbances, but this patient has symptoms that are suggestive of anxiety and depression (difficulty falling asleep and midcycle awakening).

Progestin therapy (Answer E), such as micronized progesterone, is more typically associated with drowsiness, not insomnia.

Metformin therapy (Answer C) is not associated with nocturnal hypoglycemia, and it is not a very effective drug for weight loss.

The patient reports resolution of her vasomotor symptoms, indicating that she is on appropriate, not insufficient (Answer B), hormone therapy.

EDUCATIONAL OBJECTIVE

Construct a differential diagnosis for sleep disturbances in menopausal women.

REFERENCE(S)

Caretto M, Giannini A, Simoncini T. An integrated approach to diagnosing and managing sleep disorders in menopausal women. *Maturitas.* 2019;128:1-3. PMID: 31561815

Bonanni E, Schirru A, Di Perri MC, Bonuccelli U, Maestri M. Insomnia and hot flashes. *Maturitas.* 2019;126:51-54. PMID: 31239118

7 **ANSWER: D) Oral contraceptive**

Nonclassic congenital adrenal hyperplasia (CAH) is a cause of hyperandrogenic anovulation with a clinical presentation that is similar or identical to that of polycystic ovary syndrome (hirsutism with irregular menses). The incidence varies from 1 to 10 per 20,000 live births. Nonclassic CAH is more common in those of Italian, Hispanic, Ashkenazi Jewish, and Inuit descent. In women with nonclassic CAH, basal serum 17-hydroxyprogesterone concentrations (during the follicular phase of the menstrual cycle) are usually greater than 200 ng/dL (>6.1 nmol/L) (high-normal or high). The diagnosis of nonclassic 21α-hydroxylase deficiency can be confirmed in equivocal cases by documenting stimulated levels of 17-hydroxyprogesterone greater than 1000 to 1500 ng/dL (>30.3 to 45.5 nmol/L) 30 to 60 minutes after ACTH stimulation.

Historically, dexamethasone (Answer A) (or other glucocorticoids [Answer B]) was used as first-line therapy for managing hirsutism in women with nonclassic CAH. While glucocorticoids suppress serum androgens more than combined estrogen-progestin contraceptives, oral contraceptives (Answer D) are more effective for reducing hirsutism as measured by Ferriman-Gallwey scores, and this is the best option to manage this patient's oligomenorrhea and hirsutism.

Although metformin (Answer C) has not been systematically studied in women with nonclassic CAH, it could help restore ovulatory cycles. However, it is ineffective for treating hirsutism.

Spironolactone (Answer E), an androgen receptor antagonist, can be added after 6 months if the improvement in her hirsutism in suboptimal. Spironolactone should not be used as monotherapy unless reliable contraception is used. If a patient inadvertently uses spironolactone during early pregnancy, there is a potential risk for feminization of a male fetus.

EDUCATIONAL OBJECTIVE

Recommend the best treatment of nonclassic congenital adrenal hyperplasia.

REFERENCE(S)

Martin KA, Anderson RR, Chang J, et al. Evaluation and treatment of hirsutism in premenopausal women: an Endocrine Society clinical practice guideline. *J Clin Endocrinol Metab.* 2018;103(4):1233-1257. PMID: 29522147

Krone N, Rose IT, Willis DS, et al; United Kingdom Congenital Adrenal Hyperplasia Adult Study Executive (CaHASE). Genotype-phenotype correlation in 153 adult patients with congenital adrenal hyperplasia due to 21-hydroxylase deficiency: analysis of the United Kingdom Congenital Adrenal Hyperplasia Adult Study Executive (CaHASE) cohort. *J Clin Endocrinol Metab.* 2013;98(2):E346-E354. PMID: 23337727

Finkielstain GP, Kim MS, Sinaii N, et al. Clinical characteristics of a cohort of 244 patients with congenital adrenal hyperplasia. *J Clin Endocrinol Metab.* 2012;97(12):4429-4438. PMID: 22990093

Speiser PW, Azziz R, Baskin LS, et al; Endocrine Society. Congenital adrenal hyperplasia due to steroid 21-hydroxylase deficiency: an Endocrine Society clinical practice guideline [published correction appears in *J Clin Endocrinol Metab.* 2010;95(11):5137]. *J Clin Endocrinol Metab.* 2010;95(9):4133-4160. PMID: 20823466

8 ANSWER: D) Ovarian hyperthecosis

Ovarian hyperthecosis (Answer D) or androgen-secreting ovarian or adrenal tumors can cause manifestations ranging from postmenopausal hirsutism to frank virilization. One distinguishing feature is the pace of worsening, with hyperthecosis progressing at a slower rate than tumors. Ovarian hyperthecosis occurs when high gonadotropin levels drive androgen production from the theca cells. Although it can occur in premenopausal women, it is most common in postmenopausal women. Whether women with hyperthecosis have polycystic ovary syndrome before menopause has not been clarified.

An adrenal virilizing tumor (Answer A) would present with a more rapid onset and more severe symptoms and signs. Androgen-secreting adrenal tumors are usually malignant, but benign tumors have also been described in women. Approximately 60% of adrenocortical carcinomas present with hormone excess (most with Cushing syndrome only, 25% with both Cushing syndrome and virilization, and 10% with virilization alone).

A granulosa tumor of the ovary (Answer B) would present with high estrogen levels and endometrial hyperplasia and would not cause virilization.

Obesity (Answer C) can cause hirsutism. Adipose tissue can have increased 5α-reductase activity, as well as local aromatase activity, which can cause androgenic and estrogenic effects. However, it does not usually result in such high testosterone levels or virilization. Weight loss and suppression of androgens are the goals with obesity-induced hyperandrogenism.

Ovarian tumors that cause hyperandrogenism include Sertoli-Leydig–cell tumors (Answer E), arrhenoblastomas, or hilus-cell tumors that secrete testosterone in the male normal range (>240 ng/dL [>8.3 nmol/L]) and cause virilization. Because these tumors are rare, more common causes of postmenopausal hirsutism and virilization should be considered.

EDUCATIONAL OBJECTIVE

Outline the differential diagnosis of severe hyperandrogenism in a postmenopausal woman.

REFERENCE(S)

Mamoojee Y, Ganguri M, Taylor N, Quinton R. Clinical case seminar: postmenopausal androgen excess-challenges in diagnostic work-up and management of ovarian thecosis. *Clin Endocrinol (Oxf).* 2018;88(1):13-20. PMID: 28980338

Pugeat M, Déchaud H, Raverot V, Denuzière A, Cohen R, Boudou P; French Endocrine Society. Recommendations for investigation of hyperandrogenism. *Ann Endocrinol (Paris).* 2010;71(1):2-7. PMID: 20096825

9 ANSWER: B) *FMR1* genetic testing

Fragile X premutation screening should be performed in women with primary ovarian insufficiency (menopause before age 40 years). Screening should be recommended for women who have a family history of primary ovarian insufficiency; male relatives with learning disorders, autism, or intellectual disability; or family members with ataxia and/or dementia (suggestive of fragile X–related ataxia). The screening is accomplished by *FMR1* genetic testing (Answer B). In fragile X carriers, CGG repeats are in the premutation range.

Karyotype analysis (Answer D) is now performed in all women with primary ovarian insufficiency to rule out mosaic Turner syndrome. Patients with mosaicism typically have a milder reproductive phenotype, as some girls have breast development followed by pubertal arrest, or puberty followed by secondary amenorrhea. A very small percentage of girls with Turner syndrome have normal pubertal development and regular menses. While karyotype analysis would be recommended for this patient, Turner syndrome is rarely familial; therefore, the test most likely to identify the patient's diagnosis is *FMR1* genetic testing.

Positive 21-hydroxylase antibodies (Answer C) are seen in women with autoimmune oophoritis, and they predict future risk of adrenal insufficiency as well. However, this patient does not have typical features of autoimmune oophoritis.

Thyroid antibodies (Answer E) may be positive in patients with autoimmune thyroid disease and concomitant autoimmune premature ovarian insufficiency, but an autoimmune etiology would not explain the family history of early menopause in relatives.

There is no indication to measure antimullerian hormone (Answer A), which is an indicator of follicle number and is low in premature ovarian insufficiency and high in polycystic ovary syndrome.

EDUCATIONAL OBJECTIVE

Explain the differential diagnosis of premature ovarian insufficiency and appropriately recommend fragile X carrier testing.

REFERENCE(S)

Welt CK. Primary ovarian insufficiency: a more accurate term for premature ovarian failure. *Clin Endocrinol (Oxf)*. 2008;68(4):499-509. PMID: 17970776

Wang T, Bray SM, Warren ST. New perspectives on the biology of fragile X syndrome. *Curr Opin Genet Dev*. 2012;22(3):256-263. PMID: 22382129

Hoyos LR, Thakur M. Fragile X premutation in women: recognizing the health challenges beyond primary ovarian insufficiency. *J Assist Reprod Genet*. 2017;34(3):315-332. PMID: 27995424

Hipp HS, Charen KH, Spencer JB, Allen EG, Sherman SL. Reproductive and gynecologic care of women with fragile X primary ovarian insufficiency (FXPOI). *Menopause*. 2016;23(9):993-999. PMID: 27552334

10 ANSWER: E) Primary ovarian insufficiency

Antimullerian hormone is a marker of ovarian reserve and follicular number. Infertility specialists have used it extensively in clinical practice to evaluate older women with borderline elevated FSH levels to predict response to in vitro fertilization and to diagnose primary ovarian insufficiency (Answer E) (or in its early stages, diminished ovarian reserve/occult ovarian insufficiency). Antimullerian hormone levels are lower in women with impending primary ovarian insufficiency (with higher FSH levels). Another feature suggesting primary ovarian insufficiency in this patient is her short cycles (25 to 26 days) rather than the more typical 28 days.

A woman with polycystic ovary syndrome (Answer D) would mostly likely have a high antimullerian hormone value and normal FSH value.

An FSH-secreting pituitary adenoma (Answer B) would be unusual in this age group and would be more likely to present with neurologic symptoms (headache and vision loss) than with infertility and shorter cycles.

Importantly, women with hypothalamic amenorrhea (Answer C) can also have low antimullerian hormone levels but low-normal FSH and LH levels.

Although this patient has autoimmune hypothyroidism, it is unlikely that she has autoimmune oophoritis (Answer A), an uncommon etiology for primary ovarian insufficiency. Serum LH is higher than FSH in this disorder.

EDUCATIONAL OBJECTIVE
Explain the utility of measuring antimullerian hormone in women with amenorrhea.

REFERENCE(S)

Welt CK. Primary ovarian insufficiency: a more accurate term for premature ovarian failure. *Clin Endocrinol (Oxf).* 2008;68(4):499-509. PMID: 17970776

Meczekalski B, Czyzyk A, Kunicki M, et al. Fertility in women of late reproductive age: the role of serum anti-Müllerian hormone (AMH) levels in its assessment. *J Endocrinol Invest.* 2016;39(11):1259-1265. PMID: 27300031

La Marca A, Ferraretti AP, Palermo R, Ubaldi FM. The use of ovarian reserve markers in IVF clinical practice: a national consensus. *Gynecol Endocrinol.* 2016;32(1):1-5. PMID: 26531067

Iliodromiti S, Anderson RA, Nelson SM. Technical and performance characteristics of anti-müllerian hormone and antral follicle count as biomarkers of ovarian response. *Hum Reprod Update.* 2015;21(6):698-710. PMID: 25489055

11 ANSWER: C) Estradiol, 100 mcg twice weekly, with oral micronized progesterone, 200 mg (first 12 days of the month)

Evidence suggests that recovery of normal bone metabolism requires nutritional improvement, causing bone formation, and activation of the hypothalamic-pituitary-ovarian axis, decreasing bone resorption. The best strategy to improve bone density is to increase caloric intake, reduce exercise activity, or both (Answer D). However, this patient has tried this strategy for the past 2 years with modest improvement, and it is now time to prescribe pharmacologic therapy. Physiologic estrogen (Answer C) is first-line therapy after 6 to 12 months of a reasonable trial of nutritional, psychological, and exercise intervention (it has been 2 years for this patient).

Oral contraceptive doses of estrogen (Answer B) are pharmacologic, and data suggest that compared with no treatment, they do not improve bone mineral density in young oligomenorrheic athletes.

Bisphosphonates (Answer A) are not recommended in this setting because they are incorporated into the bone for years.

EDUCATIONAL OBJECTIVE
Identify the best management strategy for patients with functional hypothalamic amenorrhea and low bone mineral density (osteoporosis).

REFERENCE(S)

Dominguez J, Goodman L, Sen Gupta S, et al. Treatment of anorexia nervosa is associated with increases in bone mineral density, and recovery is a biphasic process involving both nutrition and return of menses. *Am J Clin Nutr.* 2007;86(1):92-99. PMID: 17616767

Djokanovic N, Klieger-Grossmann C, Koren G. Does treatment with bisphosphonates endanger the human pregnancy? *J Obstet Gynaecol Can.* 2008;30(12):1146-1148. PMID: 19175968

Ackerman KE, Singhal V, Slattery M, et al M. Effects of estrogen replacement on bone geometry and microarchitecture in adolescent and young adult oligoamenorrheic athletes: a randomized trial. *J Bone Miner Res.* 2020;35(2):248-260. PMID: 31603998

Gordon CM, Ackerman KE, Berga SL, et al. Functional hypothalamic amenorrhea: an Endocrine Society clinical practice guideline. *J Clin Endocrinol Metab.* 2017;102(5):1413-1439. PMID: 28368518

12 ANSWER: D) Hemoglobin A_{1c} measurement, liver enzymes, thyroid function tests

Turner syndrome occurs in 1 in 2500 live births and is associated with growth failure, pubertal delay, and cardiac abnormalities. In addition, affected patients are at risk for a number of comorbidities, including type 2 diabetes, elevated liver enzymes, autoimmune thyroid disease, celiac disease, hearing loss, orthodontic problems, and psychosocial disorders. Cardiac MRI is the most important test because congenital cardiac abnormalities are present in up to 50% of patients and include coarctation of the aorta, bicuspid aortic valve, and partial anomalous pulmonary venous return. Echocardiography is also sometimes used as part of the routine follow-up of women with Turner syndrome (but it is not performed annually).

Current practice guidelines recommend annual visits for women with Turner syndrome. In addition to measuring blood pressure, calculating BMI, and performing a full skin examination, the following assessments are recommended: thyroid function tests, hemoglobin A_{1c} measurement, and liver enzymes (AST, ALT, γ-glutamyl transferase, alkaline phosphatase) (Answer D). Screening for other comorbidities (eg, celiac disease [Answer B] or kidney disorders [Answer E]) is performed at less frequent intervals. Complete blood cell count (Answer C) is not recommended routinely. Serum antimullerian hormone (a marker of ovarian reserve) and transvaginal ultrasonography (Answer A) are not needed. Her diagnosis of hypogonadism due to Turner syndrome is already established, and she has no current indications for pelvic imaging.

EDUCATIONAL OBJECTIVE

Recommend appropriate evaluation for girls with gonadal dysgenesis.

REFERENCE(S)

Gravholt CH, Andersen NH, Conway GS, et al; International Turner Syndrome Consensus Group. Clinical practice guidelines for the care of girls and women with Turner syndrome: proceedings from the 2016 Cincinnati International Turner Syndrome Meeting. *Eur J Endocrinol.* 2017;177(3):G1-G70. PMID: 28705803

Shankar RK, Backeljauw PF. Current best practice in the management of Turner syndrome. *Ther Adv Endocrinol Metab.* 2018;9(1):33-40. PMID: 29344338

13 ANSWER: A) Absent uterus

This patient has uterine agenesis; terms for this disorder include mullerian agenesis, vaginal agenesis, and Mayer-Rokitansky-Kuster-Hauser syndrome [MRKH]). On pelvic ultrasonography, no uterus is visualized (Answer A). She had normal adrenarche and pubertal development but presented with primary amenorrhea. Her endocrine profile and external genitalia are normal, as one would expect. On examination, she would have a blind vaginal pouch and no palpable uterus, but ovaries would be present. Mullerian agenesis is the second most common cause of primary amenorrhea after gonadal dysgenesis.

Absent uterus and ovaries (Answer B) cannot be the answer, as she has ovarian function (she developed normal secondary sexual characteristics). Absence of uterus and ovaries would be seen in a patient with complete androgen insensitivity syndrome.

Streak ovaries on ultrasonography (Answer D) would be seen with Turner syndrome or other types of gonadal dysgenesis, which this patient does not have given her normal secondary sex characteristics and normal serum FSH level.

She has no risk factors for intrauterine adhesions (Answer C), also known as Asherman syndrome, which is seen in the setting of uterine instrumentation/trauma. On ultrasonography, Asherman syndrome is characterized by absence of an endometrial stripe.

Transverse vaginal septum (Answer E) is incorrect, as she would experience cyclic pelvic pain related to her menstrual cycles.

EDUCATIONAL OBJECTIVE

Differentiate mullerian agenesis from other structural causes of primary amenorrhea by a normal endocrine profile but absent uterus on examination and ultrasonography.

REFERENCE(S)

Herlin M, Bjørn AMB, Rasmussen M, Trolle B, Petersen MB. Prevalence and patient characteristics of Mayer-Rokitansky-Küster-Hauser syndrome: a nationwide registry-based study. *Hum Reprod.* 2016;31(10):2384-2390. PMID: 27609979

Fedele L, Bianchi S, Frontino G, Ciappina N, Fontana E, Borruto F. Laparoscopic findings and pelvic anatomy in Mayer-Rokitansky-Küster-Hauser syndrome. *Obstet Gynecol.* 2007;109(5):1111-1115. PMID: 17470591

Grimbizis GF, Gordts S, Di Spiezio Sardo A, et al. The ESHRE/ESGE consensus on the classification of female genital tract congenital anomalies. *Hum Reprod.* 2013;28(8):2032-2044. PMID: 23771171

14 ANSWER: D) Recommend progestin intrauterine device and spironolactone

This patient's deep venous thrombosis is a contraindication to continuing an estrogen-progestin contraceptive, even with a lower estrogen dosage (20 mcg) (Answer A) or transdermal route (Answer E). According to the Centers for Disease Control, combined contraceptive formulations (oral, patch, and vaginal ring) represent an unacceptable health risk given that patients with a history of deep venous thrombosis/pulmonary embolism not receiving anticoagulant therapy have a higher risk factor for recurrent deep venous thrombosis/ pulmonary embolism. Higher risk is defined as having known thrombophilia; active cancer; or idiopathic, estrogen-related, pregnancy-associated, or recurrent deep venous thrombosis/pulmonary embolism.

Oral progestin-only contraception (Answer C) might be an option, but the safest method would be a nonoral route such as the progestin intrauterine device (Answer D), which would manage her bleeding, prevent endometrial hyperplasia, and provide contraception. She could then add spironolactone to manage hirsutism.

While metformin (Answer B) is a second-line therapy that might help restore normal cycles, it is unlikely to benefit her hirsutism.

EDUCATIONAL OBJECTIVE

Choose the optimal therapy for irregular menstrual cycles, hyperandrogenic symptoms, and contraception in a woman with polycystic ovary syndrome and a history of deep venous thrombosis.

REFERENCE(S)

Legro RS, Arslanian SA, Ehrmann DA, et al; Endocrine Society. Diagnosis and treatment of polycystic ovary syndrome: an Endocrine Society clinical practice guideline. *J Clin Endocriol Metab.* 2013;98(12):4565-4592. PMID: 24151290

Martin KA, Anderson RR, Chang RJ, et al. Evaluation and treatment of hirsutism in premenopausal women: an Endocrine Society clinical practice guideline. *J Clin Endocrinol Metab.* 2018;103(4):1233-1257. PMID: 29522147

Practice Committee of the American Society for Reproductive Medicine. Combined hormonal contraception and the risk of venous thromboembolism: a guideline. *Fertil Steril.* 2017;107(1):43-51. PMID: 27793376

Curtis KM, Tepper NK, Jatlaoui TC, et al. U.S. Medical eligibility criteria for contraceptive use, 2016. *MMWR Recomm Rep.* 2016;65(3):1-103. PMID: 27467196

15 ANSWER: D) Switch her regimen to a GnRH agonist with a 0.05-mg estradiol patch

In male-to-female transgender patients, estrogen therapy is needed to develop female sexual characteristics. In patients with an intact hypothalamic-pituitary-gonadal axis, the estrogen dosage needed is supraphysiologic given the need to suppress testosterone secretion. However, combined use of a GnRH agonist with estrogen allows physiologic dosages of estrogen to be used, as testosterone secretion is already suppressed. Estrogen therapy can result in marked hypertriglyceridemia. However, the lipid effects of estrogen depend on the route of administration, with the transdermal route having less effect on HDL cholesterol and triglycerides than the oral route. Given this patient's history of hypertriglyceridemia, she is not a suitable candidate for oral estrogen and the most appropriate hormone regimen would be a GnRH agonist and a low-dosage estrogen patch (Answer D), which can be titrated based on clinical response and triglyceride levels. Ethinyl estradiol (Answer B) would not be a good choice because of its negative effects on triglycerides, as well as the fact that it increases the risk of venous thromboembolism significantly more so than 17β-estradiol.

Using spironolactone alone without an estrogen (Answer C) would not provide adequate suppression and blockade of androgen action for the desired physical effects. Based on the laboratory data provided, her testosterone level was not adequately suppressed on this dosage of spironolactone even when previously combined with conjugated equine estrogen.

Adding a 5α-reductase inhibitor such as finasteride (Answer A) would neither lower testosterone nor increase estradiol levels. Finasteride can be considered in situations where spironolactone is contraindicated such as hyperkalemia or to alleviate male-pattern balding.

Given that the patient has been living as a woman for more than 2 decades, and considering the increased risk of depression and suicide in the transgender population, withholding further hormone therapy (Answer E) would most likely negatively affect her mental health.

EDUCATIONAL OBJECTIVE

Guide the hormonal care of a transgender patient with hypertriglyceridemia.

REFERENCE(S)

Hembree WC, Cohen-Kettenis PT, Gooren L, et al. Endocrine treatment of gender-dysphoric/gender-incongruent persons: an Endocrine Society clinical practice guideline. *J Clin Endocrinol Metab.* 2017;102(11):3869-3903. PMID: 28945902

Aljenedil S, Hegele RA, Genest J, Awan Z. Estrogen-associated severe hypertriglyceridemia with pancreatitis. *J Clin Lipidol.* 2017;11(1):297-300. PMID: 28391900

Lufkin EG, Ory SJ. Relative value of transdermal and oral estrogen therapy in various clinical situations. *Mayo Clin Proc.* 1994;69(2):131-135. PMID: 8309263

16 ANSWER: A) Continue current regimen

The goal of gender-affirming hormone therapy in transgender women is to promote a physical appearance that is more congruent with their gender identity. This is achieved by suppressing endogenous hormones of the biologic sex (ie, testosterone) and replacing them with those of the desired gender (ie, estradiol) and maintaining these levels in the physiologic range. For many patients, the physical change that is most desired is breast development. The regimen that the patient is currently using has resulted in the desired hormone milieu. Therefore, continuing this regimen (Answer A) and explaining to the patient that it can take 2 to 3 years for hormone therapy to have the maximum effect on breast development is the best management strategy.

Patients undergoing feminizing hormone therapy should wait a minimum of 12 months to maximize breast growth before breast augmentation surgery. Given that this patient has only been on hormone therapy for 6 months, referral for breast augmentation (Answer E) would be premature at this time.

Doubling the dosage of estrogen replacement (Answer C) when the estradiol level is already in the target range of 100 to 200 pg/mL (367-734 pmol/L) is unnecessary and places the patient at increased risk of adverse effects such as venous thromboembolism and hypertriglyceridemia.

Similarly, switching her estrogen from 17β-estradiol to ethinyl estradiol (Answer D), which is the most thrombogenic estrogen, would have a negative effect on the risk-benefit ratio, especially in a patient with obesity.

Her testosterone level is already maximally suppressed, so adding the antiandrogen spironolactone (Answer B) would not provide any additional benefit.

EDUCATIONAL OBJECTIVE

Guide the hormonal care of a transgender patient to optimize breast development.

REFERENCE(S)

Hembree WC, Cohen-Kettenis PT, Gooren L, et al. Endocrine treatment of gender dysphoric/gender incongruent persons: an Endocrine Society clinical practice guideline. *J Clin Endocrinol Metab.* 2017;102(11):1-35. PMID: 28945902

T'Sjoen G, Arcelus J, Gooren L, Klink DT, Tangpricha V. Endocrinology of transgender medicine. *Endocr Rev.* 2019;40(1):97-117. PMID: 30307546

Safer JD, Tangpricha V. Care of transgender persons. *N Engl J Med.* 2019;381(25);2451-2460. PMID: 31851801

Male Reproduction Board Review

Stephanie Page, MD, PhD

1 ANSWER: B) Add medroxyprogesterone, 5 mg daily

Continued menses can be distressing to transmen. Many transmen experience cessation of menses on testosterone alone after 2 to 6 months of therapy; however, this can require high, supraphysiologic dosing in some transmen. Such patients benefit from the temporary addition of a progestational agent such medroxyprogesterone (Answer B), a GnRH agonist, or endometrial ablation. Transmen may also still be ovulating despite physiologic levels of testosterone. If transmen are at risk for pregnancy, a progestational intrauterine device may also be considered to alleviate menses and provide contraception.

Transgender patients are often concerned regarding the time course and effectiveness of gender-normalizing hormone therapy. In this case, trough testosterone and free testosterone concentrations are in the normal male reference range. Thus, increasing the testosterone dosage (Answer D) is not an optimal choice if the goal is cessation of menses. Setting patient expectations regarding the anticipated timeline for gender-normative characteristics is a key component of care delivery. In general, after 6 months of therapy, transgender men can expect cessation of menses, worsening or development of acne/skin oiliness, increased sexual desire, and perhaps some male-pattern hair growth, all of which have occurred in this patient with the exception of cessation of menses.

When monitoring the effectiveness of gender-affirming hormone therapy, hormone concentrations also help guide therapy and should target the physiologic reference range for the transgender. When delivering hormone therapy via intramuscular injections, hormone concentrations may be assessed at the mid-dose or trough dose time intervals.

Anastrozole (Answer A) blocks the aromatization of testosterone to estradiol and may be effective in achieving amenorrhea in this setting. However, anastrozole is associated with decreases in bone density, hot flashes, and liver toxicity in some cases; therefore, progestins and GnRH antagonists are preferred.

Hemoglobin and hematocrit should be monitored every 3 months during the first year of hormone therapy in transgender men, and testosterone dosing should potentially be adjusted (Answer C) for polycythemia should it occur. Without overt polycythemia, phlebotomy (Answer E) is not indicated. With cessation of menses, there may be an increase in hemoglobin; thus, regular monitoring is indicated in this patient.

EDUCATIONAL OBJECTIVE

Achieve amenorrhea in transmen.

REFERENCE(S)

Hembree WC, Cohen-Kettenis PT, Gooren L, et al. Endocrine treatment of gender-dysphoric/gender-incongruent persons: an Endocrine Society clinical practice guideline. *J Clin Endocrinol Metab.* 2017;102(11):3869-3903. PMID: 28945902

T'Sjoen G, Arcelus J, Gooren L, Klink DT, Tangpricha V. Endocrinology of transgender medicine. *Endocr Rev.* 2019;40(1):97-117. PMID: 30307546

Safer JD, Tangpricha V. Care of transgender persons. *N Engl J Med.* 2019;381(25):2451-2460. PMID: 31851801

2 ANSWER: D) Initiate testosterone transdermal gel

This patient has both biochemical and physiologic manifestations hypogonadism (likely related to comorbidities), low testosterone and calculated free testosterone concentrations documented on 2 occasions, and elevated gonadotropins. Thus, a trial of testosterone therapy (Answer D) is indicated.

Gynecomastia may be a sign of hypogonadism; coadministration of anastrozole (Answer C) is not indicated.

He has made lifestyle changes and his testosterone is unequivocally low; thus, lifestyle changes (Answer A) will not normalize his gonadal axis.

Phosphodiesterase inhibitors (Answer B) effectively treat erectile dysfunction, but they will not improve the possible other manifestations of prolonged hypogonadism, including anemia and increased fracture risk. Also, use of nitrates is a contraindication to phosphodiesterase inhibitors.

Despite their impact on cholesterol, high-dosage statins do not significantly lower serum testosterone concentrations. His lipids are well managed on his current regimen, so switching to a PCSK9 inhibitor (Answer E) is incorrect and would not treat his hypogonadism.

There is concern that exogenous testosterone may increase the risk of cardiovascular events, particularly among individuals with a history of cardiovascular disease. This patient should be counseled regarding the uncertainty surrounding testosterone therapy and cardiovascular risk and the very recent data from the TRAVERSE study (Lincoff et al) providing reassurance regarding cardiac safety for older hypogonadal men taking testosterone doses that maintain their serum testosterone within the normal range. This discussion should also include the positive effects of androgens in hypogonadal older men from this and other studies, including improvements in anemia, walking distance, vitality, and sexual satisfaction and sex frequency. His symptomatic response to testosterone therapy should be followed over time to determine the benefits of continued therapy.

EDUCATIONAL OBJECTIVE

List the indications for testosterone replacement therapy in men with late-onset hypogonadism.

REFERENCE(S)

Bhasin S, Brito JP, Cunningham GR, et al. Testosterone therapy in men with hypogonadism: an Endocrine Society clinical practice guideline. *J Clin Endocrinol Metab.* 2018;103(5):1715-1744. PMID: 29562364

Snyder PJ. The benefits and risks of testosterone treatment in older hypogonadal men. *Endocrinol Metab Clin North Am.* 2022;51(1):149-156. PMID: 35216713

Matsumoto AM. Testosterone replacement in men with age-related low testosterone: what did we learn from the testosterone trials? *Curr Opin Endocr Metab Res.* 2019;6:34-41. PMID: 32043015

Lincoff AM, Bhasin S, Flevaris P, et al. Cardiovascular safety of testosterone-replacement therapy. *N Engl J Med.* 2023 [Online ahead of print]. PMID: 37326322

3 ANSWER: A) Refer to assisted reproductive endocrinologist for intracytoplasmic sperm injection

Male-factor infertility is common, and approximately 50% of male infertility is idiopathic. The first steps in evaluating possible male infertility are a semen analysis and evaluation of the hypothalamic/pituitary/gonadal axis. In this case, the patient has normal testosterone and gonadotropins; thus, exogenous testosterone (Answer D) is not warranted (and would impair spermatogenesis) and gonadotropin therapy (Answer C) is not indicated.

Male fertility requires effective sperm production and function. Abnormalities in sperm numbers, morphology, or motility are associated with male infertility; if more than one of these parameters is abnormal, there is increased risk for infertility. In this case, sperm motility is highly abnormal and it is unlikely (but not impossible) that a pregnancy will ensue. However, this couple is anxious because the female partner is of advanced maternal age and therefore referral for assisted reproductive technology is indicated. Since the patient has plenty of sperm in his ejaculate, testicular sperm extraction (Answer B) is not required and referral for intracytoplasmic sperm injection (Answer A) is appropriate. Referral for intracytoplasmic sperm injection is indicated when the total motile sperm count is less than 10 million (total motile sperm: ejaculate volume × sperm concentration × motility = 2.4 mL × 25 million/mL × 0.05 = 3 million, in this case).

Some weak evidence has suggested selective serotonin reuptake inhibitors may affect sperm motility, but there is no evidence of fertility impairment with serotonin and norepinephrine reuptake inhibitors and one study has examined duloxetine directly (Punjani et al). Thus, discontinuation of his antidepressant (Answer E) is not warranted.

EDUCATIONAL OBJECTIVE

Interpret seminal fluid in the evaluation and treatment of male infertility.

REFERENCE(S)

Punjani N, Kang C, Flannigan R, et al. Impact of duloxetine on male fertility: a randomised controlled clinical trial. *Andrologia.* 2021;53(10):e14207. PMID: 34374108

Anawalt BD. Approach to male infertility and induction of spermatogenesis. *J Clin Endocrinol Metab.* 2013;98(9):3532-3542. PMID: 24014811

4 ANSWER: E) Subcutaneous hCG abuse

This patient exhibits signs of androgen excess (acne, gynecomastia, erythrocytosis) and is part of a gym culture where there is a high prevalence of anabolic abuse. The marked LH suppression despite normal testosterone levels is a key feature of exogenous androgen use. Exogenous hCG (Answer E) mimics LH, causing increases in testosterone production and suppression of LH without testicular shrinkage that may occur with exogenous testosterone.

A pituitary microadenoma (Answer D) suppressing LH to this degree would not support normal testosterone production.

Erythropoietin (Answer A) increases hematocrit, but it would not suppress LH or cause stigmata of androgen excess.

Androstenedione (Answer B) can be taken orally and is a weak androgen that some athletes abuse. Androstenedione is a precursor for testosterone, and, in large quantities, it may raise serum testosterone. However, oral androgens profoundly lower HDL cholesterol and, at high enough doses to produce complete suppression of LH, would result in testicular shrinkage. Clomiphene citrate and enclomifene (Answer C) are estrogen receptor modulators that may raise serum testosterone; however, due to lack of estrogen-mediated negative feedback at the pituitary they do not suppress LH.

EDUCATIONAL OBJECTIVE

Explain the clinical and laboratory findings that reflect abuse of performance-enhancing anabolic agents.

REFERENCE(S)

King DS, Sharp RL, Vukovich MD, et al. Effect of oral androstenedione on serum testosterone and adaptations to resistance training in young men: a randomized controlled trial. *JAMA.* 1999;281(21):2020-2028. PMID: 10359391

Miller GD, Moore C, Nair V, et al. Hypothalamic-pituitary-testicular axis effects and urinary detection following clomiphene administration in males. *J Clin Endocrinol Metab.* 2019;104(3):906-914. PMID: 30295816

Anawalt BD. Diagnosis and management of anabolic androgenic steroid use. *J Clin Endocrinol Metab.* 2019;104(7):2490-2500. PMID: 30753550

5 ANSWER: C) Papanicolaou test

The schedule for cervical cancer screening for transgender men with an intact uterus is the same as it is for cisgender women (every 3 years) (Answer C). This component of health care maintenance is often overlooked in transgender men who may not have a primary care provider and see their endocrinologist as their provider for hormone therapy.

Bone density monitoring (Answer A) in transmen receiving testosterone is not indicated. Exogenous testosterone is aromatized peripherally and supports bone health in transmen.

Mammography for breast cancer screening (Answer B) in transmen who have not undergone top surgery (mastectomy) follows guidelines for cisgender women and is not indicated for individuals younger than 30 years, even for those at high risk.

Evaluation of serum testosterone levels is indicated at the initiation of gender-affirming hormone therapy. This patient has normal male serum testosterone concentrations on therapy and is not altering his treatment regimen; thus, repeated measurement of the serum free testosterone concentration (Answer E) is not indicated.

He has had cessation of menses and is exhibiting effects of androgenization (hair, acne, body composition changes). Therefore, quantification of serum estradiol (Answer D) is not warranted. The time-course for voice deepening with gender-affirming testosterone is approximately 12 months, and there is no need to check sex steroid levels due to lack of voice changes unless this a persistent concern at that time.

EDUCATIONAL OBJECTIVE

Identify the components of reproductive health care maintenance in transgender men receiving gender-affirming hormone therapy.

REFERENCE(S)

Hembree WC, Cohen-Kettenis PT, Gooren L, et al. Endocrine treatment of gender-dysphoric/gender-incongruent persons: an Endocrine Society clinical practice guideline. *J Clin Endocrinol Metab.* 2017;102(11):3869-3903. PMID: 28945902

6 ANSWER: C) Functional hypogonadotropic hypogonadism

Men who exercise excessively and/or restrict calories can develop functional hypogonadotropic hypogonadism (Answer C). This is caused by suppression of GnRH secretion and is analogous to functional hypogonadotropic hypogonadism seen in women with hypothalamic amenorrhea. Leptin has an important role in GnRH signaling, and the low levels in patients with such energy deficits are thought to mediate the suppression of the reproductive axis.

Congenital leptin deficiency (Answer B) is a rare condition due to pathogenic variants in the *LEP* gene. It is characterized by onset of severe obesity in early childhood, as well as hypogonadotropic hypogonadism resulting in absent or delayed puberty. While this patient has a very low leptin level, the fact that he is slim and well virilized indicates that his low leptin level is an acquired, rather than congenital, deficiency.

Kallmann syndrome (Answer E) is a cause of congenital hypogonadotropic hypogonadism with anosmia, and it would not explain low testosterone levels in a patient who had gone through puberty and has normal-sized testes.

A hydrocele (Answer D) is a collection of fluid between the testis and the tunica albuginea. While it can cause scrotal swelling and discomfort, it does not interfere with Leydig-cell secretion of testosterone.

Use of anabolic steroids (Answer A) could explain this patient's muscular appearance. However, patients taking anabolic steroids have undetectable LH levels due to suppression of their hypothalamic-pituitary-gonadal axis. They also tend to have hematocrit levels that are significantly higher than those in this vignette. Anabolic steroid use would also not explain the patient's low leptin level.

EDUCATIONAL OBJECTIVE

Identify stress and low body fat as causes of suppression of the hypothalamic-pituitary-gonadal axis in men.

REFERENCE(S)

Dwyer AA, Chavan NR, Lewkowitz-Shpuntoff H, et al. Functional hypogonadotropic hypogonadism in men: underlying neuroendocrine mechanisms and natural history. *J Clin Endocrinol Metab.* 2019;104(8):3403-3414. PMID: 31220265

Young J. Approach to the male patient with hypogonadotropic hypogonadism. *J Clin Endocrinol Metab.* 2012;97(3):707-718. PMID: 22392951

Montague CT, Farooqi IS, Whitehead JP, et al. Congenital leptin deficiency is associated with severe early-onset obesity in humans. *Nature.* 1997;387(6636):903-908. PMID: 9202122

7 ANSWER: E) Synkinesia

In the last decade, considerable advances have been made in unraveling the genetic basis of congenital hypogonadotropic hypogonadism, and to date, pathogenic variants have been identified in approximately 40% of cases. In familial cases such as the one described in this vignette, the mode of inheritance can be used to guide genetic testing. This pedigree is consistent with an X-linked mode of inheritance and thus a pathogenic variant in *ANOS1*. In an analysis of 219 patients with congenital hypogonadotropic hypogonadism, the following clinical features were highly associated with specific gene defects: synkinesia (*ANOS1*), dental agenesis (*FGF8/FGFR1*), digital bony abnormalities (*FGF8/FGFR1*), and hearing loss (*CHD7*). Thus, in the case described, the physical finding most likely to be encountered is synkinesia (Answer E). In addition to the important role of anosmin 1 in the neuronal migration of both the GnRH neurons and the olfactory structures, it is also important for the crossing of the neurons in the developing brain across the midline, and this accounts for the mirror movements seen in patients with pathogenic variants in *ANOS1*.

Bony abnormalities, including syndactyly (Answer D), are typically encountered in patients with pathogenic variants in genes involved in the FGF pathway such as *FGF8* or *FGFR1*.

Coloboma (Answer B) is one of the characteristic features of CHARGE syndrome due to a pathogenic variant in the *CHD7* gene.

Axillary freckling (Answer A) is a cutaneous manifestation of neurofibromatosis type 1.

A shortened fourth metacarpal (Answer C) is seen in persons with pseudohypoparathyroidism.

EDUCATIONAL OBJECTIVE

Identify synkinesia as a phenotypic feature of Kallmann syndrome due to a pathogenic variant in the *ANOS1* gene.

REFERENCE(S)

Costa-Barbosa FA, Balasubramanian R, Keefe KW, et al. Prioritizing genetic testing in patients with Kallmann syndrome using clinical phenotypes. *J Clin Endocrinol Metab.* 2013;98(5):E943-E953. PMID: 23533228

Young J, Xu C, Papadakis GE, et al. Clinical management of congenital hypogonadotropic hypogonadism. *Endocr Rev.* 2019;40(2):669-710. PMID: 30698671

8 ANSWER: B) Hypothyroidism

Several factors are known to affect the levels of circulating SHBG and therefore testosterone levels in men. This patient has an SHBG level at the lower end of the normal range. Of the answer options listed, only hypothyroidism (Answer B) causes a low SHBG level.

Topiramate (Answer E) (an enzyme inducer), liver disease (Answer C), obesity (Answer D), and estrogen (Answer A) all tend to increase SHBG levels, in which case total testosterone levels are often in the mid-normal to high range, while free testosterone levels are low-normal or low.

EDUCATIONAL OBJECTIVE

Explain the effect of hypothyroidism on SHBG levels when evaluating men for hypogonadism.

REFERENCE(S)

Dumoulin SC, Perret BP, Bennet AP, Caron PJ. Opposite effects of thyroid hormones on binding proteins for steroid hormones (sex hormone-binding globulin and corticosteroid-binding globulin) in humans. *Eur J Endocrinol.* 1995;132(5):594-598. PMID: 7749500

Bhasin S, Brito JP, Cunningham GR, et al. Testosterone therapy in men with hypogonadism: an Endocrine Society clinical practice guideline. *J Clin Endocrinol Metab.* 2018;103(5):1715-1744. PMID: 2956236

9 ANSWER: A) Perform a postejaculatory urine analysis for semen

Ejaculation is the discharge of semen from the male reproductive tract usually accompanied by orgasm. Retrograde ejaculation occurs when semen, which would normally be ejaculated via the urethra, is instead redirected to the bladder. Normally, the sphincter of the bladder contracts before ejaculation, which acts to both inhibit the release of urine and prevent a reflux of seminal fluids into the bladder during ejaculation. Any condition, medication, or surgical procedure that interferes with central control of ejaculation or the autonomic innervation to the seminal tract can cause ejaculatory dysfunction. This patient has partial retrograde ejaculation due to autonomic neuropathy from suboptimally controlled type 1 diabetes. The diagnosis, which can be suspected from the history, is confirmed by showing that sperm are present in a urine sample obtained after ejaculation (Answer A). In patients not desiring fertility, no treatment is indicated. In patients wishing to start a family, a trial of pseudoephedrine could be considered, as it improves muscle tone at the bladder neck.

There is no indication to start treatment with hCG (Answer D), given that this patient's testosterone level is just below the lower end of normal and that it is intratesticular testosterone that is most important for spermatogenesis.

Initiating testosterone therapy (Answer E) would actually suppress sperm production, so it would not be appropriate for a man trying to conceive.

Given that sperm are already present in the ejaculate, there is no need to extract them from the testis (Answer B).

Starting an α-adrenergic blocker (Answer C) would actually make the problem worse given that these drugs relax the bladder sphincter and are a common cause of retrograde ejaculation.

EDUCATIONAL OBJECTIVE

Diagnose retrograde ejaculation, characterized by reduced ejaculate volume and oligospermia, in a patient with diabetes and infertility.

REFERENCE(S)

Mehta A, Sigman M. Management of the dry ejaculate: a systematic review of aspermia and retrograde ejaculation. *Fertil Steril.* 2015;104(5):1074-1081. PMID: 26432530

10 ANSWER: A) Add FSH, 75 IU daily

For men whose infertility is due to hypogonadotropic hypogonadism as in this case, spermatogenesis can be induced with hormonal therapy in the form of either exogenous gonadotropins (hCG ± FSH) or GnRH. Gonadotropin therapy to induce spermatogenesis consists of subcutaneous administration of hCG alone or in combination with FSH. hCG bears strong structural homology to LH, and acting through the LH receptor on Leydig cells, it increases both intratesticular and systemic testosterone production. In men who become hypogonadal after normal puberty has been completed and thus have normal testicular size, treatment with hCG alone is adequate to stimulate spermatogenesis. In contrast, patients who have congenital hypogonadotropic hypogonadism and prepubertal testes (<4 mL), as in this case, need combination therapy with both hCG and FSH (Answer A) to stimulate growth of the seminiferous tubules.

The calculated half-life of hCG is 2.3 days. Therefore, it would be of no benefit to the patient to shorten the interval between injections to daily (Answer D).

In contrast, recombinant LH (Answer C) has a much shorter half-life, estimated at 1 to 5 hours. When used to trigger ovulation in women, the long serum half-life of hCG can be an undesirable characteristic in clinical practice, as residual hCG may be mistaken for early detection of de novo synthesis of hCG by a newly implanted pregnancy. However, when used to stimulate spermatogenesis, the long half-life of hCG means fewer injections for the patient and it is therefore more convenient and cheaper than recombinant LH.

This patient's trough testosterone is in the lower part of the normal range, which is where one wants it to be to avoid high estradiol levels and the development of gynecomastia, a common adverse effect when the hCG dosage is too high. Therefore, there would be no benefit to increasing the hCG dosage to 1500 IU every other day (Answer B).

Treatment with clomiphene (Answer E) requires an intact hypothalamus given that it increases LH by blocking estrogen-mediated negative feedback, so it would not be effective in a patient with congenital GnRH deficiency due to Kallmann syndrome.

EDUCATIONAL OBJECTIVE

Recommend the optimal gonadotropin regimen to stimulate spermatogenesis in Kallmann syndrome.

REFERENCE(S)

Burris AS, Rodbard HW, Winters SJ, Sherins RJ. Gonadotropin therapy in men with isolated hypogonadotropic hypogonadism: the response to human chorionic gonadotropin is predicted by initial testicular size. *J Clin Endocrinal Metab.* 1988;66(6):1144-1151. PMID: 3372679

King TFJ, Hayes FJ. Long-term outcome of idiopathic hypogonadotropic hypogonadism. *Curr Opin Endocrinol Diabetes Obes.* 2012;19(3):204-210. PMID: 22499222

Young J, Xu C, Papadakis GE, et al. Clinical management of congenital hypogonadotropic hypogonadism. *Endocr Rev.* 2019;40(2):669-710. PMID: 30698671

11 ANSWER: B) Congenital bilateral absence of the vas deferens

This couple's infertility is due to azoospermia. Absence of sperm in the ejaculate may occur because of an obstruction in the reproductive tract (obstructive azoospermia) or inadequate production of spermatozoa (nonobstructive azoospermia). The volume and pH of the seminal fluid can be used to determine in which category a patient's azoospermia falls. In this case, the low volume and low pH indicate an obstructive etiology. Obstructive azoospermia may be congenital (congenital absence of the vas deferens, idiopathic epididymal obstruction) or acquired (from infections, vasectomy, or other iatrogenic injuries to the male reproductive tract).

Congenital bilateral absence of the vas deferens (Answer B) is one of the most common causes of obstructive azoospermia. It can be diagnosed by a careful clinical examination, as the vas is normally palpable as a thin ropelike structure within the spermatic cord. The diagnosis can be confirmed by transrectal ultrasonography. Genetic testing should be performed in patients with congenital bilateral absence of the vas deferens who do not have the typical pulmonary and pancreatic manifestations of cystic fibrosis, as it is associated with compound heterozygosity for a classic (severe) *CFTR* pathogenic variant and a mild *CFTR* pathogenic variant.

All of the listed options cause nonobstructive azoospermia, in which case testis volume would be reduced because the bulk of the testis is composed of seminiferous tubules.

If this patient's azoospermia were due to anabolic steroid use (Answer A), his testosterone and gonadotropin levels would be suppressed.

Y-chromosome microdeletions (Answer E) are an important cause of nonobstructive azoospermia and typically result in reduced testicular size due to disruption of spermatogenesis and an elevated FSH level. The male-specific region on the long arm of the Y chromosome has a locus known as the azoospermia factor (AZF) that contains genes needed for spermatogenesis. This AZF locus contains 3 regions: AZFa, AZFb, and AZFc. Deletions of the entire AZFa region result in complete atrophy of the tubular compartment, with only Sertoli cells seen on testicular biopsy, making retrieval of sperm for intracytoplasmic sperm injection virtually impossible. Large deletions in the AZFb region also result in Sertoli-cell–only syndrome. Pathogenic variants in the AZFc region are the most common and account for 80% of Y-chromosome microdeletions. AZFc deletions are compatible with residual spermatogenesis, with oligospermia being a common presentation.

Patients with mosaic Klinefelter syndrome (Answer C) can present with infertility, but the patient's completely normal hormone profile, absence of gynecomastia, normal testicular size, and semen characteristics would not be consistent with this diagnosis.

Patients with a mild degree of androgen insensitivity (Answer D) can present with a low sperm count, but both testosterone and gonadotropin levels are elevated in such cases.

EDUCATIONAL OBJECTIVE

Diagnose obstructive azoospermia due to absence of the vas deferens as a cause of infertility.

REFERENCE(S)

Cooper TG, Noonan E, von Eckardstein S, et al. World Health Organization reference values for human semen characteristics. *Hum Reprod Update.* 2010;16(3):231-245. PMID: 19934213

Anawalt BD. Approach to male infertility and induction of spermatogenesis. *J Clin Endocrinol Metab.* 2013;98(9):3532-3542. PMID: 24014811

12 ANSWER: C) Measure free testosterone by equilibrium dialysis

This patient's clinical presentation with decreased libido, erectile dysfunction, and fatigue is highly suggestive of hypogonadism. His physical examination also reveals gynecomastia. Despite this, 2 total testosterone values, both measured by liquid chromatography/tandem mass spectrometry, are in the high-normal range. In such clinical scenarios, where the clinical phenotype is incongruent with biochemical results, clinicians should consider alterations in serum SHBG levels as a potential explanation. Certain clinical conditions are associated with elevated serum SHBG levels, and these include aging, liver disease, hyperthyroidism, medications (anticonvulsant drugs, estrogen), and HIV infection. Although the exact mechanism behind SHBG elevation in HIV remains unclear, increased inflammatory milieu in these patients has been posited as one of the mechanisms (SHBG is an acute-phase reactant). As longevity is increasing in persons with HIV, quality-of-life issues in this patient population are gaining considerable attention. Furthermore, the prevalence of hypogonadism in men with HIV is higher than in the general population; therefore, an accurate diagnosis is important.

Thus, in cases such as this where the history is suggestive of hypogonadism and a disorder known to impact SHBG levels is present, measurement of free testosterone (Answer C) is required to diagnose androgen deficiency. Reliable methods of free testosterone measurement include (1) measurement by equilibrium dialysis (considered the gold standard, but not routinely available in commercial laboratories); and (2) calculated free testosterone (derived from total testosterone and SHBG measurements using law of mass action equations). This patient's free testosterone level (measured by equilibrium dialysis) was low at 4.8 ng/dL (1.7 nmol/L) because of a markedly elevated SHBG level of 20.0 µg/mL (178 nmol/L), allowing a diagnosis of hypogonadism to be confirmed.

Epitestosterone is a biologically inactive 17-epimer of testosterone that is cosecreted by the Leydig cells of the testes. The urinary testosterone-to-epitestosterone ratio (Answer A) is measured in the evaluation of men when androgen abuse is suspected. However, exogenous use of testosterone by this patient would be associated with suppressed gonadotropin levels.

Men with partial androgen insensitivity syndrome resulting from pathogenic variants in the gene encoding the androgen receptor (Answer E) may also present with symptoms and signs of hypogonadism in association with an elevated serum testosterone level. However, patients with partial androgen insensitivity syndrome tend to have additional clinical manifestations, including perineoscrotal hypospadias and infertility. Importantly, gonadotropin levels in such patients are elevated due to impaired testosterone negative feedback, unlike the gonadotropin profile of patients with HIV infection who typically have secondary hypogonadism.

Measuring estradiol (Answer B) would not be very helpful in this patient, as his high SHBG levels would also tend to cause a high estradiol level. If he were taking estrogen or had an estrogen-secreting tumor as the cause of his gynecomastia, testosterone levels would be low rather than high.

Hemochromatosis, for which measuring serum ferritin (Answer D) would be the next step in the diagnostic algorithm, is a rare cause of secondary hypogonadism due to pituitary iron deposition. However, this man has normal serum gonadotropins.

EDUCATIONAL OBJECTIVE

Diagnose androgen deficiency in men with HIV who experience alterations in the concentration of serum SHBG.

REFERENCE(S)

Antonio L, Wu FC, O'Neill TW, et al; European Male Ageing Study Group. Low free testosterone is associated with hypogonadal symptoms and signs in men with normal testosterone levels. *J Clin Endocrinol Metab.* 2016;101(7):2647-2657. PMID: 26909800

Shea JL, Wong PY, Chen Y. Free testosterone: clinical utility and important analytical aspects of measurement. *Adv Clin Chem.* 2014;63:59-84. PMID: 24783351

Moreno-Pérez O, Escoín C, Serna-Candel C, et al. The determination of total testosterone and free testosterone (RIA) are not applicable to the evaluation of gonadal function in HIV-infected males. *J Sex Med.* 2010;7(8):2873-2883. PMID: 20626606

13 ANSWER: A) Congenital hypogonadotropic hypogonadism

This patient had prepubertal onset of hypogonadism as evidenced by his failure to develop secondary sexual characteristics, no increase in testicular size, and eunuchoidal proportions (arm span >5 cm above height). Laboratory tests show profound secondary hypogonadism with otherwise normal pituitary function and prolactin levels. His presentation is thus consistent with congenital hypogonadotropic hypogonadism (Answer A). Distinguishing between constitutional delay of growth and puberty (Answer B) and congenital hypogonadotropic hypogonadism can be challenging in younger adolescent boys. The fact that this patient's father was a late bloomer might lead one to suspect constitutional delay of growth and puberty. However, the absence of any signs of puberty by age 18 years, by definition, rules this out. It is important to recognize that delayed, but otherwise normal, puberty is seen in up to 12% of families with congenital hypogonadotropic hypogonadism.

Pathogenic variants in the *PROP1* gene (Answer D) are one of the most common causes of both familial and sporadic congenital combined pituitary hormone deficiency (GH, TSH, LH, FSH). Thus, the fact that the patient's pituitary hormone profile is normal apart from gonadotropin deficiency rules out an abnormality in *PROP1.*

Similarly, pathogenic variants in the *POU1F1* gene (Answer C), which were first described in 1992, cause combined pituitary hormone deficiency and are associated with GH, prolactin, and TSH deficiencies, with variable pituitary hypoplasia. Deficiencies of GH and prolactin are generally complete, but TSH deficiency is more variable. Gonadotropin deficiency is not seen in patients with *POU1F1* pathogenic variants, so it would not explain this patient's phenotype.

EDUCATIONAL OBJECTIVE

Construct the differential diagnosis of a patient with congenital hypogonadotropic hypogonadism.

REFERENCE(S)

Palmert MR, Dunkel L. Clinical practice. Delayed puberty. *N Engl J Med.* 2012;366(5):443-453. PMID: 22296078

Hayes FJ, Seminara SB, Crowley WF Jr. Hypogonadotropic hypogonadism. *Endocrinol Metab Clin North Am.* 1998;27(4):739-763. PMID: 9922906

Young J. Approach to the male patient with hypogonadotropic hypogonadism. *J Clin Endocrinol Metab.* 2012;97(3):707-718. PMID: 22392951

Costa-Barbosa FA, Balasubramanian R, Keefe KW, et al. Prioritizing genetic testing in patients with Kallmann syndrome using clinical phenotypes. *J Clin Endocrinol Metab.* 2013;98(5):E943-E953. PMID: 23533228

Turton JP, Reynaud R, Mehta A, et al. Novel mutations within the *POU1F1* gene associated with variable combined pituitary hormone deficiency. *J Clin Endocrinol Metab.* 2005;90(8):4762-4770. PMID: 15928241

14 ANSWER: E) Persistent postpubertal gynecomastia

The pathophysiology of gynecomastia involves an imbalance between free estrogen and free androgen actions in the breast tissue. During mid-to-late puberty, relatively more estrogen may be produced by the testes and peripheral tissues before testosterone secretion reaches adult levels, resulting in the gynecomastia that commonly occurs during this period. Most adolescents presenting with isolated gynecomastia have physiologic pubertal gynecomastia, which generally appears at 13 or 14 years of age, lasts for 6 months or less, and then regresses. Although the diagnosis is evident in most cases, a thorough history that includes review of medications, environmental exposures, and illicit drug use and physical examination are necessary. The case described fits the diagnosis of pubertal gynecomastia (Answer E), but unlike most cases, it has failed to regress and is causing significant psychological distress. Surgical resection should be considered for adolescents with physiologic gynecomastia that is greater than 4 cm in diameter, has not responded to medical therapy, persists for more than 1 year or after the patient is age 17 years, or is associated with embarrassment that interferes with normal daily activities.

FSH levels are invariably elevated in men with Klinefelter syndrome, even mosaic forms (Answer D), so this patient's FSH value of 4.0 mIU/mL (4.0 IU/L) effectively rules out this diagnosis.

Leydig-cell tumors (Answer B) are a rare but important cause of gynecomastia. They are frequently too small to be found on clinical examination but are usually identified on ultrasonography. They cause gynecomastia by increasing estradiol levels, so they would not explain the breast enlargement in this patient with normal estradiol levels.

A number of case reports of gynecomastia arising from inadvertent exposure to estrogens (Answer A) have been documented. If this were the case in this patient, his LH level would be suppressed, as would his endogenous estradiol.

Although there have been some case reports of marijuana smokers and gynecomastia, there is no evidence that occasional edible THC consumption causes gynecomastia (Answer C).

EDUCATIONAL OBJECTIVE

Diagnose persistent postpubertal gynecomastia.

REFERENCE(S)

Deepinder F, Braunstein GD. Drug-induced gynecomastia: an evidence-based review. *Expert Opin Drug Saf.* 2012 Sep;11(5):779-95PMID: 22862307

Guss CE, Divasta AD. Adolescent gynecomastia. *Pediatr Endocrinol Rev.* 2017;14(4):371-377. PMID: 28613047

15 ANSWER: C) Erythrocytosis

When considering testosterone replacement therapy, particularly in older men, the risks and benefits should be discussed before initiating therapy. Erythrocytosis (Answer C) is the most common adverse effect of testosterone therapy in older men. Meta-analyses of randomized controlled trials have shown that older men on testosterone are 4 to 5 times more likely to experience erythrocytosis than those on placebo. Testosterone-related erythrocytosis is dosage-dependent and is more frequently encountered in older men and in patients on injectable testosterone preparations. Androgens stimulate erythropoiesis via various mechanisms: (1) direct stimulation of erythroid cell line in the bone marrow, (2) stimulation of erythropoietin synthesis and release from the kidneys, and (3) increasing iron availability for erythropoiesis. Although the mechanism(s) explaining why older men are predisposed to erythrocytosis remains unclear, reduced metabolic clearance rate of testosterone has been posited as a cause. Anecdotal reports also suggest that men with underlying hypoxic conditions may also be more predisposed to erythrocytosis during testosterone therapy.

Before initiating testosterone therapy, baseline hematocrit should be measured. The Endocrine Society clinical practice guidelines recommend against initiating testosterone therapy in patients with a baseline hematocrit level greater than 48% (greater than 50% for men living at higher altitudes) and suggest that the underlying cause of erythrocytosis be investigated before androgen therapy is prescribed. Once testosterone therapy is initiated, it is suggested that hematocrit be assessed in 3 to 6 months and then annually. If the hematocrit level is above 54% (>0.54), testosterone therapy should be discontinued until hematocrit normalizes (and testosterone therapy can then be initiated at a reduced dosage). Such patients should be evaluated for hypoxia and sleep apnea.

PSA elevation above 4 ng/mL (>4 μg/L) (Answer E) is seen more frequently in older men on testosterone compared with rates observed in men taking placebo, but meta-analyses of randomized controlled trials show that this risk is much less common than erythrocytosis (odds ratio, 1.22).

Similarly, randomized controlled trials have not shown a higher frequency of urinary retention (Answer B) in older men.

There are no data to suggest that physiologic testosterone replacement causes aggressive behavior (Answer D) in men.

Elevated liver enzymes (Answer A) can occur in patients taking synthetic oral androgens such as methyltestosterone, which can cause jaundice, peliosis hepatitis, and hepatomas. However, hepatotoxicity is not an adverse effect of transdermal or intramuscular testosterone formulations.

EDUCATIONAL OBJECTIVE

Identify the most likely adverse effect of testosterone therapy in older men.

REFERENCE(S)

Snyder PJ, Bhasin S, Cunningham GR, et al; Testosterone Trials Investigators. Effects of testosterone treatment in older men. *N Engl J Med.* 2016;374(7):611-624. PMID: 26886521

Roy CN, Snyder PJ, Stephens-Shields AJ, et al. Association of testosterone levels with anemia in older men: a controlled clinical trial. *JAMA Intern Med.* 2017;177(4):480-490. PMID: 28241237

Calof OM, Singh AB, Lee ML, et al. Adverse events associated with testosterone replacement in middle-aged and older men: a meta-analysis of randomized, placebo-controlled trials. *J Gerontol A Biol Sci Med Sci.* 2005;60(11):1451-1457. PMID: 16339333

Shahani S, Braga-Basaria M, Maggio M, Basaria S. Androgens and erythropoiesis: past and present. *J Endocrinol Invest.* 2009;32(8):704-716. PMID: 19494706

16 ANSWER: B) Pituitary MRI

This man presents with a low-trauma fracture and symptoms of hypogonadism with onset starting at age 45 years. He was previously healthy with proven fertility and no notable medical history with the exception of a kidney stone. His laboratory values are consistent with hypogonadotropic hypogonadism and his testosterone and gonadotropins are very low with total testosterone value less than 150 ng/dL (<5.2 nmol/L) and LH and FSH levels less than 2.0 mIU/mL (<2.0 IU/L). A presumptive diagnosis of late-onset hypogonadism was made. These very low levels are not typical of late-onset hypogonadism, which is due to a combination of aging and comorbid illness. In the setting of morning testosterone levels less than 150 ng/dL (<5.2 nmol/L), Endocrine Society guidelines recommend obtaining a pituitary MRI (Answer B) to evaluate for hypothalamic-pituitary disease. In this patient, pituitary MRI was performed and a 5-mm adenoma was identified on the left side of the pituitary gland. A measurement of urinary free cortisol excretion was elevated at 310 μg/24 h (855.6 nmol/d) (6 times the upper normal limit), and Cushing disease was ultimately diagnosed as the cause of his secondary hypogonadism.

Semen analysis (Answer C) is not likely to be helpful in the evaluation of a man with central or hypogonadotropic hypogonadism.

The testosterone-to-epitestosterone ratio (Answer E) is obtained to screen for abuse of exogenous testosterone, but this patient's clinical picture is compatible with hypogonadism and not a response to anabolic steroids.

Testicular ultrasonography (Answer D) might be performed when primary hypogonadism or testicular cancer is suspected, neither of which is consistent with this patient's clinical picture.

Although he is currently hypogonadal and he may ultimately benefit from testosterone therapy, he first needs a complete workup to determine the etiology of his central hypogonadism. Treatment of his underlying pituitary disorder may allow recovery of his hypothalamic-pituitary-gonadal axis and obviate the need for testosterone therapy (Answer A). Additionally, testosterone therapy is associated with increased risk of deep venous thrombosis, which compounds his already elevated risk of due to Cushing disease.

EDUCATIONAL OBJECTIVE

Determine when to perform pituitary magnetic resonance imaging in the evaluation of secondary or hypogonadotropic hypogonadism in a middle-aged man with very low testosterone.

REFERENCE(S)

Bhasin S, Cunningham GR, Hayes FJ, et al; Task Force, Endocrine Society. Testosterone therapy in men with androgen deficiency syndromes: an Endocrine Society clinical practice guideline. *J Clin Endocrinol Metab.* 2010;95(6):2536-2559. PMID: 20525905

Obesity and Lipids Board Review

Sangeeta Kashyap, MD

1 ANSWER: D) Moderate-intensity statin daily and aspirin if lipoprotein (a) is elevated

This patient has intermediate risk of a cardiovascular disease event; her risk is greater than that indicated by her atherosclerotic cardiovascular disease (ASCVD) risk score of 8.0%. Her notable risk-enhancing factors include a family history of premature ASCVD, chronic inflammation from rheumatoid arthritis, and elevated high-sensitivity C-reactive protein. Moreover, the presence of rheumatoid arthritis elevates the relative risk of major cardiometabolic disease by 1.7. Measuring lipoprotein (a) can be considered in those with a family history of premature ASCVD. If elevated, this would make her seemingly unremarkable lipid profile more concerning for ASCVD. Nonetheless, this is a patient who would benefit from statin therapy and LDL-cholesterol reduction of 30% to 49% (Answer D).

A coronary calcium score is indicated for patients aged 40 to 70 years with risk factors for cardiovascular disease. Values greater than 100 indicate moderate plaque deposition, and in that case, a statin would be indicated, not aspirin (Answer A).

Carotid intimal thickness (Answer B) and LDL particle size (Answer C) would not add value to cardiovascular disease risk stratification. The drug of choice for this patient would be a moderate-intensity statin, not ezetimibe or a low-intensity statin.

EDUCATIONAL OBJECTIVE

Recommend a primary prevention approach for a patient with risk-enhancing factors for cardiovascular disease.

REFERENCE(S)

Sajja A, Li H-F, Spinelli KJ, et al. A simplified approach to identification of risk status in patients with atherosclerotic cardiovascular disease. *Am J Prev Cardiol.* 2021;7:100187. PMID: 34611633

Muntner P, Orroth KK, Mues KE, et al. Evaluating a simple approach to identify adults meeting the 2018 AHA/ACC Cholesterol Guideline definition of very high risk for atherosclerotic cardiovascular disease. *Cardiovasc Drugs Ther.* 2022;36(3):475-481. PMID: 33661432

2 ANSWER: C) Continue pravastatin and monitor fasting glucose and hemoglobin A_{1c} every 6 months

Although this patient is at intermediate risk based on her 10-year atherosclerotic cardiovascular disease risk score greater than 7.5%, this score does not account for the presence of metabolic syndrome, which increases the relative risk for cardiovascular disease to 1.7 compared with risk of persons who do not have metabolic syndrome. Similarly, her family history of atherosclerotic cardiovascular disease, especially her mother experiencing a premature cardiovascular event, further increases her risk by 2-fold. Although the patient is concerned about statin-associated diabetes, the effects of statins on glucose parameters are modest. Most data indicate that statin potency and dosage play a role. Specific statins appear less diabetogenic with no dose dependency. Atorvastatin, rosuvastatin, and simvastatin have the strongest associations, whereas fluvastatin, lovastatin, pitavastatin, and pravastatin have minimal or no association. Thus, continuing pravastatin and monitoring glucose parameters every 6 months (Answer C) is correct.

Changing pravastatin to rosuvastatin or fenofibrate (Answers A and B) would not be beneficial for this patient.

Eliminating statins and increasing the intensity of exercise (Answer D) would not sufficiently lower her cardiovascular disease risk.

EDUCATIONAL OBJECTIVE

Manage mixed hyperlipidemia in patients with metabolic syndrome and risk of diabetes mellitus.

REFERENCE(S)

Sattar N, Preiss D, Murray HM, et al. Statins and risk of incident diabetes: a collaborative meta-analysis of randomised statin trials. *Lancet.* 2010;375(9716):735-742. PMID: 20167359

Chou R, Dana T, Blazina I, Daeges M, Jeanne TL. Statins for prevention of cardiovascular disease in adults: evidence report and systematic review for the US Preventive Services Task Force. *JAMA.* 2016;316(19):2008-2024. PMID: 27838722

3 ANSWER: D) Low-dosage rosuvastatin twice weekly and titrate up slowly every 6 months

This patient has a mixed dyslipidemic pattern and is at intermediate risk of a primary event. His atherosclerotic cardiovascular disease risk score of 7.7% most likely underestimates his true risk because of the presence of numerous risk factors, including HIV, metabolic syndrome, persistently elevated triglycerides, and possible family history of premature atherosclerotic cardiovascular disease. According to the American College of Cardiology/American Heart Association Cholesterol Guideline, initiation of a moderate-intensity statin for an LDL-cholesterol reduction of 30% to 49% would be favored because of his risk score and multiple risk factors.

Statin-related adverse events occur in the setting of increased serum concentrations, often resulting from a drug interaction. The cytochrome P450 system has a major role in statin metabolism as it does for other drugs. Current FDA labeling indicates that lovastatin, simvastatin, and, to a lesser degree, atorvastatin are the statins most subject to drug interactions because of their high affinity for the CYP3A4 isoenzyme. Clinically relevant CYP3A4 inhibitors include azole antifungals, amiodarone, clarithromycin, erythromycin, HIV protease inhibitors, verapamil, and grapefruit juice.

Thus, for this patient, administering a high-intensity statin (rosuvastatin) less frequently is indicated, and twice-weekly administration (Answer D) is correct. Cholestyramine and ezetimibe (Answer A), fenofibrate (Answer B), lovastatin (Answer C), and omega-3 fatty acids (Answer E) would not be as effective as a high-intensity statin for lowering cardiovascular disease risk.

EDUCATION OBJECTIVE

Describe drug interactions of statins and statin-related adverse events.

REFERENCE(S)

Bellosta S, Corsini A. Statin drug interactions and related adverse reactions: an update. *Expert Opin Drug Saf.* 2018;17(1):25-37. PMID: 29058944

Feinstein MJ, Nance RM, Drozd DR, et al. Assessing and refining myocardial infarction risk estimation among patients with human immunodeficiency virus: a study by the Centers for AIDS Research Network of Integrated Clinical Systems. *JAMA Cardiol.* 2017;2(2):155-162. PMID: 28002550

4 ANSWER: C) Complete blood cell count, liver transaminases, iron, ferritin, vitamin B_{12}, and prealbumin

Multiple micronutrient deficiencies occur longitudinally after Roux-en-Y gastric bypass. This patient's symptoms are consistent with iron deficiency, and the vignette indicates that she is not adequately supplementing with iron. In patients receiving adequate supplementation per guidelines, the following is observed after bariatric surgery (compared with baseline) with a moderate level of evidence:

- Vitamin A decreases by −7.54 µg/dL (95% CI, −10.16 to −4.92 µg/dL) 12 to 23 months after Roux-en-Y gastric bypass

- Vitamin E decreases by –2.35 μg/dL (95% CI, –3.65 to –1.05 μg/dL) ≥24 months after Roux-en-Y gastric bypass
- Ferritin decreases by –54.93 μg/dL (95% CI, –77.19 to –32.67) ≥24 months after sleeve gastrectomy

Such decreases in micronutrient levels at follow-up intervals in studies with supplementation should be considered to establish a postbariatric surgery monitoring schedule for micronutrients to detect and manage micronutrient deficiencies.

Answers A, B, D, and E do not monitor the appropriate micronutrient deficiencies.

EDUCATIONAL OBJECTIVE

Monitor micronutrients after gastric bypass surgery.

REFERENCE(S)

Ha J, Kwon Y, Kwon JW, et al. Micronutrient status in bariatric surgery patients receiving postoperative supplementation per guidelines: insights from a systematic review and meta-analysis of longitudinal studies. *Obes Rev.* 2021;22(7):e13249. PMID: 33938111

5 ANSWER: E) Increased grazing and sweets consumption and binge-eating disorder

The mean weight loss after successful bariatric surgery is approximately 33% of initial body weight. However, at least one-third of patients will regain more than 25% of total weight lost, and this weight regain typically occurs within 2 to 5 years of surgery. Weight regain after bariatric surgery has the potential of adversely affecting health outcomes because of the reemergence of obesity-associated comorbidities, worsening quality of life, and increased health care costs. Therefore, it is important to recognize weight regain in patients with a history of bariatric surgery to mitigate its clinical and metabolic impact.

Disordered eating habits such as grazing and binge-eating disorder, night-eating syndrome, postsurgical eating avoidance disorder, soft-food syndrome, and eating disorders not otherwise specified have been identified as increasing the risk of weight regain after bariatric surgery (thus, Answer E is correct). It is therefore critical that patients have frequent psychological assessments for eating disorders, as well as screening for depression, which, along with other psychiatric illnesses, has been associated with increased risk of early weight plateau and weight regain.

Although anemia (Answer A) is common after bariatric surgery and is associated with fatigue and decreased physical activity, it is not associated with significant weight gain.

The antidepressant venlafaxine (Answer B) that this patient woman is taking is associated with weight loss, not weight gain.

Dilation of gastric pouch leading to increase food intake (Answer C) is incorrect because she had a normal upper gastrointestinal series that did not show this to be a cause of weight gain.

There is no evidence to suggest increased alcohol use (Answer D) as a cause for weight gain.

EDUCATIONAL OBJECTIVE

Assess weight gain in a patient after bariatric surgery.

REFERENCE(S)

Istfan NW, Lipartia M, Anderson WA, Hess DT, Apovian CM. Approach to the patient: management of the post-bariatric surgery patient with weight regain. *J Clin Endocrinol Metab.* 2021;106(1):251-263. PMID: 33119080

Livhits M, Mercado C, Yermilov I, et al. Patient behaviors associated with weight regain after laparoscopic gastric bypass. *Obes Res Clin Pract.* 2011;5(3):e169-e266. PMID: 24331108

6 ANSWER: C) Perform liver elastography and refer her to hepatology for further workup

Approximately 1 in 6 patients with type 2 diabetes has evidence of nonalcoholic steatohepatitis (NASH) on routine screening with liver biopsies. NASH can progress to cirrhosis and liver failure. Thus, current guidelines indicate that noninvasive liver scores (ie, FIB-4) should be calculated to assess this risk. This patient has intermediate risk for nonalcoholic fatty liver disease (NAFLD) and thus should be referred for imaging. Liver elastography (Answer C) provides assessment of liver stiffness; a high score indicates scarring and should prompt a referral to a hepatologist.

Liver ultrasonography (Answer A) is not specific for detecting liver fibrosis and would not be helpful in assessing for NASH risk.

Weight loss (Answer D) is certainly indicated for this patient and could reduce her risk for NAFLD, but further workup for NAFLD is indicated. Data do not support that the DASH diet would be indicated in this scenario.

Caffeine use and vitamin E (Answer B) may be helpful in persons without diabetes, but data for their usefulness in patients with type 2 diabetes do not currently exist.

EDUCATIONAL OBJECTIVE

Screen for nonalcoholic fatty liver disease.

REFERENCE(S)

Cusi K, Isaacs S, Barb D, et al. American Association of Clinical Endocrinology clinical practice guideline for the diagnosis and management of nonalcoholic fatty liver disease in primary care and endocrinology clinical settings: co-sponsored by the American Association for the Study of Liver Diseases (AASLD). *Endocr Pract.* 2022;28(5):528-562. PMID: 35569886

Lomonaco R, Godinez Leiva E, Bril F, et al. Advanced liver fibrosis is common in patients with type 2 diabetes followed in the outpatient setting: the need for systematic screening. *Diabetes Care.* 2021;44(2):399-406. PMID: 33355256

7 ANSWER: B) Dehydration, depletion of potassium, and elevated uric acid levels

The protein-sparing modified fast is a type of very low-calorie diet with high protein content and simultaneous restriction of carbohydrate and fat. It was developed in the 1970s, and since then, various permutations have been used in weight loss and health care clinics worldwide. The protein-sparing modified fast is a medically supervised diet that provides fewer than 800 kcal daily during an initial intensive phase of about 6 months, followed by the gradual reintroduction of calories during a refeeding phase of about 6 to 8 weeks. The meal plan is conducive to weight loss in patients with type 2 diabetes and results in reduced glucose parameters, improved insulin sensitivity, and lower triglyceride concentrations, and lower blood pressure (thus, Answers C and D are incorrect).

Refeeding of carbohydrates (Answer A) is incorrect because this is associated with weight gain, not weight loss. Proper counseling is required regarding the amount of carbohydrate refeeding that is required to maintain weight loss after being on ketogenic meal plans.

However, due to glycogen breakdown, there is increased osmotic diuresis, which can result in dehydration (Answer B). Elevation of uric acid occurs due to high protein intake, so this meal plan is not advised in patients with active gout.

EDUCATIONAL OBJECTIVE

Outcomes of the protein-sparing modified fast for weight loss.

REFERENCE(S)

Chang J, Kashyap SR. The protein-sparing modified fast for obese patients with type 2 diabetes: what to expect. *Cleve Clin J Med.* 2014;81(9):557-565. PMID: 25183847

Pfoh ER, Lowenthal G, Jeffers L, et al. The effect of starting the protein-sparing modified fast on weight change over 5 years. *J Gen Intern Med.* 2020;35(3):704-710. PMID: 31916212

8 ANSWER: C) Gastric bypass

This patient has class 3 obesity complicated by type 2 diabetes, nonalcoholic fatty liver disease (NAFLD), and other comorbidities worsened by obesity. Data suggest that gastric bypass (Answer C) would provide the most benefit in terms of weight loss of 25% to 30% and resolution of type 2 diabetes.

There is insufficient evidence to support use of endoscopic balloon (Answer B) or laparoscopic banding (Answer D), which elicits 15% weight loss and less benefit regarding control of type 2 diabetes and NAFLD.

Sleeve gastrectomy (Answer E) provides 20% to 25% weight loss and is inferior to gastric bypass in terms of improved metabolic control.

EDUCATIONAL OBJECTIVE

Recommend gastric bypass surgery for a patient with class 3 obesity, type 2 diabetes, and nonalcoholic fatty liver disease.

REFERENCE(S)

Mechanick JI, Apovian C, Brethauer S, et al. Clinical practice guidelines for the perioperative nutrition, metabolic, and nonsurgical support of patients undergoing bariatric procedures – 2019 update: cosponsored by American Association of Clinical Endocrinologists/American College of Endocrinology, The Obesity Society, American society for Metabolic & Bariatric Surgery, Obesity Medicine Association, and American Society of Anesthesiologists – executive summary. *Endocr Pract.* 2019;25(12):1346-1359. PMID: 31682518

Cummings DE, Rubino F. Metabolic surgery for the treatment of type 2 diabetes in obese individuals. *Diabetologia.* 2018;61(2):257-264. PMID: 29224190

9 ANSWER: A) Add alirocumab

PCSK9 inhibitors (evolocumab and alirocumab [Answer A]) are a new class of medications used to significantly lower LDL cholesterol and reduce cardiovascular disease risk. They are monoclonal antibodies that target and degrade the PCSK9 protein. PCSK9 circulates in the blood and alters the liver's handling of LDL cholesterol. Both evolocumab and alirocumab are US FDA approved for clinical atherosclerotic cardiovascular disease and heterozygous familial hyperlipidemia. PCSK9 inhibitors have been studied in statin-intolerant patients (GAUSS-1 and GAUSS-2 studies), but statin intolerance alone is not currently an approved indication in the absence of clinical atherosclerotic cardiovascular disease or familial hyperlipidemia. Clinical trials have shown that LDL cholesterol is lowered approximately 60% by evolocumab and 55% to 60% by alirocumab, which would most likely reduce this patient's LDL-cholesterol concentration below 100 mg/dL (<2.59 mmol/L). The FOURIER trial showed that evolocumab reduced LDL cholesterol 59% in patients with known coronary disease and a baseline LDL-cholesterol level of 70 mg/dL or greater (≥1.81 mmol/L) who were taking a statin compared with placebo and lowered cardiovascular event rates by 15% over 3 years (hazard ratio, 0.85; 95% CI, 0.79-0.92). Additionally, the study indicated there was added benefit at lower LDL-cholesterol levels than previously targeted.

In the ODYSSEY trial of alirocumab vs placebo after acute coronary syndrome, LDL cholesterol was lowered in the alirocumab group by 54.7% compared with LDL cholesterol in the placebo group at 48 months (mean LDL-cholesterol concentration of 53.3 mg/dL vs 101.4 mg/dL, respectively). Risk of a major cardiovascular event was lowered by 15% (hazard ratio, 0.85; 95% CI, 0.78-0.93; $P = .0003$) (preliminary results released at the American College of Cardiology – 67th Scientific Sessions, March 2010).

The newer data regarding LDL-cholesterol lowering and associated decreased cardiovascular disease risk will most likely shift the focus back to absolute LDL-cholesterol levels from the general group targets recommended in the 2013 American College of Cardiology/American Heart Association Cholesterol-Lowering Guidelines.

Niacin has been shown to lower LDL cholesterol in some trials in men, but it may also worsen this patient's glycemic control. Thus, increasing the dosage (Answer C) is incorrect.

Fenofibrate (Answer B) has not been shown to decrease cardiovascular disease event rates.

Lipopheresis (Answer E) has been used to clear LDL particles and reduce cardiovascular disease risk in some patients with heterozygous and homozygous familial hyperlipidemia, but it is invasive, not widely available, and would be an option only if all medications failed.

Increasing the pravastatin dosage to 80 mg daily (Answer D) would not effectively lower the LDL cholesterol to target in this case.

EDUCATIONAL OBJECTIVE

Explain the indications for using PCSK9 inhibitors to treat patients with hyperlipidemia.

REFERENCE(S)

Schwartz GG, Steg PG, Szarek M, et al; ODYSSEY OUTCOMES Committees and Investigators. Alirocumab and cardiovascular outcomes after acute coronary syndrome. *N Engl J Med.* 2018;379(22):2097-2107. PMID: 30403574

Sabatine MS, Giugliano RP, Keech AC, et al; FOURIER Steering Committee and Investigators. Evolocumab and clinical outcomes in patients with cardiovascular disease. *N Engl J Med.* 2017;376(18):1713-1722. PMID: 28304224

Sabatine MS, Giugliano RP, Wiviott SD, et al; Open-Label Study of Long-Term Evaluation against LDL Cholesterol (OSLER) Investigators. Efficacy and safety of evolocumab in reducing lipids and cardiovascular events. *N Engl J Med.* 2015;372(16):1500-1509. PMID: 25773607

Ajufo E, Rader DJ. Recent advances in the pharmacological management of hypercholesterolemia. *Lancet Diabetes Endocrinol.* 2016;4(5):436-446. PMID: 27012540

Steg PG, et al. Joint ACC/JACC Late-Breaking Clinical Trials. Presented at: American College of Cardiology Scientific Session; March 10-12, 2018; Orlando, FL.

10 ANSWER: D) Oral contraceptive pill use

Hypertriglyceridemia has a number of causes, including genetic pathogenic variants, medications, and other medical conditions. The described patient has both high triglycerides and high HDL-cholesterol levels. This can be observed in the setting of alcohol use or estrogen use. The vignette history lists oral contraceptive pills (Answer D) as a medication, and this is the most likely culprit. The frank hypertriglyceridemia that this patient exhibits can occur in someone with an underlying predisposition to hypertriglyceridemia who then begins oral estrogens. This typically does not occur with transdermal estrogens, but it can be associated with oral estrogens given for postmenopausal symptoms.

Lipoprotein lipase is the key enzyme in the catabolism of circulating triglyceride-rich lipoproteins VLDL and chylomicrons. Apolipoprotein C2 is a cofactor for lipoprotein lipase, so both lipoprotein lipase deficiency (Answer C) and apolipoprotein C2 deficiency (Answer A) can cause marked hypertriglyceridemia. Triglyceride levels in affected individuals are typically greater than 1000 mg/dL (>11.30 mmol/L) and can be as high as 2000 to 3000 mg/dL (22.60-33.90 mmol/L).

The enzyme cholesteryl ester transfer protein (CETP) exchanges cholesterol esters in HDL for triglyceride in VLDL and chylomicrons, resulting in increased clearance of HDL cholesterol. This process is increased when triglyceride levels are high. This explains the common association between increased triglyceride levels and decreased HDL-cholesterol levels. CETP deficiency (Answer B) is associated with very high HDL-cholesterol levels but not hypertriglyceridemia. Lipoprotein lipase deficiency and apolipoprotein C2 deficiency cause high triglyceride levels, but because of CETP, HDL-cholesterol levels are typically low.

Soy isoflavones (Answer E) do not have a clinical effect on cholesterol, including HDL cholesterol.

EDUCATIONAL OBJECTIVE

Identify the most likely cause of high triglycerides in a patient with high HDL-cholesterol levels.

REFERENCE(S)

Baksu B, Davas I, Agar E, Akyol A, Uluocak A. Do different delivery systems of estrogen therapy influence serum lipids differently in surgically menopausal women? *J Obstet Gynaecol Res.* 2007;33(3):346-352. PMID: 17578365

Brien SE, Ronksley PE, Turner BJ, Mukamal KJ, Ghali WA. Effect of alcohol consumption on biological markers associated with risk of coronary heart disease: systematic review and meta-analysis of interventional studies. *BMJ.* 2011;342:d636. PMID: 21343206

11 ANSWER: B) At increased risk because his waist circumference is greater than 35.4 in (>90 cm)

The most recent American Heart Association guidelines on the evaluation and management of obesity published in 2013 continue to advise the same BMI and waist circumference cut-points for defining overweight and obesity in white patients. However, it has become increasingly clear that these cut-points may not be appropriate for individuals from all ethnic backgrounds. In particular, the risk of diabetes is higher in persons with what would be considered modest increases in weight if they come from south Asia. The National Institute for Health Care Excellence in the United Kingdom acknowledges the increased risk for diabetes and other chronic conditions in individuals from India by using a cut-point BMI value greater than 23 kg/m^2 and a cut-point BMI value greater than 27.5 kg/m^2 for identifying those at high risk of chronic conditions (thus, Answer D is incorrect). The more widely used criteria for increased central adiposity come from the International Diabetes Federation. They suggest that cut-point waist circumference values of greater than 35.4 in (>90 cm) in men and greater than 31.5 in (80 cm) in women be used in individuals from south Asia to identify those at increased risk of metabolic diseases (thus, Answer B is correct and Answers A and E are incorrect). While the waist-to-hip ratio has been used in many studies to assess metabolic risk, it has not been widely accepted as the best way to assess regional fat distribution for purposes of risk stratification in clinical practice (thus, Answer C is incorrect).

EDUCATIONAL OBJECTIVE

Identify the ethnic differences in the relationships among weight, waist circumference, and risk for metabolic diseases.

REFERENCE(S)

International Diabetes Federation. The IDF consensus worldwide definition of the metabolic syndrome. Available at: https://www.idf.org/e-library/consensus-statements/60-idfconsensus-worldwide-definitionof-the-metabolic-syndrome.html. Accessed for verification May 2023.

National Institute for Health and Care Excellence. Obesity: identification, assessment and management. Available at: https://www.nice.org.uk/guidance/CG189. Accessed for verification May 2023.

12 ANSWER: A) Avoid alcohol

The changes in circulating triglyceride levels due to alcohol intake are sometimes dramatic. This college student most likely has underlying hypertriglyceridemia that is exacerbated by alcohol. In some patients, however, triglyceride levels are normalized without drugs. In this situation, switching to nonalcoholic beer is often the single most impactful diet change. Alcohol has several effects on liver triglyceride metabolism, including reducing fatty acid oxidation and increasing de novo triglyceride production. Thus, avoiding alcohol (Answer A) is the most important immediate lifestyle change. Several other dietary changes also reduce triglyceride levels, but the impact would probably be less dramatic than that due to elimination of alcohol.

Reducing intake of foods with simple sugars (sugar, bread, rice, potatoes, and pasta) (Answer D) and high-fat foods should lead to some triglyceride reduction.

Omega-3 fatty acids reduce triglycerides, and fruit juice is a source of free sugars (thus, Answers B and E are incorrect).

Although reducing consumption of high-fat foods, such as fried foods (Answer C), is an important dietary change, it is not the most likely culprit here.

Losing weight and exercising more are important lifestyle changes, but their effects on this patient's hypertriglyceridemia are likely to be less acute than those of avoiding alcohol.

EDUCATIONAL OBJECTIVE

Recommend avoidance of alcohol as an important lifestyle modification in a patient with severe hypertriglyceridemia.

REFERENCE(S)

Pownall HJ. Alcohol: lipid metabolism and cardioprotection. *Curr Atheroscler Rep.* 2002;4(2):107-112. PMID: 11822973

Goldberg IJ, Mosca L, Piano MR, Fisher EA. AHA Science Advisory. Wine and your heart: a science advisory for healthcare professionals from the Nutrition Committee, Council on Epidemiology and Prevention, and Council on Cardiovascular Nursing of the American Heart Association. *Stroke.* 2001;32(2):591-594. PMID: 11157206

13 ANSWER: D) Melanocortin 4 receptor (*MC4R*)

Although knowledge of the monogenic forms of severe childhood obesity is most relevant for pediatric endocrinologists, adult endocrinologists will on occasion encounter a patient with one of these syndromes, and genetic forms of obesity provide insights into important pathways that regulate body weight.

The most common monogenic form of early-onset obesity is caused by pathogenic variants in the gene than encodes the melanocortin 4 receptor (*MC4R*) (Answer D). The melanocortin 4 receptor is involved in hypothalamic signaling along the neural pathway that responds to leptin. The hypothalamus has a central role in the regulation of food intake. Leptin and insulin act on proopiomelanocortin (POMC) neurons in the arcuate nucleus to increase the expression and release of α-melanocyte–stimulating hormone, which then binds to melanocortin 4 receptors on postsynaptic cells to reduce food intake. A pathogenic variant that impairs receptor function would lead to the loss of satiety and unblocked hunger leading to hyperphagia. These patients present with childhood obesity.

Individuals who have pathogenic variants in the genes encoding leptin (Answer B) or the leptin receptor (Answer C) have hypothalamic hypogonadism and subtle impairments in GH and immune function.

A pathogenic variant in the gene encoding proopiomelanocortin (*POMC*) (Answer E) causes a rare form of early-onset, childhood obesity due to hyperphagia. POMC has an important role in regulating satiety and energy expenditure. POMC is cleaved into melanocyte-stimulating hormone and ACTH, which is necessary for normal adrenal function. Affected patients present with childhood obesity, as well as adrenal insufficiency, which may present with hypoglycemia in the neonatal period. The adrenal insufficiency is treated with glucocorticoid replacement, but the obesity is difficult to treatment. Two affected individuals were treated with setmelanotide, a melanocortin 4 receptor agonist that reduced hunger and induced weight loss of 44 to 110 lb (20-50 kg) over 12 to 42 weeks.

Pathogenic variants in the fat mass and obesity-associated protein gene (*FTO*) (Answer A) are most commonly associated with generalized obesity, not early childhood-onset obesity. The *FTO* gene, in addition to variants in more than 90 other genes, collectively explains less than 5% of the variation in BMI.

EDUCATIONAL OBJECTIVE

Identify monogenic forms of early-onset childhood obesity.

REFERENCE(S)

Kuhnen P, Clement K, Wiegand S, et al. Proopiomelanocortin deficiency treated with a melanocortin-4 receptor agonist. *N Engl J Med.* 2016;375(3):240-246. PMID: 27468060

Farooqi S, O'Rahilly S. Genetics of obesity in humans. *Endocr Rev.* 2006;27(7):710-718. PMID: 17122358

Ranadive SA, Vaisse C. Lessons from extreme human obesity: monogenic disorders. *Endocrinol Metab Clin North Am.* 2008;37(3):733-751. PMID: 18775361

Schwartz MW, Woods SC, Porte D Jr, Seeley RJ, Baskin DG. Central nervous system control of food intake. *Nature.* 2000;404(6778):661-671. PMID: 10766253

14 ANSWER: E) Tirzepatide

Obesity is an independent risk factor for cardiovascular disease, and it can adversely affect other risk factors for cardiovascular disease, including hypertension, type 2 diabetes, and dyslipidemia. Weight loss can lower cardiovascular risk for both primary and secondary prevention. Care must be taken when selecting a weight-loss medication for use in patients with a recent coronary heart disease event or who are at risk for tachyarrhythmias, as most of the currently approved weight-loss medications can affect blood pressure and heart rate. Furthermore, resting tachycardia is commonly present in patients with obesity, even in the absence of known heart disease.

Tirzepatide (Answer E) is an antidiabetes medication and a GLP-1 receptor agonist that resulted in superior glucose and weight management over 40 weeks in the SURPASS-1 trial of monotherapy in patients with type 2 diabetes. More than half of the patients achieved a hemoglobin A_{1c} value less than 5.7% (<39 mmol/mol) with weight loss of more than 11%. Of the answer options, tirzepatide is the most effective agent for glucose and body weight control. Other GLP-1 receptor agonists, including liraglutide (Answer A), are recognized as being "cardioprotective" with multiple formulations being associated with lower risk of cardiovascular events, which makes liraglutide an alternative choice in this patient. GLP-1 receptor agonists are known to increase resting heart rate, although they are not associated with increased blood pressure. Liraglutide, 3.0 mg daily, is associated with an average 2 to 3 beats/min increase in heart rate. A proportion of patients may experience an increase in resting heart rate of greater than 10 beats/min (34% compared with 19% on placebo) or greater than 20 beats/min (5% compared with 2% on placebo), but only 0.9% develop a resting heart rate higher than 100 beats/min compared with 0.3% on placebo.

Phentermine (Answer B) is a sympathomimetic agent, or stimulant, that suppresses appetite and is known to increase both blood pressure and heart rate and would thus be contraindicated in this patient. Phentermine/topiramate (Answer D) is a combination medication containing phentermine, which makes it a poor choice for weight loss in this patient.

Naltrexone/bupropion (Answer B) is contraindicated in patients with uncontrolled hypertension.

EDUCATIONAL OBJECTIVE

Select weight-loss medications for a patient with a history of cardiovascular disease and arrhythmic potential.

REFERENCE(S)

Frias JP, Nauck MA, Van J, et al. Efficacy and safety of LY3298176, a novel dual GIP and GLP-1 receptor agonist, in patients with type 2 diabetes: a randomised, placebo-controlled and active comparator-controlled phase 2 trial. *Lancet.* 2018;392(10160):2180-2193. PMID: 30293770

Apovian CM, Aronne LJ, Bessesen DH, et al; Endocrine Society. Pharmacological management of obesity: an Endocrine Society clinical practice guideline. *J Clin Endocrinol Metab.* 2015;100(2):342-362. PMID: 25590212

Yanovski SZ, Yanovski JA. Long-term drug treatment for obesity: a systematic and clinical review. *JAMA.* 2014;311(1):74-86. PMID: 24231879

Pi-Sunyer X, Astrup A, Fujioka K, et al; SCALE Obesity and Prediabetes NN8022-1839 Study Group. A randomized, controlled trial of 3.0 mg of liraglutide in weight management. *N Engl J Med.* 2015;373(1):11-22. PMID: 26132939

15 ANSWER: B) Atorvastatin

Many commonly prescribed medications are associated with weight gain. Of the available antihypertensive medications, β-adrenergic blockers (Answer A) are associated with weight gain, while ACE inhibitors, angiotensin receptor blockers, calcium-channel blockers, and diuretics are not.

Many diabetes medications are associated with weight gain, up to 10 to 20 lb (4.5-9.1 kg) in the first 6 to 12 months, including the anabolic hormone insulin, insulin secretagogues (eg, sulfonylureas (Answer E), meglitinides), and thiazolidinediones.

Metformin is weight neutral in general, although it is associated with mild weight loss in some patients.

DPP-4 inhibitors and α-glucosidase inhibitors are weight neutral, and GLP-1 receptor agonists promote weight loss in addition to blood glucose control.

SGLT-2 inhibitors are associated with mild weight loss in the context of glucosuria and water loss. More recently, antihistamines (Answer C) have been recognized as weight promoting. The more potent the antihistamine, the more likely the patient is to gain weight with long-term use. H1-antihistamines such as cetirizine are the most likely to be associated with weight gain.

Inhaled glucocorticoids (Answer D) are associated with weight gain.

Other medication classes that can lead to weight gain include glucocorticoids, antidepressants, antipsychotic agents, and hormonal contraceptives.

Statins (Answer B) are not associated with significant weight gain.

EDUCATIONAL OBJECTIVE

Identify weight-promoting and weight-neutral medications among commonly prescribed medications for adults.

REFERENCE(S)

Apovian CM, Aronne LJ, Bessesen DH, et al; Endocrine Society. Pharmacological management of obesity: an Endocrine Society clinical practice guideline. *J Clin Endocrinol Metab.* 2015;100(2):342-362. PMID: 25590212

16 ANSWER: B) Add evolocumab

Given that this patient had progressive coronary disease while on high-intensity statin therapy (atorvastatin, 80 mg daily), with an LDL-cholesterol concentration of 109 mg/dL (2.82 mmol/L), he would benefit from the addition of a PCSK9 inhibitor (Answer B) to target an LDL-cholesterol concentration less than 70 mg/dL (<1.81 mmol/L). Thus, advising no further treatment (Answer E) is incorrect. PCSK9 is a hepatic-produced protein that is secreted, binds to cell-surface LDL receptors, and mediates their intracellular degradation. Antibodies to PCSK9 prevent this and lead to increased LDL-receptor levels, which in turn reduce circulating LDL-cholesterol levels. Up-regulation of LDL receptors is also the mechanism for statin-mediating LDL-cholesterol reductions because inhibition of de novo cholesterol biosynthesis increases sterol-responsive element–binding protein (SREBP)–mediated transcription of the LDL receptor. Oligonucleotide inhibition of apolipoprotein B and inhibition of microsomal triglyceride transfer protein are therapies recently approved for treatment of the rare homozygous form of familial hypercholesterolemia.

Current indications for PCSK9 inhibitors include heterozygous familial hyperlipidemia and clinical atherosclerotic cardiovascular disease such as acute coronary syndromes, stable and unstable angina, myocardial infarction, peripheral vascular disease, history of coronary or other arterial revascularization, transient ischemic attack, and stroke for secondary prevention.

Icosapent ethyl (Answer C) is a purified n-3 fatty acid that lowers triglycerides and the risk of cardiovascular events in studies of individuals with coronary disease who have optimized their LDL-cholesterol levels to less than 100 mg/dL (<2.59 mmol/L) but have residually elevated triglycerides between 135 and 499 mg/dL (1.53-5.64 mmol/L), commonly with type 2 diabetes. This patient does have type 2 diabetes, but his triglycerides are not persistently elevated. Also, given that his LDL cholesterol is not yet optimized, the addition of a PCSK9 inhibitor is the best next treatment, not icosapent ethyl.

Although bempedoic acid (Answer A) is associated with modest LDL-cholesterol reduction, it would not be as effective as evolocumab in lowering this patient's cardiovascular risk.

Changing atorvastatin to rosuvastatin (Answer D) would not significantly lower his LDL cholesterol or alter his cardiovascular risk as compared with the lipid-lowering effect of evolocumab.

EDUCATIONAL OBJECTIVE

List the indications for addition of PCSK9 inhibitors to statin therapy to reduce risk of cardiovascular disease events.

REFERENCE(S)

Sabatine MS, Giugliano RP, Keech AC, et al; FOURIER Steering Committee and Investigators. Evolocumab and clinical outcomes in patients with cardiovascular disease. *N Engl J Med.* 2017;376(18):1713-1722. PMID: 28304224

Sabatine MS, Giugliano RP, Wiviott SD, et al; Open-Label Study of Long-Term Evaluation against LDL Cholesterol (OSLER) Investigators. Efficacy and safety of evolocumab in reducing lipids and cardiovascular events. *N Engl J Med.* 2015;372(16):1500-1509. PMID: 25773607

Ajufo E, Rader DJ. Recent advances in the pharmacological management of hypercholesterolaemia. *Lancet Diabetes Endocrinol.* 2016;4(5):436-446. PMID: 27012540

17 ANSWER: D) Hypobetalipoproteinemia

This patient has hypobetalipoproteinemia (Answer D) with a reduction in production of both LDL (cholesterol) and VLDL (triglyceride). This condition is most often due to a defect in liver production of apolipoprotein B–containing lipoproteins because of defective production of apolipoprotein B. With apolipoprotein B, a defective protein is associated with lower than one-half normal LDL-cholesterol levels. In hypobetalipoproteinemia, inability to efficiently secrete lipoproteins from the liver can lead to nonalcoholic fatty liver disease.

Hypobetalipoproteinemia should be distinguished from abetalipoproteinemia (Answer A), a rare autosomal recessive disorder caused by a pathogenic variant in the gene encoding the microsomal transfer protein causing low levels of apolipoproteins used in the synthesis and export of chylomicrons and VLDL. LDL-cholesterol and triglyceride levels are much lower in this setting, and affected patients develop deficiencies of fat-soluble vitamins with neurologic symptoms, including weakness and balance problems as adults. This profile can also be the result of drugs that inhibit microsomal triglyceride transfer protein or antisense therapies to reduce apolipoprotein B secretion.

Dysbetalipoproteinemia (Answer B) is an autosomal recessive disorder associated with an *APOE*E2/APOE*E2* genotype and clinically characterized by palmar xanthomas with roughly equal and significant elevations in both total cholesterol and triglycerides, not low levels. This is the same genetic locus that is associated with risk for Alzheimer disease (*APOE*E4/APOE*E4* genotype).

Persons with hypoalphalipoproteinemia (Answer C), also known as apolipoproteinemia A1 deficiency, lack a structural protein associated with HDL and consequently have very low HDL-cholesterol levels but the other lipid fractions are not as low as in this vignette.

EDUCATIONAL OBJECTIVE

Identify conditions characterized by very low cholesterol levels and associated health risks.

REFERENCE(S)

Musunuru K, Pirruccello JP, Do R, et al. Exome sequencing, ANGPTL3 mutations, and familial combined hypolipidemia. *N Engl J Med.* 2010;363(23):2220-2227. PMID: 20942659

Cuchel M, Bloedon LT, Szapary PO, et al. Inhibition of microsomal triglyceride transfer protein in familial hypercholesterolemia. *N Engl J Med.* 2007;356(2):148-156. PMID: 17215532

Tanoli T, Yue P, Yablonskiy D, Schonfeld G. Fatty liver in familial hypobetalipoproteinemia: roles of the APOB defects, intra-abdominal adipose tissue, and insulin sensitivity. *J Lipid Res.* 2004;45(5):941-947. PMID: 14967820

Mahley RW, Huang Y, Rall SC Jr. Pathogenesis of type III hyperlipoproteinemia (dysbetalipoproteinemia). Questions, quandaries, and paradoxes. *J Lipid Res.* 1999;40(11):1933-1949. PMID: 10552997

18 ANSWER: C) Apolipoprotein *E2/E2*

The apolipoprotein *E2/E2* phenotype (Answer C) is present in patients with dysbetalipoproteinemia, which is also referred to as type III hyperlipidemia. Classic skin manifestations include tuberoeruptive lesions at the elbows and palmar xanthomas as observed in this patient. The apolipoprotein *E2/E2* phenotype occurs in about 1 per 100 persons, but the development of characteristic dyslipidemia is infrequent and usually appears later in life due to acquired medical conditions such as hypothyroidism, obesity, diabetes mellitus, or estrogen replacement therapy. The lipoprotein that accumulates is a remnant of triglyceride metabolism (beta VLDL) and is associated with an increased risk of atherosclerotic vascular disease. Although the calculated LDL-cholesterol level is increased in this patient, it is spurious due to accumulation of the beta VLDL. This remnant is cholesterol ester–enriched and has "balanced" concentrations of cholesterol and triglyceride, which accounts for the "near-equal" serum cholesterol and triglyceride levels.

ABCA1 is a protein involved in moving cholesterol from peripheral tissues onto HDL particles. Deficiency of this protein results in the condition known as Tangier disease, characterized by very low HDL-cholesterol levels (<20 mg/dL [<0.52 mmol/L]), and the classic physical examination finding of orange tonsils, which this patient does not have. Thus, ABCA1 deficiency (Answer A) is incorrect.

LDL-receptor deficiency (Answer D) results in the condition known as familial hyperlipidemia. Patients with familial hyperlipidemia have very high LDL-cholesterol levels but not triglycerides unless there is an additional defect. They present with tendinous xanthomas and premature coronary artery disease. Lipoprotein lipase is an enzyme that acts in the vascular bed to hydrolyze triglycerides.

Lipoprotein lipase deficiency (Answer E) results in very high triglyceride levels (>1000 mg/dL [>11.30 mmol/L]), which this patient does not have.

Apolipoprotein CII is a cofactor for lipoprotein lipase. Deficiency of apolipoprotein CII (Answer B) results in marked hypertriglyceridemia such as that seen in lipoprotein lipase deficiency, typically greater than 1000 mg/dL (>11.30 mmol/L).

EDUCATIONAL OBJECTIVE

Identify the clinical features of dysbetalipoproteinemia.

REFERENCE(S)

Garg A, Simha V. Update of dyslipidemia. *J Clin Endocrinol Metab.* 2007;92(5):1581-1589. PMID: 17483372

Walden CC, Hegele RA. Apolipoprotein E in hyperlipidemia. *Ann Intern Med.* 1994;120(12):1026-1036. PMID: 8185134

Marais AD, Solomon GA, Blom DJ. Dysbetalipoproteinaemia: a mixed hyperlipidaemia of remnant lipoproteins due to mutations in apolipoprotein E. *Crit Rev Clin Lab Sci.* 2014;51(1):46-62. PMID: 24405372

19 ANSWER: B) Accumulation of lipoprotein X

Primary biliary cirrhosis is a progressive liver disease that most commonly presents in older women and can be associated with marked elevation of serum lipid levels. Elevated total cholesterol levels in these patients are most often due to the presence of an abnormal LDL-like particle named lipoprotein X (Answer B). Lipoprotein X is made up in part by biliary lipids that are not being excreted by the liver. Several clinical series do not show an increased risk of coronary artery disease in these patients, despite high levels of what would be considered LDL cholesterol if the Friedewald formula were used to estimate LDL-cholesterol levels. Individuals with high levels of lipoprotein X can develop coronary artery disease, and they do have a reduction in cholesterol levels with statins, but they just do not appear to have a degree of risk for coronary artery disease that would be expected given the high level of "LDL-like" lipoprotein particles.

Lecithin-cholesterol acyltransferase (LCAT) is the enzyme that converts free cholesterol to cholesterol esters, thereby trapping the cholesterol in HDL to be taken to the liver. LCAT deficiency (Answer D) is a genetic disorder that is associated with very low levels of HDL cholesterol, hemolytic anemia, corneal opacities, renal insufficiency, and, uncommonly, atherosclerosis. While LCAT deficiency may be part of the pathogenesis of lipoprotein X production, it is not the only mechanism at work.

Lipoprotein (a) (Answer A) is an LDL particle that has apolipoprotein (a) covalently attached to apolipoprotein B, which is the structural backbone of LDL. It is not associated with primary biliary cirrhosis.

Ursodeoxycholic acid treatment (Answer C) does not worsen serum lipids in patients with primary biliary cirrhosis; in fact, data suggest that cholesterol levels fall with the use of this medication. Liver disease is a secondary cause of hyperlipidemia that should routinely be screened for when caring for a patient with hyperlipidemia.

Increased production of apolipoprotein B is the underlying cause of hyperlipidemia in familial combined hyperlipidemia. However, increased production of apolipoprotein B (Answer E) is not typical in primary biliary cirrhosis and would not be expected to increase total cholesterol levels to the degree seen in this patient.

EDUCATIONAL OBJECTIVE

Identify the lipid abnormalities associated with primary biliary cirrhosis.

REFERENCE(S)

Sorokin A, Brown JL, Thompson PD. Primary biliary cirrhosis, hyperlipidemia, and atherosclerotic risk: a systematic review. *Atherosclerosis.* 2007;194(2):293-299. PMID: 17240380

Longo M, Crosignani A, Battezzati PM, et al. Hyperlipidaemic state and cardiovascular risk in primary biliary cirrhosis. *Gut.* 2002;51(2):265-269. PMID: 12117892

20 ANSWER: D) Switch metoprolol to amlodipine

Patients with collagen-vascular disease can develop severe hyperlipidemias. On occasion, these are due to the production of antibodies that can inhibit lipoprotein lipase or heparin (and lipase binding to endothelium). Antibodies can also be directed to apolipoproteins: antibodies to apolipoprotein B lead to hypobetalipoproteinemia, and antibodies to apolipoprotein AI lead to low HDL-cholesterol levels. Several medications in this setting, as well as in patients without collagen-vascular disease, can exacerbate hypertriglyceridemia. One such class of medications is β-adrenergic blockers. Thus, substituting a calcium-channel blocker for metoprolol (Answer D) is correct.

Changing from one steroid to another (Answer E) should not affect the hypertriglyceridemia.

Neither infliximab nor lisinopril affects triglyceride levels (thus, Answers A and C are incorrect).

Apremilast (Answer C) is a treatment for plaque psoriasis, not lupus.

Although thiazide diuretics increase triglycerides, so does chlorthalidone (Answer B).

EDUCATIONAL OBJECTIVE

Advise patients on medications, such as β-adrenergic blockers, that increase triglyceride levels.

REFERENCE(S)

Stone NJ. Secondary causes of hyperlipidemia. *Med Clin North Am.* 1994;78(1):117-141. PMID: 8283927

Dinu AR, Merrill JT, Shen C, Antonov IV, Myones BL, Lahita RG. Frequency of antibodies to the cholesterol transport protein apolipoprotein A1 in patients with SLE. *Lupus.* 1998;7(5):355-360. PMID: 9696140

21 ANSWER: B) Cholesterol ester transfer protein (CETP) deficiency

HDL-cholesterol levels are highly genetically determined. Deficiencies of both cholesterol ester transfer protein (CETP) and hepatic lipase lead to increased plasma HDL cholesterol. CETP deficiency is most commonly seen in patients of Japanese ancestry (thus, Answer B is the most likely explanation). The protective value of this very high HDL cholesterol is unclear; however, these patients do not have premature disease. Pharmacologic inhibition of CETP is being studied as a method to raise HDL cholesterol, and these inhibitors also reduce plasma LDL cholesterol and lipoprotein (a). It should be noted that the first generation of these drugs increased blood pressure and, unexpectedly, cardiac events.

Hepatic lipase deficiency (Answer C) is very rare. Aside from increased HDL cholesterol (not usually to this degree), affected patients also have increased cholesterol and triglycerides, suggestive of an accumulation of remnant lipoproteins. Moreover, they have premature coronary artery disease.

The SR-B1 receptor is associated with delivery of HDL cholesterol to the liver, and its deficiency (Answer E) has been rarely reported (not in Asian patients) and is associated with increased HDL cholesterol, although not to this degree. Carriers of pathogenic variants in the gene encoding SR-B1 have higher HDL-cholesterol levels than noncarriers (70.4 mg/dL [1.82 mmol/L] vs 53.4 mg/dL [1.38 mmol/L]).

The other options lead to reduced HDL-cholesterol levels. Lecithin cholesterol acyltransferase (LCAT) is needed to esterify cholesterol and create spherical HDL (thus, Answer D is incorrect). ABCA1 transports cholesterol from hepatocytes and enterocytes to mature, newly formed HDL (thus, Answer A is incorrect).

EDUCATIONAL OBJECTIVE

Describe the metabolic role of enzymes affecting HDL cholesterol.

REFERENCE(S)

Cannon CP, Shah S, Dansky HM, et al; Determining the Efficacy and Tolerability Investigators. Safety of anacetrapib in patients with or at high risk for coronary heart disease. *N Engl J Med.* 2010;363(25):2406-2415. PMID: 21082868

Nicholls SJ, Brewer HB, Kastelein JJ, et al. Effects of the CETP inhibitor evacetrapib administered as monotherapy or in combination with statins on HDL and LDL cholesterol: a randomized controlled trial. *JAMA.* 2011;306(19):2099-2109. PMID: 22089718

Barter PJ, Caulfield M, Eriksson M, et al; ILLUMINATE Investigators. Effects of torcetrapib in patients at high risk for coronary events. *N Engl J Med.* 2007;357(21):2109-2122. PMID: 17984165

Hegele RA, Tu L, Connelly PW. Human hepatic lipase mutations and polymorphisms. *Hum Mutat.* 1992;1(4):320-324. PMID: 1301939

Vergeer M, Korporaal SJ, Franssen R, et al. Genetic variant of the scavenger receptor BI in humans. *N Engl J Med.* 2011;364(2):136-145. PMID: 21226579

22 ANSWER: D) A reduction in energy expended from physical activity and an increase in ghrelin

In epidemiologic studies, shortened sleep time has been associated with weight gain, obesity, and type 2 diabetes. Experimental studies have tried to unravel the mechanisms that underlie this association. Because sleep is a time of reduced energy expenditure, reducing the time spent sleeping could increase total daily energy expenditure. An increase in total daily energy expenditure was in fact found in several studies using whole-room indirect calorimetry to examine the effects of shortened sleep time on energy expenditure. However, shortened sleep time could also reduce spontaneous physical activity, which would result in reduced energy expended in physical activity. Studies examining this hypothesis have come to a variety of conclusions. It is clear, however, that total energy expenditure measured by indirect calorimetry or doubly labeled water either stays the same or increases with shortened sleep time, it does not go down (thus, Answers A and B are incorrect). In addition, a number of studies have shown that shortened sleep time results in an increased drive to eat associated with increases in ghrelin levels (thus, Answer D is correct). Some studies have shown a fall in leptin levels, but others have not (thus, Answer E is incorrect). While cortisol levels and insulin resistance increase with shortened sleep time, Answer C is incorrect because ghrelin levels increase.

EDUCATIONAL OBJECTIVE

List the responses to shortened sleep time that predispose to weight gain.

REFERENCE(S)

Jung CM, Melanson EL, Frydendall EJ, Perreault L, Eckel RH, Wright KP. Energy expenditure during sleep, sleep deprivation and sleep following sleep deprivation in adult humans. *J Physiol.* 2011;589(Pt 1):235-244. PMID: 21059762

Markwald RR, Melanson EL, Smith MR, et al. Impact of insufficient sleep on total daily energy expenditure, food intake, and weight gain. *Proc Natl Acad Sci U S A.* 2013;110(14):5695-5700. PMID: 23479616

Spiegel K, Leproult R, Van Cauter E. Impact of sleep debt on metabolic and endocrine function. *Lancet.* 1999;354(9188):1435-1439. PMID: 10543671

23 ANSWER: B) Corneal arcus

Premature development of corneal arcus (Answer B) (<age 40 years per the Dutch Lipid Criteria for diagnosis of familial hyperlipidemia) is one of the signature signs of familial genetic hypercholesterolemia. The cardinal feature of the disorder on physical examination is tendon xanthoma affecting either the Achilles tendon or

the tendons on the dorsum of the hands. The reason why lipid accumulates in the tendons is not completely understood, but it is thought to be secondary to recurrent inflammation and macrophage recruitment to where the tendon interacts with its overlying sheath. Tendon xanthomas are usually most prominent in the Achilles tendon. Some patients with familial hypercholesterolemia do not have tendon xanthomas but do have premature corneal arcus. In current practice, many patients with heterozygous familial hyperlipidemia do not exhibit these 2 signs, as they have been on lipid-lowering therapy for years before their specific genetic disorder is diagnosed.

Most often, patients with familial hypercholesterolemia have a heterozygous pathogenic variant in the gene encoding the LDL receptor. Defective apolipoprotein B, the ligand for the receptor, and a defect in an intracellular adaptor protein cause a similar phenotype. Persons who are heterozygous have total cholesterol concentrations of 350 to 600 mg/dL (9.06-15.54 mmol/L), LDL-cholesterol concentrations greater than 250 mg/dL (>6.48 mmol/L), premature coronary artery disease, and aortic stenosis.

This patient is being treated with atorvastatin, 80 mg daily; his off-therapy LDL-cholesterol concentration is most likely around 300 mg/dL (7.77 mmol/L). The homozygous form of this disease leads to atherosclerosis before age 20 years (sometimes before age 10 years). Liver transplant is often the treatment. Genetic testing does not alter therapy and is not usually performed.

Lipemia retinalis (Answer D) is the milky appearance of the retina and retinal vessels that accompanies severe hypertriglyceridemia.

Eruptive xanthomas (Answer C) are acne-like papules that are found on extensor surfaces of the arms and on the back and buttocks. They are also a sign of severe hypertriglyceridemia.

Palmar xanthomas (Answer E) are lipid depositions in the creases of the palms that occur with dysbetalipoproteinemia (formerly called type 3 hyperlipoproteinemia).

Arthropathy (Answer A) is not a sign of a dyslipoproteinemia.

EDUCATIONAL OBJECTIVE

Identify physical findings of hyperlipidemias.

REFERENCE(S)

Semenkovich CF, Goldberg IJ. Disorders of lipid metabolism. In: Melmed S, Auchus RJ, Goldfine AB, Koenig RJ, Rosen CJ, eds. *Williams Textbook of Endocrinology.* 14th ed. Elsevier Saunders; 2019:1581-1621.

24 ANSWER: A) Continue atorvastatin and add fenofibrate

This patient has known cardiovascular disease in the context of type 2 diabetes and mixed hyperlipidemia, with both elevated LDL cholesterol and triglycerides. She is at very high risk for another cardiovascular event and would benefit from continuing the statin for cardiovascular risk reduction (thus, Answers E is incorrect). The most common inherited lipid disorder in type 2 diabetes is familial combined hyperlipidemia, which has a very variable clinical phenotype regarding LDL-cholesterol and triglyceride elevations that can shift over time within the same patient. This patient most likely had a triglyceride concentration greater than 1000 mg/dL (>11.3 mmol/L), as she had several episodes of pancreatitis. Her current fasting triglyceride concentration of 760 mg/dL (8.59 mmol/L) while on a statin does put her at risk for pancreatitis. The 2013 American College of Cardiology/American Heart Association Guidelines on the Treatment of Blood Cholesterol to Reduce Atherosclerotic Cardiovascular Risk in Adults recommend treating triglycerides as a secondary target when levels remain above 500 mg/dL (>5.65 mmol/L). She would benefit from lipid-lowering therapy targeted at lowering triglycerides.

Gemfibrozil (Answer B) and fenofibrate (Answer A) effectively lower triglycerides, but gemfibrozil is contraindicated due to concurrent use of a statin because of the increased risk of muscle-related adverse effects, including myositis and rhabdomyolysis. Adding fenofibrate to a statin is the safer choice for additional triglyceride lowering.

Niacin (Answer C) may help to lower triglycerides, but it would also most likely worsen her diabetes and is therefore not the best choice.

Incremental dose elevation of atorvastatin (Answer D) would not be as effective in triglyceride lowering as adding fenofibrate.

EDUCATIONAL OBJECTIVE

Recommend when and how to treat hypertriglyceridemia in patients with cardiovascular disease.

REFERENCE(S)

Stone NJ, Robinson JG, Lichtenstein AH, et al; American College of Cardiology/American Heart Association Task Force on Practice Guidelines. 2013 ACC/AHA guideline on the treatment of blood cholesterol to reduce atherosclerotic cardiovascular risk in adults: a report of the American College of Cardiology/American Heart Association Task Force on Practice Guidelines [published correction appears in *Circulation.* 2014;129(25 Suppl 2):S46-S48]. *Circulation.* 2014;129(25 Suppl 2):S1-S45. PMID: 24222016

Stone NJ, Robinson JG, Lichtenstein AH, et al; 2013 ACC/AHA Cholesterol Guideline Panel. Treatment of blood cholesterol to reduce atherosclerotic cardiovascular disease risk in adults: synopsis of the 2013 American College of Cardiology/American Heart Association cholesterol guideline. *Ann Intern Med.* 2014;160(5):339-343. PMID: 24474185

Berglund L, Brunzell JD, Goldberg AC, et al; Endocrine Society. Evaluation and treatment of hypertriglyceridemia: an Endocrine Society clinical practice guideline. *J Clin Endocrinol Metab.* 2012;97(9):2969-2989. PMID: 22962670

25 ANSWER: C) Fenofibrate therapy

For unknown reasons, peroxisome proliferator–activated receptor (PPAR) α agonists sometimes lead to a marked reduction in HDL cholesterol, as is seen in this patient. This is especially the case when a PPARα drug such as fenofibrate (Answer C) is given to a patient who is treated with a PPARγ agonist (pioglitazone or rosiglitazone); the paradoxical HDL-cholesterol reduction occurs in 1.39% of patients on this drug combination. The correct approach is to stop the fenofibrate; his HDL-cholesterol level will presumably return to baseline.

Problems with HDL production such as lecithin cholesterol acyltransferase deficiency (also known as fish-eye disease) (Answer A) or defective apolipoprotein AI production could lead to similarly low HDL-cholesterol levels; however, HDL-cholesterol concentration would not change significantly over time.

ABCA1 defects are the cause of Tangier disease and low HDL cholesterol. ABCA1 is responsible for allowing cholesterol transport out of cells, including the liver and peripheral macrophages, but it is not inhibited by metformin (Answer D). Impaired diabetes control increases triglycerides and reduces HDL cholesterol, but not to this level.

Statins do not generally reduce HDL cholesterol, although atorvastatin dosages of 40 to 80 mg daily sometimes do, but only by approximately 10% (Answer E).

HDL cholesterol is measured as the residual cholesterol in the blood after precipitation of apolipoprotein B lipoproteins (VLDL and LDL). Although laboratory errors (Answer B) can occur, PPAR agonist–induced HDL-cholesterol reduction is more likely.

EDUCATIONAL OBJECTIVE

Identify causes of hypoalphalipoproteinemia.

REFERENCE(S)

Keidar S, Guttmann H, Stam T, Fishman I, Shapira C. High incidence of reduced plasma HDL cholesterol in diabetic patients treated with rosiglitazone and fibrate. *Pharmacoepidemiol Drug Saf.* 2007;16(11):1192-1194. PMID: 17636555

Semenkovich CF, Goldberg IJ. Disorders of lipid metabolism. In: Melmed S, Auchus RJ, Goldfine AB, Koenig RJ, Rosen CJ, eds. *Williams Textbook of Endocrinology.* 14th ed. Elsevier Saunders; 2019:1581-1621.

Roshan B, Ganda OP, Desilva R, et al. Homozygous lecithin:cholesterol acyltransferase (LCAT) deficiency due to a new loss of function mutation and review of the literature. *J Clin Lipidol.* 2011;5(6):493-499. PMID: 22108153

26 ANSWER: B) Apolipoprotein E genotyping

Increased triglycerides commensurate with increased cholesterol occur in 2 situations: familial combined hyperlipidemia and dysbetalipoproteinemia. The former is due to an increase in both VLDL and LDL and is a relatively common dyslipidemia, especially in patients with diabetes. However, the cholesterol concentration in this patient and her lack of obesity or thyroid disorder suggest that she has a primary genetic abnormality. She has palmar xanthomas and cholesterol and triglyceride levels greater than 600 mg/dL (>15.54 mmol/L and >6.78 mmol/L, respectively) that are approximately equal. This finding occurs in dysbetalipoproteinemia, a disorder that is usually associated with an *APOE*E2/APOE*E2* genotype (thus, Answer B is correct). This molecular defect is autosomal recessive, but it occurs in 1% of the population. However, only 1 in 10,000 patients present with the phenotype of this disease. Therefore, it is assumed that there must be an additional underlying factor that leads to its manifestation.

Apolipoprotein E is needed to clear many lipoprotein particles by the liver, and presumably a high-fat diet leads to large numbers of circulating remnant lipoproteins that are not efficiently cleared (*see figure*). Unlike LDL, the shortened apolipoprotein B_{48} in chylomicrons is unable to serve as a ligand for liver lipoprotein receptors, and remnant lipoproteins produced in the intestine use apolipoprotein E as the primary ligand for receptor-mediated uptake by the liver. As an alternative to genotyping, centrifugation analysis of VLDL particles should show that they are cholesterol enriched. Patients with dysbetalipoproteinemia respond well to fibric acids. Untreated, the disorder is associated with a marked increase in both cardiovascular and peripheral vascular disease. Of note, this is the same genetic locus that is associated with risk for Alzheimer disease (the *APOE*E4/APOE*E4* genotype).

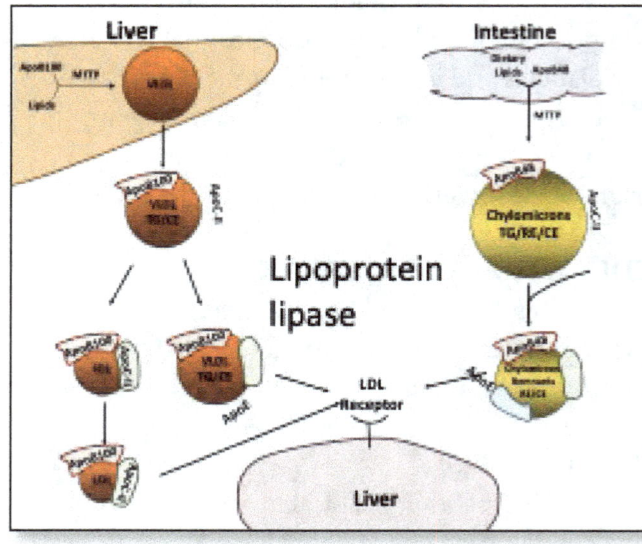

Measurements of apolipoprotein AI (Answer A) would not be useful.

LDL particle size (Answer C) is not useful in this circumstance, although the phenotyping might uncover increased numbers of circulating large remnant lipoproteins.

Lipoprotein(a) is another risk factor for cardiovascular disease, but genotyping (Answer D) is not helpful in making the definitive diagnosis in this patient.

EDUCATIONAL OBJECTIVE

Evaluate mixed hyperlipidemia and diagnose dysbetalipoproteinemia.

REFERENCE(S)

Chahil TJ, Ginsberg HN. Diabetic dyslipidemia. *Endocrinol Metab Clin North Am.* 2006;35(3):491-510. PMID: 16959582

Mahley RW, Huang Y, Rall SC Jr. Pathogenesis of type III hyperlipoproteinemia (dysbetalipoproteinemia). Questions, quandaries, and paradoxes. *J Lipid Res.* 1999;40(11):1933-1949. PMID: 10552997

Berglund L, Brunzell JD, Goldberg AC, et al; Endocrine Society. Evaluation and treatment of hypertriglyceridemia: an Endocrine Society clinical practice guideline. *J Clin Endocrinol Metab.* 2012;97(9):2969-2989. PMID: 22962670

Pituitary Board Review

John D. Carmichael, MD

1 **ANSWER: E) Restart levothyroxine, 125 mcg daily**

TSH values should not be used to guide levothyroxine dosage adjustment in patients with central hypothyroidism. In this case, undetectable TSH reflects this patient's panhypopituitarism and does not indicate overreplacement with levothyroxine. TSH values are also not helpful in determining whether a patient has developed endogenous hypersecretion of thyroid hormones. With a normal free T_4 value and no symptoms to suggest thyrotoxicosis, the decision to decrease the levothyroxine dosage has led to fatigue. Serum free T_4 levels should be used to determine dosing of thyroid hormone replacement, with a goal of keeping the concentration within the upper half of the reference range. Thus, levothyroxine should be restarted at a dosage of 125 mcg daily (Answer E).

Treatment with methimazole (Answer B) is unwarranted because the free T_4 concentration is normal and there is no clinical evidence of thyrotoxicosis.

Similarly, a radioactive iodine uptake and scan (Answer D) is not helpful without evidence of hyperthyroidism.

Measuring T_3 (Answer C) would be more appropriate in the setting of clinical hyperthyroidism to help explain suppression of TSH with normal serum T_4 levels. However, in the setting of hypopituitarism, this explanation for the undetectable TSH is far less likely.

Changing estrogen from an oral formulation to the patch (Answer A) may help with effects on thyroid-binding globulin and reduce interactions with other pituitary hormone replacement. However, the oral estrogen effect of increasing thyroid-binding globulin and total T_4 do not explain the undetectable TSH, and proper replacement of thyroid hormone deficiency is a higher priority.

EDUCATIONAL OBJECTIVE

Identify the correct analyte to monitor for adequate thyroid hormone dosing and educate patients about thyroid hormone replacement in central hypothyroidism.

REFERENCE(S)

Beck-Peccoz P, Rodari G, Giavoli C, Lania A. Central hypothyroidism - a neglected thyroid disorder. *Nat Rev Endocrinol.* 2017;13(10):588-598. PMID: 28549061

Persani L, Bonomi M, Radin R, Beck-Peccoz P. Diagnostic and therapeutic challenges of acquired thyrotropic deficiency. *Ann Endocrinol (Paris).* 2012;73(2):138-140. PMID: 2254199

2 **ANSWER: B) Initiate levothyroxine, 100 mcg daily**

This patient has presented with thyrotroph hyperplasia in response to primary hypothyroidism that began approximately 8 months ago in the postpartum state. As a compensatory response to low levels of circulating T_4, thyrotropin-releasing hormone (TRH) and TSH are both elevated. Elevation of TRH stimulates both TSH and prolactin secretion and is one of the causes of hyperprolactinemia associated with primary hypothyroidism. Prolactin may also be elevated due to a lack of clearance by the kidney secondary to hypothyroidism. Treatment of primary hypothyroidism with levothyroxine (Answer B) should lower TRH and TSH levels and reduce thyroid hyperplasia. Treatment of the underlying cause avoids the need for unnecessary surgery (Answer E).

Because this patient has hypothyroidism, uptake of radioactive iodine (Answer D) would be very low despite the TSH elevation. Radioactive iodine testing is not helpful in patients with hypothyroidism.

Measurement of α-subunit (Answer C) is more helpful in determining the difference between a TSH-secreting adenoma and thyroid hormone resistance. The low free T_4 concentration in this vignette makes both of these diagnoses highly unlikely.

While cabergoline (Answer A) may improve her hyperprolactinemia and symptoms directly associated with prolactin elevation, the primary treatment of hypothyroidism will resolve the hyperprolactinemia and make cabergoline treatment unnecessary.

EDUCATIONAL OBJECTIVE

Identify thyrotroph hyperplasia as a manifestation of primary hypothyroidism and recommend appropriate treatment.

REFERENCE(S)

Kocova M, Netkov S, Sukarova-Angelovska E. Pituitary pseudotumor with unusual presentation reversed shortly after the introduction of thyroxine replacement therapy. *J Pediatr Endocrinol Metab.* 2001;14(9):1665-1669. PMID: 11795659

Joshi AS, Woolf PD. Pituitary hyperplasia secondary to primary hypothyroidism: a case report and review of the literature. *Pituitary.* 2005;8(2):99-103. PMID: 16195776

Shukla P, Bulsara KR, Luthra P. Pituitary hyperplasia in severe primary hypothyroidism: a case report and review of the literature. *Case Rep Endocrinol.* 2019;2019:2012546. PMID: 31341683

3 ANSWER: D) Refer to neurosurgery for transsphenoidal surgery

This patient has an incidentally discovered pituitary tumor with no symptoms. Incidental pituitary tumors are common, with an estimated prevalence of 10%. Retrospective data suggest that solid tumors are more likely to grow than cystic lesions, and solid macroadenomas have a higher propensity for growth than solid microadenomas. While initial management of incidentalomas can take many forms, repeated imaging of macroadenomas is recommended. In this case, the patient returns for imaging and is now symptomatic with hormonal deficiency, either from mild hyperprolactinemia consistent with stalk effect or compressive hypogonadotropic hypogonadism. His tumor has increased in size and abuts the optic chiasm. While there are no evidence-based recommendations for surgery based on growth rate alone, a growth rate exceeding 1 mm per year with threat to vision indicates a recommendation for surgical resection (Answer D).

Although cabergoline (Answer A) could be offered as treatment of hyperprolactinemia from stalk effect, a history of tumor growth and threat to vision makes this choice incorrect. Cabergoline has not demonstrated any favorable effect on tumor size of nonfunctioning adenomas and would not be an effective treatment for this tumor.

Testosterone replacement (Answer B) would not be the best choice, as it would not correct the underlying problem of tumor growth, and it would be potentially problematic with the recent discovery of a prostate mass and elevated PSA.

Similarly, surgery to remove the prostate mass (Answer C) may not be indicated for possibly benign prostate disease and would also not address the problem of tumor growth and possible future optic chiasm compression.

Stereotactic radiosurgery (Answer E) is helpful to control residual disease after pituitary surgery, but it is not indicated as a primary treatment of choice for nonfunctioning pituitary adenomas. The proximity to the chiasm also eliminates this possibility due to risk of optic nerve damage.

EDUCATIONAL OBJECTIVE

Identify the need for surgery during monitoring of incidentally discovered pituitary adenomas.

REFERENCE(S)

Langlois F, Fleseriu M. What to do with incidentally discovered pituitary abnormalities? *Med Clin North Am.* 2021;105(6):1081-1098. PMID: 34688416

Karavitaki N, Collison K, Halliday J, et al. What is the natural history of nonoperated nonfunctioning pituitary adenomas? *Clin Endocrinol (Oxf).* 2007;67(6):938-943. PMID: 17692109

Fernández-Balsells MM, Murad MH, Barwise A, et al. Natural history of nonfunctioning pituitary adenomas and incidentalomas: a systematic review and metaanalysis. *J Clin Endocrinol Metab.* 2011;96(4):905-912. PMID: 21474687

4 ANSWER: D) Stop topical testosterone, begin hCG, 2000 IU subcutaneous injection 3 times weekly

This patient initially presented during puberty with pubertal arrest. His features and findings suggest he has anosmic idiopathic hypogonadotropic hypogonadism (IHH). There are normosmic forms and anosmic forms of IHH, and the anosmic form is referred to as Kallmann syndrome. The genetics of Kallmann syndrome include pathogenic variants in the *ANOS1* gene, which are inherited in an X-linked recessive manner. Kallmann syndrome is thus far more common in males than in females. Genetic testing could be considered for patients prior to initiation of fertility, but this was not provided as an answer choice.

The clinical phenotype of patients with Kallmann syndrome varies; some individuals present with absent pubertal development, while others start puberty, but it does not progress. Presenting features prior to puberty may be cryptorchidism and microphallus. Presentation at puberty may include some testicular development, with eunuchoid habitus and absent sense of smell. Secondary sexual characteristics are generally absent. Pubic hair may be absent or scant due to adrenal androgens, and testes are usually prepubertal in size.

Treatment of hypogonadism without a goal of fertility consists of testosterone replacement. Since the hypogonadism caused by Kallmann syndrome is associated with decreased levels of gonadotropins, induction of fertility can be accomplished with hCG injections (Answer D). Testosterone replacement does not result in spermatogenesis since this treatment does not stimulate Leydig-cell production of local testosterone in the testes, where a much higher testosterone level is required than the circulating testosterone resulting from testosterone replacement. Continued testosterone (Answers A and E), regardless of switching formulations, is insufficient to stimulate spermatogenesis.

Anastrozole (Answer A) is not helpful in promoting fertility, but it is sometimes used for the treatment of gynecomastia in patients with other forms of hypogonadism.

Clomiphene citrate (Answer C) would not be helpful for this patient in that the defect in gonadal function lies in the hypothalamus. Clomiphene blocks negative feedback to the hypothalamus, increasing GnRH and, in turn, gonadotropin secretion. Without GnRH stimulation, clomiphene would be ineffective.

Referral for testicular sperm extraction (Answer B) may be beneficial if medical induction of fertility is inadequate, but it would be considered premature or potentially unsuccessful without first attemting medical induction of spermatogenesis.

EDUCATIONAL OBJECTIVE

Identify patients with congenital GnRH deficiency who require sex steroid replacement and treatment with centrally acting medications for fertility.

REFERENCE(S)

Boehm U, Bouloux P-M, Dattani MT, et al. Expert consensus document: European Consensus Statement on congenital hypogonadotropic hypogonadism--pathogenesis, diagnosis and treatment. *Nat Rev Endocrinol.* 2015;11(9):547-564. PMID: 26194704

Pitteloud N, Hayes FJ, Boepple PA, et al. The role of prior pubertal development, biochemical markers of testicular maturation, and genetics in elucidating the phenotypic heterogeneity of idiopathic hypogonadotropic hypogonadism. *J Clin Endocrinol Metab.* 2002;87(1):152-160. PMID: 11788640

5 ANSWER: B) Recommend exercise, calorie counting, and nutrition referral

This patient presents with mildly decreased total testosterone levels and a clear history of weight gain over the past few years. His history consists of an abrupt change in exercise, and his overall presentation is consistent with features of metabolic syndrome. His initial testosterone measurement was low due to concomitant opioid and corticosteroid medications, but these are reversible causes. His testosterone abnormality now is due to a low level of SHBG caused by obesity. Reductions in SHBG decrease serum total testosterone levels without reducing circulating free testosterone. Free testosterone is a challenge to measure and should either be calculated or measured by equilibrium dialysis. Gonadotropins remain normal when obesity lowers total testosterone. In this case, the best advice is to recommend exercise, calorie counting, and nutrition referral (Answer B) because the issue is not diminished testosterone secretion, but weight-related changes in binding proteins. Weight loss improves SHBG and total testosterone levels.

This patient does not currently meet clear criteria for testosterone replacement (Answer E), and his symptom of fatigue would be unlikely to improve with this treatment.

Similarly, clomiphene (Answer C), which would increase gonadotropin secretion and subsequently raise testosterone, is not indicated given his normal pituitary function. Additionally, clomiphene would not correct the underlying issue of low SHBG.

hCG (Answer D) is intended to treat infertility associated with hypogonadotropic hypogonadism, which is not present in this case.

Pituitary MRI (Answer A) is not the best choice in this scenario because there is little indication that a pituitary mass is causing low testosterone levels. His prolactin concentration is normal, gonadotropin concentrations are normal, and the low testosterone value noted in the past has improved with the discontinuation of offending medications.

EDUCATIONAL OBJECTIVE

Identify patients with low testosterone and nonspecific symptoms who are not candidates for testosterone replacement as first-line treatment and recognize obesity's role in changes related to the gonadal axis.

REFERENCE(S)

Anawalt BD, Matsumoto AM. Aging and androgens: physiology and clinical implications. *Rev Endocr Metab Disord.* 2022;23(6):1123-1137. PMID: 36459352

Wu FCW. Ageing male (part 2): management of functional hypogonadism in older men, a patient-centric holistic approach. *Best Pract Res Clin Endocrinol Metab.* 2022;36(4):101626. PMID: 35461757

Bhasin S, Brito JP, Cunningham GR, et al. Testosterone therapy in men with hypogonadism: an Endocrine Society clinical practice guideline. *J Clin Endocrinol Metab.* 2018;103(5):1715-1744. PMID: 29562364

6 ANSWER: C) Measurement of morning plasma ACTH

This patient presents with signs and symptoms consistent with Cushing syndrome with symptoms starting about 1 year ago. Her presentation has many cardinal features of hypercortisolemia, making the pretest probability of Cushing syndrome high. This patient has been screened with 3 different methods of cortisol assessment, with each test providing an abnormal result. Combined with the high pretest probability, the unequivocal results of testing (cortisol >2 to 3 times the upper normal limit), and no identified cause for nontumoral hypercortisolemia, the diagnosis of Cushing syndrome is confirmed. However, the next step in diagnosis is to determine whether the etiology is an ACTH-dependent or -independent cause. Thus, morning plasma ACTH should be measured (Answer C). ACTH secretion remains pulsatile, even in patients who have ACTH-dependent Cushing syndrome, so 2 samples are recommended. A value greater than 20 pg/mL (>4.4 pmol/L) is consistent with ACTH-dependent disease, limiting the etiology to a pituitary source or an ectopic source. A low ACTH value, typically suppressed below 5 pg/mL (<1.1 pmol/L), is consistent with a non–ACTH-dependent adrenal source.

Imaging of the adrenal or pituitary (Answers A and E) is premature without measurement of ACTH to narrow the etiology.

Inferior petrosal sinus sampling (Answer B) should only be done once hypercortisolemia from an ACTH-dependent source is confirmed. Overlap among healthy individuals, those with nontumoral hypercortisolemia, and those with Cushing disease makes this test only useful to determine the source of ACTH, and not helpful in determining whether hypercortisolemia is from a tumoral or nontumoral source.

The 8-mg overnight dexamethasone-suppression test (Answer D) is also meant to help determine the source of an ACTH-dependent elevation of cortisol and has been largely replaced by inferior petrosal sinus sampling. When inferior petrosal sinus sampling is not available, the 8-mg test can be used to help make the diagnosis.

EDUCATIONAL OBJECTIVE

Recommend the initial step in the differential diagnosis of Cushing syndrome.

REFERENCE(S)

Fleseriu M, Auchus R, Bancos I, et al. Consensus on diagnosis and management of Cushing's disease: a guideline update. *Lancet Diabetes Endocrinol.* 2021;9(12):847-875. PMID: 34687601

Findling JW, Raff H. Cushing's syndrome: important issues in diagnosis and management. *J Clin Endocrinol Metab.* 2006;91(10):3746-3753. PMID: 16868050

Nieman LK. Cushing's syndrome: update on signs, symptoms and biochemical screening. *Eur J Endocrinol.* 2015;173(4):M33-M38. PMID: 26156970

7 ANSWER: C) Desmopressin-stimulation test

This patient presents with mild hypercortisolism on some tests (while others are negative) and a history and physical examination findings suggesting nonneoplastic hypercortisolism (pseudo-Cushing syndrome). Her history suggests a possible source of this cortisol elevation (untreated depression) Psychiatric disease, alcohol abuse, and obesity are among chronic conditions that can cause cortisol elevations that are not due to tumors secreting ACTH or cortisol and must be distinguished from tumoral sources to avoid unnecessary treatment. Of the answer choices, desmopressin-stimulation testing (Answer C) is the only test that would be appropriate at this stage of the workup. Tests to distinguish Cushing syndrome from pseudo-Cushing syndrome include the dexamethasone–corticotropin-releasing hormone test and the desmopressin test. Both tests have a high degree of accuracy. With limited access to corticotropin-releasing hormone, the desmopressin test is the preferred assessment in this situation. Inferior petrosal sinus sampling (Answer A) and the 8-mg dexamethasone-suppression test (Answer E) are both used to determine the source of ACTH-dependent Cushing syndrome and are not appropriate without a clear demonstration of hypercortisolemia.

Similarly, the ^{68}Ga-DOTATATE scan (Answer D) is used for localization and not diagnosis. It is helpful in determining the location of ectopic ACTH sources in patients with ACTH-dependent Cushing syndrome.

Chest CT (Answer B) is also used to locate an ectopic ACTH source and would not be appropriate without other testing to first confirm both hypercortisolemia and an ectopic ACTH source.

EDUCATIONAL OBJECTIVE

Identify nontumoral causes of hypercortisolemia in the differential diagnosis and determine a diagnostic approach for further investigation and discrimination between causes of elevated cortisol.

REFERENCE(S)

Fleseriu M, Auchus R, Bancos I, et al. Consensus on diagnosis and management of Cushing's disease: a guideline update. *Lancet Diabetes Endocrinol.* 2021;9(12):847-875. PMID: 34687601

Rollin GAF, Costenaro F, Gerchman F, Rodrigues TC, Czepielewski MA. Evaluation of the DDAVP test in the diagnosis of Cushing's disease. *Clin Endocrinol (Oxf).* 2015;82(6):793-800. PMID: 25376361

8 ANSWER: B) Dopamine agonist

Some points cannot be overemphasized, and this is one. No one can state, legitimately, that a sellar mass is a particular type of lesion. In a teenager, a cystic suprasellar mass, especially one with calcifications, is often a craniopharyngioma, but not always. A serum prolactin concentration greater than 200 ng/mL (>8.7 nmol/L) is too high to be considered secondary to stalk effect or medication use. The patient's serum prolactin concentration is the clue that the mass is more likely a lactotroph adenoma. In this case, a misdiagnosis led to transcranial surgery, permanent partial loss of vision, and permanent panhypopituitarism. As with all prolactinomas, a dopamine agonist (Answer B) should be the initial treatment. The other modalities listed (Answers A, C, D, and E) are reserved for patients who do not respond to dopamine agonist therapy, for cases in which the lesion is largely cystic and there is visual field compromise, or for true craniopharyngiomas.

EDUCATIONAL OBJECTIVE

Distinguish between hyperprolactinemia resulting from hypothalamic/stalk dysfunction and tumor production and recommend the best management.

REFERENCE(S)

Freda PU, Post KD. Differential diagnosis of sellar masses. *Endocrinol Metab Clin North Am.* 1999;28(1):81-117. PMID: 10207686

Lucas JW, Zada G. Imaging of the pituitary and parasellar region. *Semin Neurol.* 2012;32(4):320-331. PMID: 23361479

9 ANSWER: A) Another MRI in 12 months

This 48-year-old patient has been found incidentally to have a microadenoma of the pituitary gland. Because this is a microadenoma without associated symptoms or biochemical demonstration of hormone excess or deficiency, there is no indication for surgery (Answer C) or irradiation (Answer B). Appropriate management would simply be to perform serial monitoring and assess for a change in tumor size in 12 months with another MRI (Answer A). Tumors such as this one grow quite slowly (0.6 mm/y on average), so he is in no imminent danger from tumor growth. If the MRI had shown significant suprasellar extension with abutment of the optic chiasm, then visual field testing (Answer D) should have been performed; otherwise, it should not.

EDUCATIONAL OBJECTIVE

Manage a pituitary incidentaloma.

REFERENCE(S)

Molitch ME. Pituitary tumours: pituitary incidentalomas. *Best Pract Res Clin Endocrinol Metab.* 2009;23(5):667-675. PMID: 19945030

Freda PU, Beckers AM, Katznelson L, et al; Endocrine Society. Pituitary incidentalomas: an Endocrine Society clinical practice guideline. *J Clin Endocrinol Metab.* 2011;96(4):894-904. PMID: 21474686

Scangas GA, Laws ER Jr. Pituitary incidentalomas. *Pituitary.* 2014;17(5):486-491. PMID: 24052242

10 ANSWER: C) Metastasis

The key features in this patient are the rapid growth of the mass and the presence of arginine vasopressin deficiency, formerly known as diabetes insipidus. This is most consistent with metastasis (Answer C). Metastasis to the sella is most commonly seen in patients with a known primary cancer and is uncommonly the first manifestation of a metastatic neoplasm. Arginine vasopressin deficiency occurs because the metastasis involves the posterior pituitary. The most common cancers causing such metastases are breast cancer in women and lung cancer in men. This patient's history of breast cancer makes this the most likely diagnosis.

Clinically nonfunctioning pituitary adenomas (Answer A) are usually slow growing and are rarely associated with arginine vasopressin deficiency.

Prolactinoma (Answer E) is unlikely given the modestly elevated serum prolactin, the rapid increase in tumor size, and the presence of arginine vasopressin deficiency (rarely associated).

Craniopharyngioma (Answer B) can also be associated with arginine vasopressin deficiency, but lesions are cystic and affected patients usually present at a younger age.

There is no clinical evidence of sarcoidosis (Answer D) based on history or chest imaging.

EDUCATIONAL OBJECTIVE

Differentiate metastases from other pituitary mass lesions.

REFERENCE(S)

Al-Aridi R, El Sibai K, Fu P, Khan M, Selman WR, Arafah BM. Clinical and biochemical characteristic features of metastatic cancer to the sella turcica: an analytical review. *Pituitary.* 2014;17(6):575-587. PMID: 24337713

Ariel D, Sung H, Coghlan N, Dodd R, Gibbs IC, Katznelson L. Clinical characteristics and pituitary dysfunction in patients with metastatic cancer to the sella. *Endocr Pract.* 2013;19(6):914-919. PMID: 23757610

Cai H, Liu W, Feng T, Li Z, Liu Y. Clinical presentation and pathologic characteristics of pituitary metastasis from breast carcinoma: cases and a systematic review of the literature. *World Neurosurg.* 2019;S1878-S8750(18)32949-8. PMID: 30630045

11 ANSWER: B) Measurement of HAMA (human anti-mouse antibodies)

The typical patient with hyperthyroidism, including Graves disease, has autonomous production of thyroid hormone by the thyroid with resultant suppression of TSH levels. In a hyperthyroid patient, when TSH levels are normal or elevated in the setting of elevated T_4 and T_3 levels, the most common cause is a TSH-producing tumor. Therefore, MRI is often done next. In this case, the MRI was normal. In patients with TSH-secreting tumors, there is commonly an imbalance in the secretion of α-subunit, resulting in a relative increase in α-subunit disproportionate to the TSH level (not β subunit [Answer A]). The free α-subunit test was not an answer choice in this vignette.

An alternative explanation for elevated TSH in a patient such as this one is that the TSH measurement is artifactually high due to the presence of heterophile antibodies. These antibodies are directed against specific animal immunoglobulins, usually human anti-mouse antibodies (HAMA) (Answer B). In this case, a commercial laboratory detected the presence of HAMA antibodies. When specific HAMA-blocking reagents were added, the patient's TSH concentration was documented to be less than 0.01 mIU/L. The patient works in an animal laboratory and was exposed to mice, which may have elicited this response.

A T_3-suppression test (Answer E) is now rarely done in patients with toxic nodular goiters.

Petrosal sinus sampling (Answer D) is done primarily to distinguish between pituitary vs ectopic ACTH secretion in patients with Cushing syndrome. However, ectopic TSH secretion outside the cranium has actually never been reported in TSH-dependent hyperthyroidism.

EDUCATIONAL OBJECTIVE

Evaluate patients with hyperthyroidism who have nonsuppressed TSH levels.

REFERENCE(S)

Beck-Peccoz P, Lania A, Beckers A, Chatterjee K, Werneau JL. 2013 European Thyroid Association guidelines for the diagnosis and treatment of thyrotropin-secreting pituitary tumours. *Eur Thyroid J.* 2013;2(2):76-82. PMID: 24783044

Després N, Grant AM. Antibody interference in thyroid assays: a potential for clinical misinformation. *Clin Chem.* 1998;44(3):440-454. PMID: 9510847

12 ANSWER: A) Add pegvisomant, 40 mg subcutaneously weekly

Although studies do show that increasing the somatostatin analogue dosage or increasing the dose frequency, such as every 21 days (Answer B) may be beneficial, these regimens are not generally adopted and are demonstrated to have less than 50% efficacy in small studies.

Cabergoline (Answer D) can be useful in the setting of modest acromegaly, and it may show benefit in combination with octreotide. However, this regimen is effective in less than half of patients and is unlikely to be effective in this patient who has active disease.

Radiation therapy (Answer C) often takes several years to be effective, and it is therefore unlikely to be effective within 6 months.

The addition of weekly pegvisomant (Answer A) is the most effective treatment in this timeframe, with response rates of 60% to 90% with various combination regimens.

Pasireotide (Answer E) is more effective than either octreotide or lanreotide, and switching affords an improvement in approximately 25% of patients. However, this improvement is not clearly as effective as the combination of a somatostatin analogue and weekly pegvisomant.

EDUCATIONAL OBJECTIVE

Recommend the best therapeutic approach in a patient with acromegaly who has had a partial response to adjuvant therapy with somatostatin analogue therapy.

REFERENCE(S)

Fleseriu M, Langlois F, Lim DST, Varlamov EV, Melmed S. Acromegaly: pathogenesis, diagnosis, and management. *Lancet Diabetes Endocrinol.* 2022;10(11):804-826. PMID: 36209758

Bonert V, Mirocha J, Carmichael J, Yuen KCJ, Araki T, Melmed S. Cost-effectiveness and efficacy of a novel combination regimen in acromegaly: a prospective, randomized trial. *J Clin Endocrinol Metab.* 2020;105(9):dgaa444. PMID: 32754748

13 ANSWER: A) An adverse effect of cabergoline

Several studies have shown that dopamine agonists, both cabergoline and bromocriptine, can cause impulse control disorders, including hypersexuality compulsive behavior, in 15% to 20% of treated patients (Answer A). The effect appears to be somewhat dosage dependent, so lowering the dosage, if not discontinuing the dopamine agonist, may be helpful.

This patient's tumor is probably not large enough to cause substantial hypothalamic damage (Answer C).

Increasing the serum testosterone to the normal range (Answer D) should not lead to impulse control behavior.

While a behavior change unrelated to this tumor or treatment (Answer B) is possible, an adverse effect of cabergoline is the most likely explanation.

EDUCATIONAL OBJECTIVE

Describe potential adverse effects of dopamine agonist treatment in patients with prolactinomas.

REFERENCE(S)

Ioachimescu AG, Fleseriu M, Hoffman AR, Vaughan TB, Katznelson L. Psychological effects of dopamine agonist treatment in patients with hyperprolactinemia and prolactin-secreting adenomas. *Eur J Endocrinol.* 2019;180(1):31-40. PMID: 30400048

Bancos I, Nannenga MR, Bostwick JM, Silber MH, Erickson D, Nippoldt TB. Impulse control disorders in patients with dopamine agonist-treated prolactinomas and nonfunctioning pituitary adenomas: a case-control study. *Clin Endocrinol (Oxf).* 2014;80(6):863-868. PMID: 24274365

De Sousa SMC, Baranoff J, Rushworth RL, et al. Impulse control disorders in dopamine agonist-treated hyperprolactinemia: prevalence and risk factors. *J Clin Endocrinol Metab.* 2020;105(3):dgz076. PMID: 31580439

14 ANSWER: C) Lanreotide depot monthly

Somatostatin analogues are effective in managing acromegaly and are often used as first-line medical therapy. Somatostatin analogues are also very useful in patients with headache. Therefore, lanreotide depot, a somatostatin analogue, given monthly (Answer C) should be the initial treatment choice in this patient. Octreotide LAR (long-acting release) is another somatostatin analogue with similar efficacy and adverse effect profile to that of lanreotide depot.

Of medical therapies, pegvisomant has the highest likelihood of normalizing this patient's IGF-1 levels. However, in the most recent Endocrine Society guidelines, pegvisomant was recommended to be considered as first-line medical therapy when administered as daily, not weekly, dosing (Answer D). Also, somatostatin analogues may be superior to pegvisomant in the setting of significant headache.

Repeated surgery (Answer A) is probably not indicated if the residual tumor is within the cavernous sinus, as additional surgery is unlikely to be curative.

Although cabergoline (Answer B) may be useful in selected patients, it is mostly useful for patients with mildly elevated IGF-1. This patient has a more significantly elevated IGF-1 concentration.

EDUCATIONAL OBJECTIVE

Manage persistent acromegaly after transsphenoidal surgery.

REFERENCE(S)

Katznelson L, Laws ER Jr, Melmed S, et al. Acromegaly: an Endocrine Society clinical practice guideline. *J Clin Endocrinol Metab.* 2014;99(11):3933-3951. PMID: 25356808

Giustina A, Chanson P, Kleinberg D, et al; Acromegaly Consensus Group. Expert consensus document: a consensus on the medical treatment of acromegaly. *Nat Rev Endocrinol.* 2014;10(4):243-248. PMID: 24566817

15 **ANSWER: A) Craniopharyngioma**

The key feature in this vignette is that the patient has arginine vasopressin deficiency, which indicates a primarily hypothalamic origin of his tumor. Craniopharyngiomas (Answer A) can occur in children and teenagers, and there is a distinct second peak in older adults (age 50-74 years). The presence of a cystic tumor in this man, as well as arginine vasopressin deficiency, points to a craniopharyngioma. Craniopharyngiomas are typically described on MRI as calcified, solid, and/or cystic lesions, usually with a lobular shape and diameter of 20 to 40 mm. The solid elements are often isointense or hypointense on T1-weighted images, exhibit inhomogeneous high intensity on T2-weighted images, and heterogeneously enhance after gadolinium administration.

Arginine vasopressin deficiency is very uncommon in patients with pituitary adenomas (gonadotroph adenoma [Answer B], prolactinoma [Answer D], and silent corticotroph adenoma [Answer E]). The very mild prolactin elevation in this case is from hypothalamic damage rather than from a prolactinoma and could accompany any of these other tumors/lesions.

Langerhans cell histiocytosis (Answer C) usually presents as an infiltrative disease of the hypothalamus and stalk with stalk thickening on MRI rather than as a mass lesion.

EDUCATIONAL OBJECTIVE

Differentiate among hypothalamic and pituitary mass lesions.

REFERENCE(S)

Bogusz A, Müller HL. Childhood-onset craniopharyngioma: latest insights into pathology, diagnostics, treatment, and follow-up. *Expert Rev Neurother.* 2018;18(10):793-806. PMID: 30257123

Müller HL. Craniopharyngioma. *Endocr Rev.* 2014;35(3):513-543. PMID: 24467716

Zada G, Lin N, Ojerholm E, Ramkissoon S, Laws ER. Craniopharyngioma and other cystic epithelial lesions of the sellar region: a review of clinical, imaging, and histopathological relationships. *Neurosurg Focus.* 2010;28(4):E4. PMID: 20367361

Erfurth EM, Holmer H, Fjalldal SB. Mortality and morbidity in adult craniopharyngioma. *Pituitary.* 2013;16(1):46-55. PMID: 22961634

16 **ANSWER: C) Increase lanreotide dosage to 120 mg and extend the time between lanreotide depot doses to every 6 weeks**

The serum half-lives of both octreotide LAR and lanreotide depot are considerably longer than 4 weeks. Studies have now shown that in selected patients who have acromegaly that is well controlled on low dosages of these somatostatin analogues, the dosing frequency can be gradually spaced out to longer than every 4 weeks while still maintaining control of GH and IGF-1 levels. In fact, some patients can be tapered off the somatostatin analogue altogether. The US FDA has approved lanreotide for an extended dosing interval using the 120-mg dose with intervals of every 6 or 8 weeks. Studies have also been performed extending octreotide LAR. Although the current dosage could certainly be continued

(Answer B), it would be cost-effective to try decreasing the dosing frequency (Answer C).

Because this patient has responded so well to the somatostatin analogue, there is no reason to switch to pegvisomant (Answer E), add cabergoline (Answer A), or to perform stereotactic radiotherapy (Answer D).

EDUCATIONAL OBJECTIVE

Manage acromegaly with somatostatin analogue therapy.

REFERENCE(S)

Turner HE, Thornton-Jones VA, Wass JA. Systematic dose-extension of octreotide LAR: the importance of individual tailoring of treatment in patients with acromegaly. *Clin Endocrinol (Oxf).* 2004;61(2):224-231. PMID: 15272918

Abrams P, Alexopoulou O, Abs R, Maiter D, Verhelst J. Optimalization and cost management of lanreotide- Autogel therapy in acromegaly. *Eur J Endocrinol.* 2007;157(5):571-577. PMID: 17984236

Ronchi CL, Rizzo E, Lania AG, et al. Preliminary data on biochemical remission of acromegaly after somatostatin analogs withdrawal. *Eur J Endocrinol.* 2008;158(1):19-25. PMID: 18166813

17 ANSWER: A) Decrease the GH dosage

Oral estrogens can decrease the responsiveness of the liver to GH with respect to IGF-1 production. Therefore, to maintain a steady level of IGF-1, the GH dosage may actually need to be decreased in this setting (thus, Answer A is correct and Answer C is incorrect). Interestingly, estrogens also stimulate hepatic thyroxine-binding globulin, so increases in levothyroxine dosages are sometimes needed and, presumably, the converse is also true (thus, Answer E is incorrect). Although increasing the hydrocortisone dosage (Answer D) could be considered useful given that GH may metabolize cortisol and lead to relative adrenal insufficiency, the first step for this patient would be to reduce the GH dosage. Stopping estrogen has no effect on hydrocortisone dosage requirements, so decreasing the hydrocortisone dosage (Answer B) is incorrect.

EDUCATIONAL OBJECTIVE

Describe interactions among hormonal replacement therapies.

REFERENCE(S)

Glynn N, Kenny H, Quisenberry L, et al. The effect of growth hormone replacement on the thyroid axis in patients with hypopituitarism: in vivo and ex vivo studies. *Clin Endocrinol (Oxf).* 2017;86(5):747-754. PMID: 27809356

Birzniece V, Ho KKY. Sex steroids and the GH axis: implications for the management of hypopituitarism. *Best Pract Res Clin Endocrinol Metab.* 2017;31(1):59-69. PMID: 28477733

Fleseriu M, Hashim IA, Karavitaki N, et al. Hormonal replacement in hypopituitarism in adults: an Endocrine Society clinical practice guideline. *J Clin Endocrinol Metab.* 2016;101(11):3888-3921. PMID: 27736313

18 ANSWER: E) Start dopamine agonist therapy and repeat MRI in 6 months

This 75-year-old man with known coronary artery disease, hypertension, and mild kidney insufficiency was found to have an incidental macroadenoma. His pituitary function is notable for a decrease in total testosterone, which may be due to prolactin interference with the gonadal axis. He has hyperprolactinemia, and the prolactin value is in the range consistent with stalk effect and would be expected to be higher in the presence of a macroprolactinoma. Thus, this patient most likely has a clinically nonfunctioning adenoma. Given the lack of local mass effects, there is no immediate indication for surgery (Answer B) or irradiation (Answer C), but he should be assessed for change in tumor size in 6 months with a repeated MRI. Such tumors grow quite slowly (0.6 mm/y on average), so he is in no imminent danger from tumor growth. If the MRI showed clinically significant suprasellar extension with abutment of the optic chiasm, then visual field testing (Answer A) should be performed; otherwise, it should not. Although there are reports of tumor shrinkage with dopamine agonists, these agents are not consistently found to be useful in reducing the size of nonfunctioning pituitary macroadenomas.

However, this patient may benefit from reduction in prolactin and restoration of the gonadal axis (by starting a dopamine agonist), with planned surveillance of his nonfunctioning adenoma (Answer E). While surveillance with MRI at 6 months alone (Answer D) would be adequate to monitor for growth, it would leave a reversible cause of hypogonadism untreated.

EDUCATIONAL OBJECTIVE

Manage pituitary incidentalomas.

REFERENCE(S)

Freda PU, Beckers AM, Katznelson L, et al; Endocrine Society. Pituitary incidentaloma: an Endocrine Society clinical practice guideline. *J Clin Endocrinol Metab.* 2011;96(4):894-904. PMID: 21474686

Molitch ME. Nonfunctioning pituitary tumors. *Handb Clin Neurol.* 2014;124:167-184. PMID: 25248587

19 ANSWER: B) DDAVP, 0.1 mg orally as needed for polyuria and hypernatremia

This patient has acute onset of arginine vasopressin deficiency. In this setting, the cause is central, due to deficiency of vasopressin. The goal of therapy is to control the free water depletion from polyuria, as well as maintain comfort. DDAVP should be administered in a short-acting regimen with avoidance of prescheduled dosing given the risk of hyponatremia from syndrome of inappropriate antidiuretic hormone secretion (SIADH) in the subsequent days as part of the triphasic response following surgery. Therefore, DDAVP should be administered as needed (0.1 mg orally, and higher doses of 0.2 to 0.3 mg may be necessary) (Answer B) or as subcutaneous aqueous DDAVP, 0.5 to 1.0 mcg (not offered as an option in this vignette).

Scheduled dosing (Answer D) should be avoided. Administration of DDAVP immediately following endonasal surgery should be given through oral or parenteral routes. Intranasal administration (Answer C) would not be absorbed sufficiently given trauma to the mucosal membranes from surgery, but it may be considered in the future if arginine vasopressin deficiency persists and the mucosal membranes have healed.

Fluid restriction (Answer A) is contraindicated in these patients who are prone to dehydration and is used to treat hyponatremia.

Tolvaptan (Answer E) is an oral vasopressin receptor antagonist used for the treatment of severe hyponatremia, which is not present in this patient.

EDUCATIONAL OBJECTIVE

Manage arginine vasopressin deficiency following pituitary surgery.

REFERENCE(S)

Woodmansee WW, Carmichael J, Kelly D, Katznelson L; AACE Neuroendocrine and Pituitary Scientific Committee. American Association of Clinical Endocrinologists and American College of Endocrinology disease state clinical review: postoperative management following pituitary surgery. *Endocr Pract.* 2015;21(7):832-838. PMID: 26172128

Fleseriu M, Hashim IA, Karavitaki N, et al. Hormonal replacement in hypopituitarism in adults: an Endocrine Society clinical practice guideline. *J Clin Endocrinol Metab.* 2016;101(11):3888-3921. PMID: 27736313

20 ANSWER: A) Increase in polyuria and polydipsia

Cortisol and thyroid hormone deficiencies increase the sensitivity of vasopressin receptors to vasopressin. Thus, when these hormones are replaced, the small amount of vasopressin still being secreted in a patient with partial arginine vasopressin deficiency may no longer be sufficient to effect water reabsorption, and subclinical arginine vasopressin deficiency may manifest with polyuria and polydipsia (Answer A). This is particularly the case with administration of glucocorticoids. The converse of excessive vasopressin secretion with hyponatremia (Answer C) is certainly not going to occur.

While headache is a common finding with Rathke cleft cyst, replacement of deficient hormones would not exacerbate or worsen the headache (Answer D), especially at physiologic doses used in standard hormone replacement.

Institution of steroids should not cause orthostatic hypotension (Answer B). Administration of levothyroxine alone without glucocorticoids could cause hypotension if it unmasks adrenal insufficiency.

EDUCATIONAL OBJECTIVE

Explain the effects of thyroid hormone and cortisol on vasopressin action.

REFERENCE(S)

Iida M, Takamoto S, Masuo M, Makita K, Saito T. Transient lymphocytic panhypophysitis associated with SIADH leading to diabetes insipidus after glucocorticoid replacement. *Intern Med.* 2003;42(10):991-995. PMID: 14606714

Huang CH, Chou KJ, Lee PT, Chen CL, Chung HM, Fang HC. A case of lymphocytic hypophysitis with masked diabetes insipidus unveiled by glucocorticoid replacement. *Am J Kidney Dis.* 2005;45(1):197-200. PMID: 15696461

Sala E, Moore JM, Amorin A, et al. Natural history of Rathke's cleft cysts: a retrospective analysis of a two centres experience. *Clin Endocrinol (Oxf).* 2018;89(2):178-186. PMID: 29781512

Lin M, Wedemeyer MA, Bradley D, et al. Long-term surgical outcomes following transsphenoidal surgery in patients with Rathke's cleft cysts. *J Neurosurg.* 2018;130(3):831-837. PMID: 29775155

21 ANSWER: C) Pseudotumor cerebri (benign, idiopathic, intracranial hypertension)

Empty sella is a common incidental finding on MRI performed for other reasons. Some series suggest that some degree of hypopituitarism is present in up to 35% of patients with empty sellas. Pseudotumor cerebri (benign, idiopathic, intracranial hypertension) (Answer C) is commonly associated with a partially empty sella. Recent MRI studies suggest that empty sella is due more to enlargement of the sella itself than to a decrease in pituitary size. Such changes are thought to be caused by chronically elevated cerebrospinal fluid pressure with pressure pulsation that results in enlargement of the sella and some compression of the pituitary.

Acute trauma causing pituitary infarction (Answer D) would show blood in the pituitary with pituitary enlargement rather than a small pituitary.

Sarcoidosis (Answer A) and Langerhans cell histiocytosis (Answer B) are infiltrative diseases of the hypothalamus and pituitary stalk and might present with stalk thickening rather than an empty sella. Both entities usually present with arginine vasopressin deficiency.

EDUCATIONAL OBJECTIVE

Construct the differential diagnosis of an empty sella.

REFERENCE(S)

Ranganathan S, Lee SH, Checkver A, et al. Magnetic resonance imaging finding of empty sella in obesity related idiopathic intracranial hypertension is associated with enlarged sella turcica. *Neuroradiology.* 2013;55(8):955-961. PMID: 23708942

Guitelman M, Garcia Basavilbaso N, et al. Primary empty sella (PES): a review of 175 cases. *Pituitary.* 2013;16(2):270-274. PMID: 22875743

Sala E, Moore JM, Amorin A, et al. Natural history of Rathke's cleft cysts: a retrospective analysis of a two centres experience. *Clin Endocrinol (Oxf).* 2018;89(2):178-186. PMID: 29781512

Lin M, Wedemeyer MA, Bradley D, et al. Long-term surgical outcomes following transsphenoidal surgery in patients with Rathke's cleft cysts. *J Neurosurg.* 2018;130(3):831-837. PMID: 29775155

22 ANSWER: E) Transsphenoidal surgery now

All of these treatment modalities can improve Cushing disease, and treatment during pregnancy is advocated because it results in better fetal outcomes. Transsphenoidal surgery has a cure rate of 80% to 90% in expert neurosurgical hands, with very low complication and fetal loss rates when done in the second trimester. Surgery now (Answer E) should be strongly considered in this patient. Because of the presence of active Cushing disease, it is not safe for either the fetus or the mother to have uncontrolled hypercortisolism through the rest of the pregnancy. Thus, delaying surgery until after delivery (Answer D) is not acceptable.

Mifepristone (Answer B) was originally developed as a progesterone receptor blocker and is a potent abortifacient (RU486); therefore, its use in pregnancy is absolutely contraindicated.

There is experience with only about 50 cases in which somatostatin analogues have been used to treat acromegaly during pregnancy, with relatively minor adverse effects. However, somatostatin analogues cross the placenta and have unknown effects on the fetus. There is no documented experience with pasireotide (Answer C) during pregnancy, and it would be expected to worsen glucose tolerance in this population susceptible to gestational diabetes.

Although cabergoline (Answer A) is safe when stopped after conception, there is little experience when used throughout pregnancy, and its ability to normalize cortisol levels in Cushing disease is only modest.

EDUCATIONAL OBJECTIVE

Guide treatment of Cushing disease during pregnancy.

REFERENCE(S)

Marions L. Mifepristone dose in the regimen with misoprostol for medical abortion. *Contraception.* 2006;74(1):21-25. PMID: 16781255

Lindsay JR, Jonklaas J, Oldfield EH, Nieman LK. Cushing's syndrome during pregnancy: personal experience and review of the literature. *J Clin Endocrinol Metab.* 2005;90(5):3077-3083. PMID: 15705919

Cohen-Kerem R, Railton C, Oren D, Lishner M, Koren G. Pregnancy outcome following non-obstetric surgical intervention. *Am J Surgery.* 2005;190(3):467-473. PMID: 16105538

Thyroid Board Review

Jacqueline Jonklaas, MD, PhD, MPH

1 ANSWER: B) Free radiolabeled iodine reaching the thyroid gland

Iodine 131–labeled ligands have been used to treat several malignancies. In the case of radioactive ^{131}I MIBG, this compound resembles norepinephrine and can be used to target and destroy tissues that have norepinephrine transporters. Tumors expressing norepinephrine transporters, such as pheochromocytomas, paragangliomas, and neuroblastomas, may allow sufficient therapeutic ^{131}I MIBG uptake into malignant cells to cause tumor destruction. A small amount of ^{131}I dissociates from MIBG and as unbound ^{131}I enters the thyroid via the sodium-iodide transporter and concentrates within thyroid tissue. Following organification into thyroglobulin, the radioisotope is trapped inside thyroid cells and the emitted β radiation leads to DNA damage. The affected cells undergo apoptosis, resulting in ablation of the thyroid tissue. As a consequence of thyroid tissue damage, hypothyroidism ensues (thus, Answer B is correct). Radiolabeled ligands are being evaluated for other malignancies, such as prostate-specific membrane antigen-targeted radioligand therapy for prostate cancer.

Multiple regimens have been used for thyroid prophylaxis in children after ^{131}I MIBG treatment, and they typically involve cold iodine and sometimes methimazole and levothyroxine administration. These regimens are repeated after each radiolabeled MIBG treatment. Despite this prophylaxis, overt hypothyroidism occurs at a median of 12 months and develops in 17% to 56% of treated patients.

There is no need to consider a pathogenic variant in the gene encoding the sodium-iodide transporter (Answer D) to explain ^{131}I transport into thyroid tissue.

Metastatic neuroblastoma to the thyroid (Answer C) is vanishingly rare.

TPO antibody–negative Hashimoto thyroiditis (Answer E) is a known entity, but this is not the best explanation when postablative hypothyroidism is well described after use of ^{131}I MIBG.

Failure to escape from the Wolff-Chaikoff (Answer A) describes the lack of reversal of the acute autoregulatory inhibition of thyroid hormone synthesis that occurs following an iodine load. If the inhibition of thyroid hormone synthesis is longstanding, rather than the acute autoregulatory phenomenon, this results in hypothyroidism, as might occur in an individual with Hashimoto thyroiditis. Such an effect is not being observed here, as this patient does not have Hashimoto thyroiditis and he would not be expected to be susceptible to this effect of cold iodine.

EDUCATIONAL OBJECTIVE

Describe the therapeutic effect of targeted ^{131}I ligands and their potential thyroid toxicity.

REFERENCE(S)

Kotwal A, McLeod DSA. Thyroid dysfunction from treatments for solid organ cancers. *Endocrinol Metab Clin North Am.* 2022;51(2):265-286. PMID: 35662441

Clement SC, van Rijn RR, van Eck-Smit BL, et al. Long-term efficacy of current thyroid prophylaxis and future perspectives on thyroid protection during 131I-metaiodobenzylguanidine treatment in children with neuroblastoma. *Eur J Nucl Med Mol Imaging.* 2015;42(5):706-715. PMID: 25512056

Bombardieri E, Giammarile F, Aktolun C, et al; European Association for Nuclear Medicine. 131I/123I-metaiodobenzylguanidine (mIBG) scintigraphy: procedure guidelines for tumour imaging. *Eur J Nucl Med Mol Imaging.* 2010;37(12):2436-2446. PMID: 20644928

2 ANSWER: D) Spot urine iodine

This vignette illustrates the differential diagnosis that should be considered when encountering hyperthyroidism associated with low iodine uptake seen on an ^{123}I thyroid scan and uptake. Thyroiditis is definitely one of the potential diagnoses to be considered. The fact that the patient had no neck tenderness makes this less likely, and thyroiditis would have been expected to respond to prednisone. Furthermore, the lengthy duration of the hyperthyroidism also makes the diagnosis of thyroiditis less tenable, as the damaged thyroid should not be able to synthesize thyroid hormone for a several-month period. Testing for COVID infection (Answer B) or antibodies to COVID (Answer A) is unlikely to be helpful because thyroiditis associated with COVID infection or vaccination generally responds to steroid therapy and is of self-limited duration.

If thyroiditis is excluded, remaining considerations are an exogenous iodine load and exogenous thyroid hormone consumption. Exogenous thyroid hormone consumption is unlikely because of the patient's thyroglobulin concentration of 60 ng/mL. A random urinary iodine measurement (Answer D) was, in fact, revealing in this patient's case and showed an elevated level of 1000 µg/dL. The patient did not provide a history of amiodarone use or iodinated contrast exposure, but further investigation revealed that he was taking nasal drops for sinusitis, which, at the dosage he was using, were believed to provide 12 mg iodine daily. With cessation of the nasal drops and reinstitution of methimazole, the patient's hyperthyroidism, which was thought to be due to a toxic multinodular goiter, gradually resolved.

A whole-body iodine scan (Answer E) is usually performed to rule out struma ovarii in which there are functional thyroid components occurring in a teratoma or dermoid tumor in the ovary. This would be unlikely in this male patient.

hCG-induced thyrotoxicosis can be caused by a variety of germ-cell tumors that produce sufficiently high hCG levels to stimulate thyroid hormone production by thyroid tissue. In this setting, ^{123}I uptake would be anticipated to be elevated when imaging with a thyroid scan and uptake is performed. Therefore, this could not provide a single diagnosis in this patient, as an iodine load would have to be present concomitantly to account for the low uptake seen with his thyroid scan and uptake. Measuring serum hCG (Answer C) is incorrect.

EDUCATIONAL OBJECTIVE

Differentiate among the potential causes of hyperthyroidism in the setting of low uptake documented with a ^{123}I thyroid scan and uptake.

REFERENCE(S)

Ross DS, Burch HB, Cooper DS, et al. 2016 American Thyroid Association guidelines for diagnosis and management of hyperthyroidism and other causes of thyrotoxicosis. *Thyroid.* 2016;26(10):1343-1421. PMID: 27521067

Praw SS, Brent GA. Approach to the patient with a suppressed TSH. *J Clin Endocrinol Metab.* 2023;108(2):472-482. PMID: 36329632

3 ANSWER: C) Pathogenic variant in the gene encoding the chloride-iodide cotransporter in the thyroid, inner ear, and kidney

The described patient appears to have Pendred syndrome, which is due to pathogenic variants in the pendrin gene that codes a multifunction anion exchanger with an affinity for chloride, iodine, and bicarbonate (Answer C). The pendrin gene, *SLC26A4*, maps to chromosome 7q31. The pendrin protein is expressed in the thyroid, inner ear, and kidney. Within the thyroid gland, pendrin is necessary for iodine efflux into the follicular lumen. Despite the partial impairment of iodine organification that ensues, affected individuals usually have a goiter but are most commonly euthyroid. In the inner ear, pendrin is necessary for endolymphatic fluid resorption, acid-base balance, and normal inner ear function. Affected individuals have dilation of the endolymphatic sacs within the auditory canals and dysplastic cochlea. Bilateral sensorineural deafness is usually seen. The defects in pendrin protein in the kidney can place patients at risk for developing metabolic alkalosis.

Diagnosis of Pendred syndrome starts with the appropriate clinical presentation and can be confirmed by testing for pathogenic variants in the *SLC26A4* gene, in which at least 150 pathogenic variants have been found. The mode of transmission is autosomal recessive, not autosomal dominant (Answer A). Both of this patient's parents were heterozygous, and she and her brother would each have had a 25% chance of having Pendred syndrome.

If performed, results of a perchlorate test (Answer B) would be abnormal. In this test, radioactive iodine is administered and once sufficient time has elapsed for organification to occur, perchlorate is administered to displace nonorganified iodide. In individuals with normal iodide organification, there is little iodide discharge following perchlorate administration. A loss of more than 10% indicates an organification defect, as there will be more nonorganified iodine discharged compared with that associated with a normal thyroid gland.

MRI of the auditory canal (Answer E) should show the characteristic Mondini deformity seen in Pendred syndrome. This consists of marked bilateral dilation of the endolymphatic sacs, a dysplastic cochlea, with coalescence of the apical and middle turns and mildly enlarged vestibules.

Although autoimmune thyroid disease (Answer D) can coexist with Pendred syndrome, it is not characteristic.

EDUCATIONAL OBJECTIVE

Describe abnormalities in the chloride-iodide anion exchanger that can be responsible for iodine organification defects in the thyroid gland and impaired formation of the cochlea and vestibule of the inner ear.

REFERENCE(S)

Wémeau JL, Kopp P. Pendred syndrome. *Best Pract Res Clin Endocrinol Metab.* 2017;31(2):213-224. PMID: 28648509

Kopp P, Pesce L, Solis-S JC. Pendred syndrome and iodide transport in the thyroid. *Trends Endocrinol Metab.* 2008;19(7):260-268. PMID: 18692402

4 ANSWER: E) Thymic tissue

A significant amount of thymic tissue (Answer E) may be present in young persons and other individuals with thymic hyperplasia, such as those with Graves disease. The thymus can be a source of "false-positive" radioiodine uptake on either pretherapy or posttherapy whole-body scans. Visualization of thymic tissue is believed to be secondary to functional sodium-iodide symporter expression in thymic cells and iodine concentration within Hassall bodies. One report suggests that innocent iodine uptake in the thymus may be seen in 3.4% of patients. In one study, 6 of 175 patients had visualization of thymus on a combination of diagnostic scans and posttherapy scans. Proof that the thymus is responsible for the uptake could be provided by resection or biopsy of the mass. In this patient's case, the resected tissue was, in fact, hyperplastic thymic tissue. Other findings suggestive of this cause (as opposed to metastatic thyroid cancer to the thymus or a mediastinal lymph node) are young age, visualization of thymus on CT, and a low serum thyroglobulin concentration. Visualization of a patient's radioiodine-avid thymus using fused SPECT and CT images are shown (*see images*).

Axial fused SPECT and CT images

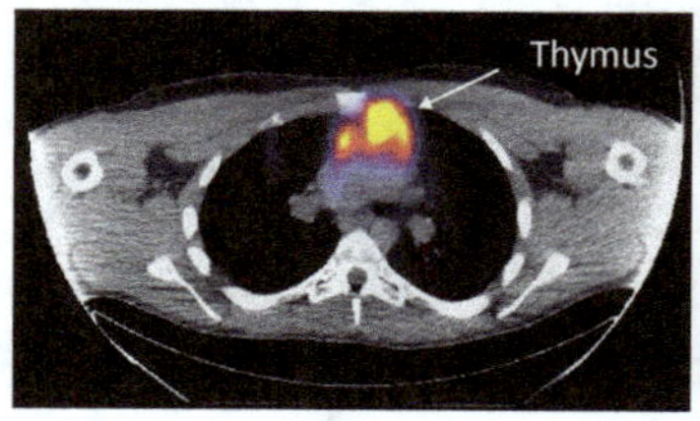

Coronal fused SPECT CT images

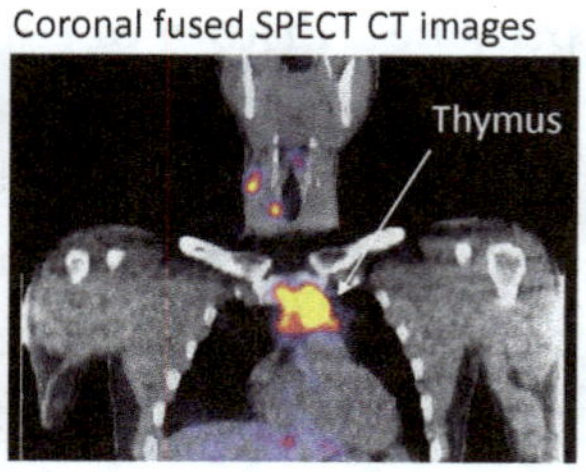

Ectopic thyroid tissue (Answer A) within the thymus has been reported and likely reflects the origin of both tissues from the primordial pharynx. Separated fragments of ectopic thyroid tissue may come to rest anywhere in the midline along the pathway of the embryologic descent of the heart and great vessels. However, ectopic thyroid tissue within the thymus is an uncommon finding.

Similarly, rare cases of thyroid cancer metastatic to the thymus (Answer B) have been reported. In this scenario, the serum thyroglobulin might be more elevated.

Parathyroid tissue (Answer D) can be found in ectopic locations, including within thymic tissue in the anterior mediastinum. However, parathyroid tissue would not take up iodine and would not be visualized on iodine scanning.

Normal lymph nodes (Answer C) would not accumulate radioiodine due to the absence of the sodium-iodide symporter in lymph tissue.

EDUCATIONAL OBJECTIVE

Describe how some areas of uptake seen on iodine scanning may be false-positive findings, rather than thyroid or thyroid cancer tissue, and thymic tissue is one example of such a false-positive.

REFERENCE(S)

Oh JR, Ahn B-C. False-positive uptake on radioiodine whole-body scintigraphy: physiologic and pathologic variants unrelated to thyroid cancer. *Am J Nucl Med Mol Imaging.* 2012;2(3):362-385. PMID: 23133823

Davidson J, McDougall IR. How frequently is the thymus seen on whole-body iodine-131 diagnostic and post-treatment scans? *Eur J Nucl Med.* 2000;27(4):425-430. PMID: 10805116

Kim MJ, Oh SW, Youn H, et al. Thyroid-related protein expression in the human thymus. *Int J Endocrinol.* 2017;2017:8159892. PMID: 28386277

Veronikis IE, Simkin P, Braverman LE. Thymic uptake of iodine-131 in the anterior mediastinum. *J Nucl Med.* 1996;37(6):991-992. PMID: 8683329

5 ANSWER: E) The patient's older age

Small papillary thyroid carcinomas often have an indolent course, and some may not cause any consequences during a patient's lifetime. In such cases, it is reasonable to elect not to undergo surgery, but to follow the patient to determine whether surgery becomes advisable. If choosing active surveillance rather than immediate surgical management for papillary thyroid carcinoma, certain criteria should be met. These criteria have been used in clinical trials of active surveillance of patients with low-risk papillary thyroid cancer conducted primarily in Japan, Korea, and the United States. These clinical trials have typically enrolled patients with papillary thyroid cancers smaller than 1 cm and have used serial monitoring by ultrasonography, initially every 6 months and then yearly.

Criteria for immediate surgery include lymph node metastasis (thus, Answer D is incorrect) and significant extrathyroidal extension of the papillary thyroid cancer (thus, Answer A is incorrect). Patients with minimal extrathyroidal extension may possibly still be candidates for active surveillance according to a recent Japanese consensus statement, but careful imaging by ultrasonography and/or CT is necessary.

Another contraindication to active surveillance is invasion into the recurrent laryngeal nerve or trachea or other compromise of these structures. Patient with new-onset hoarseness are not good candidates for active surveillance until the source of the hoarseness has been attributed to causes other than laryngeal nerve involvement (thus, Answer C is incorrect).

Other potential reasons not to delay surgery include evidence of an aggressive subtype of papillary thyroid cancer based on cytologic examination or other thyroid or parathyroid disease that would require surgery. A diagnosis of hyperparathyroidism with a serum calcium concentration of 11 mg/dL (2.75 mmol/L) may well be best managed with surgery (thus, Answer B is incorrect).

The clinical trials of active surveillance have provided information about the growth patterns of papillary microcarcinomas. They mostly grow slowly or are stable, some tumors shrink, and only a few grow rapidly. Tumors with initial enlargement in maximal diameter greater than 3 mm and increase in tumor volume greater than 50% sometimes demonstrate a slowing of growth rate after an initial increase in size. Therefore, it is suggested that surgery may not be immediately necessary after an initial increase in size has been observed. When examining increase in size of papillary microcarcinomas according to age, increased size and development of cervical lymph node metastases may be seen more frequently in younger patients. Older patients (Answer E) are ideal candidates for active surveillance.

Active surveillance of low-risk papillary thyroid carcinomas has become more acceptable in clinical practice in many countries, with some practitioners also using active surveillance for tumors measuring 1 to 2 cm.

EDUCATIONAL OBJECTIVE

Identify features that suggest that a small papillary thyroid cancer may be safely followed and thus support a decision for active surveillance.

REFERENCE(S)

Sugitani I, Ito Y, Takeuchi D, et al. Indications and strategy for active surveillance of adult low-risk papillary thyroid microcarcinoma: consensus statements from the Japan Association of Endocrine Surgery Task Force on Management for Papillary Thyroid Microcarcinoma. *Thyroid.* 2021;31(2):183-192. PMID: 33023426

Miyauchi A, Ito Y, Oda H. Insights into the management of papillary microcarcinoma of the thyroid. *Thyroid.* 2018 Jan;28(1):23-31. PMID: 28629253

Ito Y, Miyauchi A, Kihara M, Higashiyama T, Kobayashi K, Miya A. Patient age is significantly related to the progression of papillary microcarcinoma of the thyroid under observation. *Thyroid.* 2014;24(1):27-34. PMID: 24001104

Tuttle RM, Fagin J, Minkowitz G, et al. Active surveillance of papillary thyroid cancer: frequency and time course of the six most common tumor volume kinetic patterns. *Thyroid.* 2022;32(11):1337-1345. PMID: 36178355

6 ANSWER: E) Composition, almost completely solid; echogenicity, hypoechoic; margin, ill-defined; echogenic foci, punctate echogenic foci

Several systems have been used for the purposes of stratifying the risk of malignancy in thyroid nodules. These include several versions of TI-RADS (ACR TI-RADS, European TI-RADS, Korean TI-RADS, Artificial Intelligence TI-RADS) and the American Thyroid Association scoring system. TI-RADS uses several sonographic features as follows: composition, echogenicity, shape, margin, and echogenic foci. Points are assigned for subcategories within each feature, and the summation of the points can be used to determine the risk of malignancy divided into 5 risk levels. By extension, the risk levels can be used to assign a recommended size criterion for proceeding to FNA biopsy. The size cutoffs for FNA biopsy differ among the different TI-RADS categorization systems, resulting in different performance characteristics for each system. ACR TI-RADS generally recommends fewer FNA biopsies than other risk stratification systems because of the higher size thresholds for biopsy. However, it also recommends a follow-up plan based on nodule size.

The nodule depicted in this image is best described by Answer E. It is almost completely solid (2 points), is hypoechoic (2 points), has an ill-defined margin (0 points), has a wider than tall shape (0 points), and has punctate echogenic foci (3 points). Thus, this nodule earns a total of 7 points and falls into TI-RADS risk level 5. FNA biopsy would be recommended for this highly suspicious nodule if it were 1.0 cm or larger, whereas follow-up would be recommended if it were 0.5 cm or larger. The dimensions of this nodule were 0.8 × 0.9 × 0.6 cm; thus, follow-up without immediate FNA biopsy would be recommended based on ACR TI-RADS.

The other answer options can be eliminated based on their failure to accurately describe the nodule. The nodule is not mixed cystic and solid. Although it has some small cystic areas, these probably occupy less than 5% of the volume. Spongiform nodules have at least 50% of their volume occuped by cystic spaces. For spongiform nodules, these are not assigned points from the other categories. The nodule is not isoechoic (not the same reflectivity as adjacent thyroid tissue). The nodule does not have smooth margins, extrathyroidal extension, or peripheral calcifications.

EDUCATIONAL OBJECTIVE

Describe the sonographic features associated with the commonly used ACR TI-RADS risk stratification system.

REFERENCE(S)

Tessler FN, Middleton WD, Grant EG, et al. ACR Thyroid Imaging, Reporting and Data System (TI-RADS): white paper of the ACR TI-RADS Committee. *J Am Coll Radiol.* 2017;14(5):587-595. PMID: 28372962

Tessler FN, Middleton WD, Grant EG. Thyroid Imaging Reporting and Data System (TI-RADS): a user's guide. *Radiology.* 2018;287(1):29-36. PMID: 29558300

Hoang JK, Middleton WD, Tessler FN. Update on ACR TI-RADS: successes, challenges, and future directions, from the *AJR* Special Series on Radiology Reporting and Data Systems. *AJR Am J Roentgenol.* 2021;216(3):570-578. PMID: 33112199

Hoang JK, Asadollahi S, Durante C, Hegedüs L, Papini E, Tessler FN. An international survey on utilization of five thyroid nodule risk stratification systems: a needs assessment with future implications. *Thyroid.* 2022;32(6):675-681. PMID: 35229624

7 ANSWER: E) At least 150 mcg levothyroxine daily

There are 2 issues to consider with treating this patient's hypothyroidism. One is restoring euthyroidism in a severely hypothyroid patient. The other is restoring euthyroidism during the first trimester of pregnancy, a time when optimal fetal development requires transplacental transfer of maternal thyroid hormone. As the patient is at 8 weeks' gestation, rendering her euthyroid requires a higher dosage of thyroid hormone than would be needed in the nonpregnant state. Most patients with hypothyroidism who are euthyroid before pregnancy require approximately a 30% increase in their levothyroxine dosage. This is particularly true in individuals who have little residual thyroid function, as may be the case in this patient who was treated with ^{131}I to ablate her previously overactive thyroid. The increased levothyroxine requirement is due to factors such as increased levels of thyroxine-binding globulin and increased blood volume during pregnancy.

Treating the patient with a lower levothyroxine dosage (63 mcg [Answer A] and 112 mcg [Answer B]) than the dosage of 125 mcg daily that rendered her euthyroid in the nonpregnant state is incorrect. These options also do not account for the higher dosage of levothyroxine that would be needed to sustain euthyroidism during pregnancy. Similarly, the dosage of 125 mcg daily (Answer C) is also insufficient, as although it normalized her TSH value when she was not pregnant, it does not account for the increased thyroid hormone requirement during pregnancy.

Restoring euthyroidism in this patient is a matter of urgency. Inadequately treated hypothyroidism in the first trimester is associated with impaired fetal neurodevelopment, including reduced intelligence quotient. Hypothyroidism later in pregnancy can be associated with preeclampsia, placental abruption, low birth weight, and fetal death. Despite this patient's severe hypothyroidism, cautious initiation of thyroid hormone should not be the strategy. She is relatively young, does not appear to have cardiac pathology (despite her previous symptoms associated with thyroid hormone treatment) and a full treatment dosage of levothyroxine is imperative for optimizing her fetal and pregnancy outcomes. Therefore, starting at least 150 mcg daily (Answer E) is the best choice. Although not documented and tested as a potential approach, it may also be reasonable to provide this patient with several days of a loading dose of levothyroxine (eg, twice her anticipated dose) to facilitate a more rapid trajectory towards euthyroidism.

Triiodothyronine (Answer D) does not cross the placenta. Therefore, combination therapy with both levothyroxine and liothyronine is not recommended during pregnancy because this may result in inadequate provision of thyroid hormone to the fetus.

EDUCATIONAL OBJECTIVE

Promptly restore euthyroidism during pregnancy and account for the increased thyroid hormone requirement manifesting early in pregnancy.

REFERENCE(S)

Lee SY, Pearce EN. Testing, monitoring, and treatment of thyroid dysfunction in pregnancy. *J Clin Endocrinol Metab.* 2021;106(3):883-892. PMID: 33349844

Alexander EK, Pearce EN, Brent GA, et al. 2017 guidelines of the American Thyroid Association for the diagnosis and management of thyroid disease during pregnancy and the postpartum. *Thyroid.* 2017;27(3):315-389. PMID: 28056690

8 ANSWER: C) Low free T_3 and high reverse T_3

This patient has been hospitalized with a serious illness for a prolonged period. She has also undergone surgery that has likely resulted in an insult to her hypothalamus and pituitary. The diagnoses of nonthyroidal illness syndrome and central hypothyroidism are each potential explanations for the patient's abnormal thyroid test results.

Nonthyroidal illness is a condition characterized by low concentrations of serum T_3, most typically elevated concentrations of reverse T_3, and generally low levels of T_4 and TSH. This syndrome is thought to be due to a complex set of changes in the hypothalamic-pituitary axis and to alterations in thyroid hormone metabolism at the organ and tissue level. Regarding the hypothalamic-pituitary axis, there is failure to mount an elevated TSH response to low thyroid hormone levels, suggesting down-regulation of the axis, perhaps via reduced thyrotropin-releasing hormone expression mediated, in turn, by altered deiodinase expression (reduced type 2 deiodinase and increased type 3 deiodinase). Reduction in type 1 deiodinase in the liver may also contribute to changes in T_3 availability. T_4 may be preferentially inactivated to reverse T_3. These changes may be exacerbated by lack of nutritional support. Whether the nonthyroidal illness syndrome is adaptive or maladaptive is hotly debated.

Central hypothyroidism due to damage to the hypothalamic pituitary axis might have several laboratory features in common with nonthyroidal illness syndrome. TSH, T_4, free T_4, T_3, and free T_3 would all be low. One discriminating feature could be that reverse T_3 would be predicted to be low in central hypothyroidism, when T_4 would be preferentially converted to T_3 and high in nonthyroidal illness when T_4 might be inactivated to reverse T_3. Thus, a high reverse T_3 favors nonthyroidal illness, although it is not definitive, as sometimes reverse T_3 can be normal. Reviewing the answer choices, low free T_3 and high reverse T_3 (Answer C) most favors a diagnosis of nonthyroidal illness.

A high FSH concentration (Answers A and B) in this patient would suggest an intact gonadotroph axis, which does not discriminate between nonthyroidal illness and central hypothyroidism. Although a low FSH concentration would suggest a deficient gonadotroph axis (and perhaps also a damaged thyroid axis), this is not definitive because illness could temporarily dampen the FSH response to estrogen deficiency.

Low free T_3 and a negative TPO antibody titer (Answer D) is not a good discriminator. A low free T_3 concentration plus positive TPO antibodies (Answer E) would suggest primary hypothyroidism if an elevated TSH concentration had initially been observed.

A low free T_3 and low reverse T_3 concentration (an answer combination not given) would be consistent with central hypothyroidism due to hypothalamic pituitary damage.

EDUCATIONAL OBJECTIVE

Describe the thyroid hormone profile that characterizes nonthyroidal illness syndrome and central hypothyroidism and distinguish between these 2 entities.

REFERENCE(S)

Fliers E, Boelen A. An update on non-thyroidal illness syndrome. *J Endocrinol Invest.* 2021;44(8):1597-1607. PMID: 33320308

Fliers E, Bianco AC, Langouche L, Boelen A. Thyroid function in critically ill patients. *Lancet Diabetes Endocrinol.* 2015;3(10):816-825. PMID: 26071885

Langouche L, Jacobs A, Van den Berghe G. Nonthyroidal illness syndrome across the ages. *J Endocr Soc.* 2019;3(12):2313-2325. PMID: 31745528

Van den Berghe G. Non-thyroidal illness in the ICU: a syndrome with different faces. *Thyroid.* 2014;24(10):1456-1465. PMID: 24845024

9 ANSWER: C) *PTEN* hamartoma tumor syndrome

Both the patient's history and her family history are highly suggestive of *PTEN* hamartoma tumor syndrome (also known as Cowden syndrome) (Answer C). *PTEN* hamartoma tumor syndrome is an autosomal dominant syndrome in which a germline *PTEN* pathogenic variant predisposes individuals to both hamartomas and increased risk of malignancy. Affected persons usually present in the second to third decade of life with mucocutaneous lesions such as clusters of papillomatous papules near the eyelids, forehead, nose, mouth, hands, or feet; flesh-colored hamartomas at the hairline (trichilemmomas); and acral keratoses. There are both major and minor diagnostic criteria for this syndrome, and the 2021 revised clinical diagnostic criteria permit diagnosis in an individual with 3 or more major criteria, 1 of which must be macrocephaly, Lhermitte–Duclos disease, or gastrointestinal hamartomas, or in an individual with a combination of 2 major and 3 minor criteria.

Major criteria for diagnosis of *PTEN* hamartoma syndrome include the previously mentioned mucocutaneous lesions, breast cancer, endometrial cancer, follicular thyroid cancer, gastrointestinal hamartomas, macrocephaly, and Lhermitte–Duclos disease. Lhermitte–Duclos disease is characterized by a dysplastic gangliocytoma of the cerebellum, which presents with headaches, cerebellar ataxia, and visual problems.

In addition to breast, endometrial, and thyroid cancers, other associated cancers are colon cancer and renal cell carcinoma. This patient's qualifying diagnoses are breast cancer, thyroid cancer, mucocutaneous lesions, lipoma, and thyroid structural lesions. Papillary thyroid cancer is considered one of the minor criteria. The importance of recognizing this diagnosis is not only for surveillance of additional features in the patient but also for screening her family members and subsequent surveillance for associated malignancies.

Familial adenomatous polyposis (Answer A) is caused by inactivating germline *APC* pathogenic variants and is characterized by multiple colorectal adenomatous polyps; a high risk of colorectal, thyroid, and other cancers; and desmoid tumors. This does not describe the patient's phenotype.

Werner syndrome (Answer E) is an autosomal recessive disease with genetic instability and cancer predisposition. Symptoms typically start at about 20 years of age, and the syndrome is characterized by premature graying and/or thinning of scalp hair, bilateral ocular cataracts, chronic ulcers involving the ankles, and short stature.

Both a serum TSH concentration that is above the reference range (Answer D) and Hashimoto thyroiditis (Answer B) are associated with an increased risk of thyroid cancer. However, the increased risk associated with *PTEN* hamartoma tumor syndrome (standardized incidence ratio of approximately 50), is far greater than the increased risk seen with elevated TSH levels (increased odds ratio of 1.6 for each 1.0 mIU/L increase in TSH) and Hashimoto thyroiditis (relative risk, 1.6).

EDUCATIONAL OBJECTIVE

Identify the characteristics of *PTEN* hamartoma tumor syndrome, including its association with thyroid cancer.

REFERENCE(S)

Dragoo DD, Taher A, Wong VK, et al. PTEN hamartoma tumor syndrome/Cowden syndrome: genomics, oncogenesis, and imaging review for associated lesions and malignancy. *Cancers (Basel).* 2021;13(13):3120. PMID: 34206559

Pilarski R, Burt R, Kohlman W, Pho L, Shannon KM, Swisher E. Cowden syndrome and the PTEN hamartoma tumor syndrome: systematic review and revised diagnostic criteria. *J Natl Cancer Inst.* 2013;105(21):1607-1616. PMID: 24136893

Tan MH, Mester JL, Ngeow J, Rybicki LA, Orloff MS, Eng C. Lifetime cancer risks in individuals with germline PTEN mutations. *Clin Cancer Res.* 2012;18(2):400-407. PMID: 22252256

Cameselle-Teijeiro JM, Mete O, Asa SL, LiVolsi V. Inherited follicular epithelial-derived thyroid carcinomas: from molecular biology to histological correlates. *Endocr Pathol.* 2021;32(1):77-101. PMID: 33495912

10 **ANSWER: D) Serum T_3**

This patient's history suggests well-established Hashimoto hypothyroidism with a requirement for replacement thyroid hormone during her 3 pregnancies. Her thyroid gland appears atrophic on imaging, suggesting that she may have little functional thyroid tissue. Currently, she is not taking prescribed thyroid hormone and her laboratory testing suggests thyrotoxicosis. There are patients who have both thyroid inhibitory and thyroid-stimulating antibodies and oscillate between hyperthyroidism and hypothyroidism. However, these cases are relatively rare and such patients usually retain palpable thyroid tissue that supports the reemergence of hyperthyroidism. Although an elevated thyroid-stimulating immunoglobulin level (Answer E) would support such a hypothesis, this is not the simplest explanation.

Assessment of the patient's TPO antibody titer (Answer A) also would not be helpful. It has likely declined since the patient's initial diagnosis and would not explain current hyperthyroidism.

Serum selenium (Answer C) might be elevated if the patient has been taking a selenium-containing supplement, but it would not cause hyperthyroidism in the setting of minimal functional thyroid tissue.

Similarly, if one of the patient's supplements has significant iodine content, this would lead to elevated urinary iodine (Answer B). However, there has to be functioning thyroid tissue to use the iodine for endogenous thyroid hormone synthesis.

The patient provided a photograph of one of her current supplements. Its contents included the following: selenium, iodine, kelp, l-tyrosine, lyophilized bovine hypothalamus, lyophilized bovine pituitary, and lyophilized bovine thyroid. Her serum T_3 concentration (Answer D) was found to be significantly elevated at 400 ng/dL (6.16 nmol/L). This finding is most consistent with iatrogenic thyrotoxicosis caused by the consumption of bovine tissue that contains both T_4 and T_3, with a higher ratio of T_3 to T_4 than is seen with normal human thyroid functioning. The lyophilized bovine hypothalamus and pituitary would not have contributed to the thyrotoxicosis, as they contain peptide hormones that would be digested in the gastrointestinal tract.

Reports of over-the-counter supplements causing thyrotoxicosis abound in the literature. These products are not regulated by the US FDA, so it is difficult to ascertain the exact thyroid hormone content. This patient's supplement listed 200 mg lyophilized bovine thyroid in its contents, but it did not list its T_4 and T_3 content. One study, which measured the T_4 and T_3 content of selected "thyroid health" supplements, found "clinically relevant amounts of T_4 and T_3, some of which exceeded common treatment doses for hypothyroidism."

EDUCATIONAL OBJECTIVE

Explain that over-the-counter health supplements may contain thyroid hormones and can be responsible for iatrogenic thyrotoxicosis.

REFERENCE(S)

Kang GY, Parks JR, Fileta B, Chang A, Abdel-Rahim MM, Burch HB, Bernet VJ. Thyroxine and triiodothyronine content in commercially available thyroid health supplements. *Thyroid.* 2013;23(10):1233-1237. PMID: 23758055

Hoang TD, Mai VQ, Clyde PW, Shakir MK. Over-the-counter-drug-induced thyroid disorders. *Endocr Pract.* 2013;19(2):268-274. PMID: 23529350

Irwig MS, Fleseriu M, Jonklaas J, et al. Off-label use and misuse of testosterone, growth hormone, thyroid hormone, and adrenal supplements: risks and costs of a growing problem. *Endocr Pract.* 2020;26(3):340-353. PMID: 32163313

11 ANSWER: D) His TSH value is normal for octogenarians

This elderly patient has an asymptomatic, mild TSH elevation. An analysis of the NHANES-III population survey (Third National Health and Nutrition Examination Survey) has shown that normal older patients without goiter or serologic evidence of Hashimoto thyroiditis have a rightward shift in the upper normal limit for TSH, with the upper 95% confidence interval ranging to approximately 7.5 mIU/L in octogenarians (thus, Answer D is correct). The best management option in this asymptomatic octogenarian is no intervention.

Apathetic hyperthyroidism, but not hypothyroidism (Answer B), has been described in older patients.

Levothyroxine treatment (Answer E) is not indicated in the absence of true hypothyroidism.

Some studies have shown improved survival in elderly patients with mild serum TSH elevation, without a decrement in cognitive function, depression, or other disability in daily living. The reason for this finding is unclear, but it may be related to avoidance of the higher risk of arrhythmia that occurs with lower TSH values. However, improved survival has not been confirmed in all studies.

Increased cardiovascular disease has been observed in association with increased serum TSH values in a recent study, with the cardiovascular disease mediating increased mortality. This association might be explained by such effects of low thyroid hormone levels as causing dyslipidemia, increasing systemic vascular resistance, and inducing endothelial dysfunction. A slightly high TSH value might be associated with increased systemic vascular resistance, not decreased systemic vascular resistance (Answer A). The association between TSH and mortality was not seen in other studies, including a study of individuals older than 60 years.

Although there can be increases in LDL cholesterol even with TSH values in the upper part of the reference range, a statin (Answer C) is not indicated without measuring cholesterol.

EDUCATIONAL OBJECTIVE

Explain age-specific normal ranges for serum thyrotropin.

REFERENCE(S)

Surks MI, Boucai L. Age- and race-based serum thyrotropin reference limits. *J Clin Endocrinol Metab.* 2010;95(2):496-502. PMID: 19965925

Gussekloo J, van Exel E, de Craen AJ, Meinders AE, Flolich M, Westendorp RG. Thyroid status, disability and cognitive function, and survival in old age. *JAMA.* 2004;292(21):2591-2599. PMID: 15572717

Rodondi N, den Elzen WP, Bauer DC, et al; Thyroid Studies Colloraboration. Subclinical hypothyroidism and the risk of coronary heart disease and mortality. *JAMA.* 2010;304(12):1365-1374. PMID: 20858880

Wang Y, Liu C, Liu L, et al. Association of elevated thyroid stimulating hormone with atherosclerotic cardiovascular disease and its mortality in elderly community-dwelling Chinese. *Clin Interv Aging.* 2022;17:1139-1150. PMID: 35942336

Inoue K, Ritz B, Brent GA, Ebrahimi R, Rhee CM, Leung AM. Association of subclinical hypothyroidism and cardiovascular disease with mortality. *JAMA Netw Open.* 2020;3(2):e1920745. PMID: 32031647

12 ANSWER: D) Start hydrocortisone, start SSKI, and optimize β-adrenergic blockade before surgery

This patient has experienced hepatotoxicity while taking methimazole. Although hepatic dysfunction on methimazole is frequently described as cholestatic in nature, a hepatocellular destructive pattern manifested by transaminitis may also occur. In 1 series of methimazole-induced hepatic dysfunction, 11 of 30 cases involved noncholestatic hepatocellular injury. In this particular case, the patient's regimen cannot be switched to the alternative antithyroid drug, propylthiouracil, because of his marked hepatic transaminase elevation. His refusal to consider radioiodine leaves only thyroidectomy. Because he has moderate thyrotoxicosis, he will require preoperative preparation for thyroidectomy to reduce the risk of perioperative morbidity. Corticosteroids such as hydrocortisone and dexamethasone are potent inhibitors of T_4-to-T_3 conversion. Supersaturated potassium iodide (SSKI) acutely inhibits thyroid hormone synthesis and release. Thus, starting hydrocortisone, starting SSKI, and optimizing β-adrenergic blockade before surgery (Answer D) is the best approach. At some centers, cholestyramine, which interferes with the enterohepatic circulation of thyroid hormone, is added in this setting as well.

The remaining options are not as attractive. Resuming methimazole at a lower dosage (Answer C) or starting propylthiouracil (Answer E) would expose the patient to continued hepatotoxicity.

Patients treated with SSKI experience an escape from the acute inhibition of thyroid hormone synthesis (ie, they escape from the Wolff-Chaikoff effect), frequently after 10 to 14 days of therapy, so a prolonged course (Answer A) is not acceptable.

Therapy with a β-adrenergic blocker (Answer B) as a single agent will not sufficiently contribute to attempts to lower the thyroid hormone level and is insufficient to prevent perioperative morbidity.

EDUCATIONAL OBJECTIVE

Devise a preoperative approach to a patient with thyrotoxicosis who cannot take antithyroid drugs because of hepatotoxicity.

REFERENCE(S)

Langley RW, Burch HB. Perioperative management of the thyrotoxic patient. *Endocrinol Metab Clin North Am.* 2003;32(2):519-534. PMID: 12800544

Ross DS, Burch HB, Cooper DS, et al. 2016 American Thyroid Association guidelines for diagnosis and management of hyperthyroidism and other causes of thyrotoxicosis. *Thyroid.* 2016;26(10):1343-1421. PMID: 27521067

13 ANSWER: E) Nephrotic syndrome

Nephrotic syndrome (Answer E) is the cause of this patient's progressive increase in levothyroxine dosage requirement, due largely to loss of thyroid-binding proteins (with thyroid hormone still bound to them) in the urine. Clues to this etiology include her lower-extremity edema, low albumin, and high lipid levels. This case and similar cases have been reported in the literature. In the setting of reversible nephrotic syndrome, levothyroxine dosage requirements return to baseline as the proteinuria resolves. In a study of 9 patients, the mean age was 43 years and serum TSH increased from a baseline of 2.1 mIU/L prior to development of nephrotic syndrome to 8.2 mIU/L after diagnosis, resulting in a need for an 18% increase in the levothyroxine dosage. Remission of nephrotic syndrome was associated with a 15% decrease in the levothyroxine dosage needed to maintain normal thyroid function.

Other sources of unexpected changes in levothyroxine dosage requirements include starting new medications that interfere either with absorption (iron, calcium, and binding resins) or with clearance (phenytoin, phenobarbital, and possibly sertraline) of thyroid hormone, significant weight gain or weight loss, and, of course, nonadherence to therapy.

Metformin therapy (Answer D) is associated with a slight decrease in serum TSH concentrations in levothyroxine-treated patients. It is one of the few medications that lowers serum TSH levels in contrast to the multiple medications that raise TSH levels. It does not increase the levothyroxine dosage requirement.

Although medication nonadherence (Answer C) and celiac disease (Answer A) could both increase the levothyroxine dosage requirement, they would not explain the clinical stigmata of nephrotic syndrome described in the vignette.

The patient is not acutely ill, so euthyroid sick syndrome (Answer B) is not pertinent, and even if it were, this syndrome does not result in an increased thyroid hormone dosage requirement.

EDUCATIONAL OBJECTIVE

Explain the effect of thyroid-binding protein loss in urine on the thyroid hormone dosage requirement.

REFERENCE(S)

Karethimmaiah H, Sarathi V. Nephrotic syndrome increases the need for levothyroxine replacement in patients with hypothyroidism. *J Clin Diagn Res.* 2016;10(12):OC10-OC12. PMID: 28208903

Halma C. Thyroid function in patients with proteinuria. *Neth J Med.* 2009;67(4):153. PMID: 19581660
Fukata S, Ito M, Nishikawa M, et al. Hypothyroidism due to nephrotic syndrome: a notable clinical entity. *Endocr J.* 2022;69(3):307-311. PMID: 34615836

14 ANSWER: D) Repeat complete blood cell count with differential

This patient has most likely developed agranulocytosis due to antithyroid drug therapy, which would be confirmed by repeating the complete blood cell count with differential (Answer D). His normal complete blood cell count 2 weeks earlier should not be considered reassuring because this disorder can develop rapidly and unpredictably. A recent large review of agranulocytosis cases in Japan showed that more than half of agranulocytosis cases occur within 2 weeks of a previously normal granulocyte count. Therefore, patients receiving antithyroid drugs should be reminded at each clinical interaction of the need to seek medical attention immediately for fever or sore throat, for the explicit purpose of excluding this rare complication, which affects approximately 1 in 200 patients treated. A recent study suggests that there may be a genetic predisposition to thionamide-induced agranulocytosis, as the risk of agranulocytosis was increased with several HLA haplotypes for methimazole and propylthiouracil, with certain haplotypes being more specific to methimazole-induced agranulocytosis.

After a diagnosis of antithyroid drug–related agranulocytosis, patients should not receive any form of thionamide therapy again (thus, Answers B and E are incorrect).

A throat culture (Answer C), even if positive, does not prove agranulocytosis.

There is no clinical evidence of thyroid storm (Answer A) in this patient.

Thionamide antithyroid drugs are associated with other important minor and major adverse effects. The most common minor adverse effect is a pruritic rash that affects 3% to 5% of treated patients. This may require antihistamines or switching to the alternative antithyroid drug. Major adverse effects include hepatotoxicity, antineutrophil cytoplasmic antibodies (ANCA)–positive vasculitis (more common with propylthiouracil), and agranulocytosis, as illustrated in this vignette.

EDUCATIONAL OBJECTIVE

Diagnose agranulocytosis and review appropriate management.

REFERENCE(S)

Nakamura H, Miyauchi A, Miyawaki N, Imagawa J. Analysis of 754 cases of antithyroid drug-induced agranulocytosis over 30 years in Japan. *J Clin Endocrinol Metab.* 2013;98(12):4776-4783. PMID: 24057289
Ross DS, Burch HB, Cooper DS, et al. 2016 American Thyroid Association guidelines for diagnosis and management of hyperthyroidism and other causes of thyrotoxicosis. *Thyroid.* 2016;26(10):1343-1421. PMID: 27521067
Chen WT, Chi C-C. Associations of HLA genotypes with antithyroid drug-induced agranulocytosis: a systematic review and meta-analysis of pharmacogenomics studies. *Br J Clin Pharmacol.* 2019;85(9):1878-1887. PMID: 31108563

15 ANSWER: E) Type 3 deiodinase

Type 3 deiodinase (DIO3) (Answer E) is an inactivating enzyme located in the placenta, brain, skin, and fetal liver. This enzyme inactivates T_4 to reverse T_3 and to 3,3'-T2 and most likely has a major role in modulating the thyroid hormone status of the early fetus. The considerably elevated reverse T_3 levels in this patient point to high levels of type 3 deiodinase. In contrast to the type 3 deiodinase, both type 1 and type 2 deiodinases (DIO1 and DIO2) are activating enzymes, converting T_4 to T_3. Ectopic or paraneoplastic expression of DIO3 has been described in highly vascularized hemangiomas in children, and gastrointestinal stromal tumors, hepatic hemangiomas, and a few other tumor types in adults. Patients with paraneoplastic synthesis of this enzyme require very large amounts of exogenous T_4 and T_3 to keep up with the enhanced deactivation occurring through tumor expression of

DIO3. This process has been referred to as "consumptive hypothyroidism." Therapy with liothyronine can also be initiated to treat this disorder.

Tumoral production of the other entities has not been described. Ectopic production of the sodium-iodide transporter (Answer C), the protein responsible for iodine transport, would not be expected to result in consumptive hypothyroidism.

Tumor production of monocarboxylase transporter 8 (Answer A), the transmembrane protein responsible for intracellular transport of thyroid hormone, could in theory decrease circulating thyroid hormone levels, but this has not been described.

TPO (Answer D) in thyroid follicular cells catalyzes the oxidation of iodide and is required for thyroid hormone organification. Defects in the gene encoding TPO are a common cause of congenital hypothyroidism, but they would not explain this patient's presentation and TPO production from tumor cells has not been reported.

Pendrin (Answer B) is a multifunctional anion exchanger that is believed to mediate iodine efflux from the apical membrane of thyroid follicular cells. Tumor production of pendrin has not been described.

EDUCATIONAL OBJECTIVE

Explain the consequences of overexpression of the type 3 deiodinase.

REFERENCE(S)

Huang SA, Tu HM, Harney JW, et al. Severe hypothyroidism caused by type 3 iodothyronine deiodinase in infantile hemangiomas. *N Engl J Med.* 2000;343(3):185-189. PMID: 10900278

Huang SA, Dorfman DM, Genest DR, Salvatore D, Larsen PR. Type 3 iodothyronine deiodinase is highly expressed in the human uteroplacental unit and in fetal epithelium. *J Clin Endocrinol Metab.* 2003;88(3):1384-1388. PMID: 1269133

Huang SA, Fish SA, Dorfman DM, et al. 21-year-old woman with consumptive hypothyroidism due to a vascular tumor expressing type 3 iodothyronine deiodinase. *J Clin Endocrinol Metab.* 2002;87(10):4457-4461. PMID: 12364418

Maynard MA, Marino-Enriquez A, Fletcher JA, et al. Thyroid hormone inactivation in gastrointestinal stromal tumors. *N Engl J Med.* 2014 Apr 3;370(14):1327-1334. PMID: 24693892

16 ANSWER: E) Vandetanib therapy

The tyrosine kinase inhibitors are a group of drugs that affect several proteins involved in the modulation of cell growth. Receptor kinases are involved in both normal cellular function and pathologic processes such as oncogenesis, metastasis, tumor angiogenesis, and maintenance of the tumor microenvironment. Tyrosine kinase inhibitors are small, orally active molecules that inhibit phosphorylation of tyrosine molecules at key ATP-binding sites. Affected targets include VEGF receptors 2 and 3, platelet-derived growth factor receptor, Flt-3, c-kit, and RET. On the basis of phase 3 trials showing beneficial effects, 2 tyrosine kinase inhibitors, vandetanib (Answer E) and cabozantinib, have been approved for treatment of medullary thyroid cancer in patients with extensive local disease or distant metastases. Although complete remission is very rare with these agents, disease stabilization and prolongation of progression-free survival have been found when compared with placebo (30.5 vs 19.3 months for vandetanib; 11.2 vs 4 months for cabozantinib in phase 3 trials). Palliative therapy is another option for this patient, given the limited, albeit improved, response duration for tyrosine kinase inhibitors. There are additional agents, selpercatinib and pralsetinib, that are FDA-approved for *RET*-associated medullary thyroid cancer.

There is no role for radioactive iodine therapy (Answer C) in medullary cancer. Similarly, there is no role for TSH suppression therapy and a patient's TSH can be kept in the normal range.

Cytotoxic chemotherapy (Answer A) has been applied as therapy for metastatic medullary thyroid cancer with limited utility; most regimens involve dacarbazine combined with a second agent.

Focal radiotherapy (Answer D) would not delay the systemic progression of metastatic disease in this patient.

There is no role for somatostatin analogue therapy (Answer B) in this case.

Table. Tyrosine Kinase Inhibitors Currently Approved for Use in Advanced Medullary Thyroid Cancer.

Tyrosine kinase Inhibitor	Targets of inhibition	Progression-free survival*
Vandetanib	RET, VEGFR, EGFR	30.5 vs 19.3 months (**compared with placebo**)
Cabozantinib	RET, VEGFR2, MET	11.2 vs 4 months (**compared with placebo**)
Selpercatinib	RET	1 year progression free survival 64%-92% (phase 1-2 trial)
Pralsetinib	RET	1 year progression free survival 75%-81% (phase 1-2 trial)

*Note: enrolled populations were different; efficacy cannot be compared directly across studies.

EDUCATIONAL OBJECTIVE

List indications for tyrosine kinase inhibitor therapy in advanced medullary thyroid cancer.

REFERENCE(S)

Wells SA Jr, Asa SL, Dralle H, et al; American Thyroid Association Guidelines Task Force on Medullary Thyroid Carcinoma. Revised American Thyroid Association guidelines for the management of medullary thyroid carcinoma. *Thyroid.* 2015;25(6):567-610. PMID: 25810047

Haddad RI, Bischoff L, Ball D, et al. Thyroid carcinoma, version 2.2022, NCCN clinical practice guidelines in oncology. *J Natl Compr Canc Netw.* 2022;20(8):925-951. PMID: 35948029

Matrone A, Gambale C, Prete A, Elisei R. Sporadic medullary thyroid carcinoma: towards a precision medicine. *Front Endocrinol (Lausanne).* 2022;13:864253. PMID: 35422765

Elisei R, Schlumberger MJ, Müller SP, et al. Cabozantinib in progressive medullary thyroid cancer. *J Clin Oncol.* 2013;31(29):3639-3646. PMID: 24002501

Wells SA Jr, Robinson BG, Gagel RF, et al. Vandetanib in patients with locally advanced or metastatic medullary thyroid cancer: a randomized, double-blind phase III trial. *J Clin Oncol.* 2012;30(2):134-141. PMID: 22025146

17 ANSWER: B) Referral for total thyroidectomy

In the Bethesda classification system for reporting thyroid cytopathology, nodules with indeterminate results, which include Bethesda category III (atypia of uncertain significance/follicular lesion of uncertain significance [AUS/FLUS]), category IV (follicular neoplasm/suspicious for follicular neoplasm [FN/SFN]), and category V (suspicious for malignancy [SM]), are sometimes selected for molecular testing. They have a predicted probability of cancer of 10% to 30%, 25% to 40%, and 50% to 75%, respectively.

Testing using a specific panel of pathogenic variants known to be associated with thyroid cancer is most helpful when a variant or rearrangement is present (higher positive predictive value) and is generally not helpful when no variant is identified (lower negative predictive value) because many cancers do not contain the limited set of abnormalities sought in the testing. In this patient with a large nodule (>4 cm), a follicular neoplasm on FNA biopsy, and a positive finding of a *RET/PTC* rearrangement, there is a high enough risk of thyroid cancer (80%-90%) that total thyroidectomy (Answer B) is recommended. The *RET/PTC* gene rearrangement, found in 20% to 70% of papillary thyroid cancers, causes constitutive activation of transcription of the RET tyrosine-kinase domain in follicular cells, leading to uncontrolled cell proliferation.

An example of how genetic testing can be used to guide clinical decision-making is shown in the figure from a study of one of the original genetic testing panels.

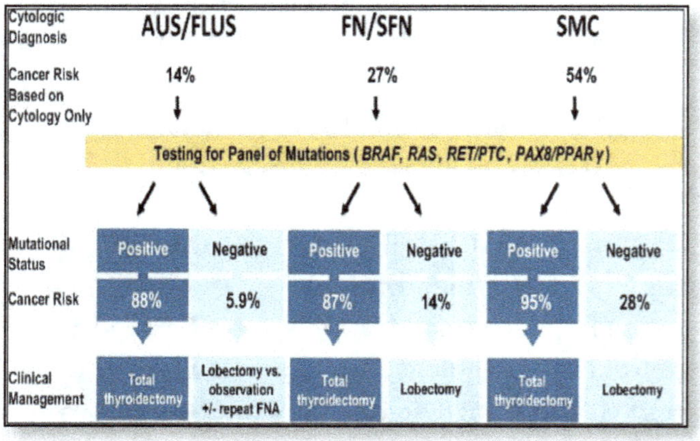

Reprinted from Nikiforov YE et al. *J Clin Endocrinol Metab*, 2011; 96(11):3390-3397. © The Endocrine Society.

Two major types of molecular testing have been developed. One is a microarray-based test with a proprietary algorithm that analyzes the mRNA expression of a panel of genes. This has been refined and augmented through various iterations to improve its ability to aid surgical decision-making for indeterminate nodules. Similarly, the other type of panel uses next-generation sequencing and assays for a panel of gene point mutations, insertions, deletions, copy number alterations, fusions, and gene expression alterations associated with thyroid cancer. These tests are continually being revised and expanded.

Lobectomy (Answer A) is inappropriate because of the high risk of malignancy. Given that his nodule is larger than 4 cm, a completion thyroidectomy would most likely be required when pathologic examination confirms a malignant nodule.

Although total thyroidectomy seems advisable, bilateral neck dissection (Answer C) is not warranted given the absence of suspicious lymph nodes on ultrasonography.

Performing thyroid ultrasonography (Answer E) or FNA biopsy (Answer D) again in 6 months would incorrectly defer thyroid surgery.

EDUCATIONAL OBJECTIVE

Apply molecular testing to thyroid nodule evaluation.

REFERENCE(S)

Steward DL, Carty SE, Sippel RS, et al. Performance of a multigene genomic classifier in thyroid nodules with indeterminate cytology: a prospective blinded multicenter study. *JAMA Oncol.* 2019;5(2):204-212. PMID: 30419129

Alexander EK, Kennedy GC, Baloch ZW, et al. Preoperative diagnosis of benign thyroid nodules with indeterminate cytology. *N Engl J Med.* 2012;367(8):705-715. PMID: 22731672

Nikiforov YE. Role of molecular markers in thyroid nodule management: then and now. *Endocr Pract.* 2017;23(8):979-988. PMID: 28534687

Nikiforov YE, Ohori NP, Hodak SP, Carty SE, LeBeau SO, Ferris RL, et al. Impact of mutational testing on the diagnosis and management of patients with cytologically indeterminate thyroid nodules: a prospective analysis of 1056 FNA samples. *J Clin Endocrinol Metab.* 2011;96(11):3390-3397. PMID: 21880806

Silaghi CA, Lozovanu V, Georgescu CE, et al. Thyroseq v3, Afirma GSC, and microRNA panels versus previous molecular tests in the preoperative diagnosis of indeterminate thyroid nodules: a systematic review and meta-analysis. *Front Endocrinol (Lausanne).* 2021;12:649522. PMID: 34054725

18 ANSWER: E) Repeated blood tests after stopping biotin for 7 days

The recommended daily intake for biotin is 300 mcg daily, but dosages that are orders of magnitude higher than requirements are available in many nutritional supplements. The use of biotin supplements can cause artifactual interference with commonly used biotin-streptavidin immunoassays for TSH, thyroid hormone, and TSH receptor antibodies. High circulating biotin levels cause falsely low measurements in immunometric sandwich assays (such as that for TSH), but falsely high measurements for competitive immunoassays (such as those for free T_4, T_3, and thyroid-stimulating immunoglobulin).

Thus, euthyroid patients taking biotin may have laboratory results identical to those found in Graves hyperthyroidism. Artifactual thyroid function results have been reported in patients taking at least 1500 mcg of biotin daily. Test results normalize 2 to 7 days after stopping the biotin. Therefore, the best next step is to repeat blood tests after stopping biotin for 7 days (Answer E).

Measurement of serum thyroid-stimulating immunoglobulin (Answer C) may be misleading while this patient is still taking biotin, as it could be falsely positive, although the result should be reliable, and presumably negative, once the patient has been off biotin.

Radioactive iodine uptake and scan (Answer D) would be diagnostic if this patient truly had Graves disease, but it would not be warranted if her blood tests normalize after ceasing biotin.

Finally, starting methimazole (Answer A) will not be indicated if this patient's laboratory values normalize once off biotin.

Patients frequently take biotin because of hair loss, but other hair products (Answer B) have not been documented to precipitate hyperthyroidism.

EDUCATIONAL OBJECTIVE

Describe the potential for biotin interference with thyroid function and thyroid antibody assays.

REFERENCE(S)

Kummer S, Hermsen D, Distelmaier F. Biotin treatment mimicking Graves' disease. *N Engl J Med.* 2016;375(7):704-706. PMID: 27532849

Elston MS, Sehgal S, Du Toit S, Yarndley T, Conaglen JV. Factitious Graves' disease due to biotin immunoassay interference-a case and review of the literature. *J Clin Endocrinol Metab.* 2016;101(9):3251-3255. PMID: 27362288

Barbesino G. Misdiagnosis of Graves' disease with apparent severe hyperthyroidism in a patient taking biotin megadoses. *Thyroid.* 2016;26(6):860-863. PMID: 27043844

19 ANSWER: E) TSH, 0.01 mIU/L; total T_4, 5.0 μg/dL (64.4 nmol/L); total T_3, 70 ng/dL (1.1 nmol/L); free T_4, 2.8 ng/dL (36.0 pmol/L)

This patient, previously euthyroid on a stable levothyroxine dosage, has recently started taking anabolic steroids. Unlike estrogens, which increase thyroxine-binding globulin values, androgens substantially decrease thyroxine-binding globulin. Euthyroid patients who are not taking levothyroxine would be expected to develop decreased serum total T_4 and T_3 levels while on high-dosage androgens, but, due to hypothalamic-pituitary-thyroid axis feedback, would be able to maintain normal free T_4 and serum TSH values (Answer D). However, a patient taking a fixed dosage of levothyroxine has the potential to become hyperthyroid when starting high-dosage androgens. Given marked variability in the ability of different androgens to aromatize, exact changes in thyroid function values are difficult to predict. However, Answer E is the only available choice that shows both a downward shift in total T_4 and T_3 values and a lack of compensation. A classic description of patients with hypothyroidism developing hyperthyroidism while on stable levothyroxine dosages can be found in a 1994 article in which women given androgen therapy for breast cancer required a 25% to 50% reduction in their thyroid hormone dosages to maintain euthyroidism.

In patients starting estrogens instead of androgens, opposite patterns might be observed: an increase in thyroxine-binding globulin driving increased total thyroid hormone values in which euthyroidism might be maintained in someone who was euthyroid at baseline (Answer B), but which might lead to hypothyroidism (Answer A) in a patient taking levothyroxine. Clinically, it is important to measure TSH 6 to 8 weeks after initiating estrogen or androgen therapy in patients on thyroid hormone replacement.

EDUCATIONAL OBJECTIVE

Diagnose androgen excess as a cause of a decrease in thyroxine-binding globulin and altered thyroid hormone requirements.

REFERENCE(S)

Tahboub R, Arafah BM. Sex steroids and the thyroid. *Best Pract Res Clin Endocrinol Metab.* 2009;23(6):769-780. PMID: 19942152

Arafah BM. Decreased levothyroxine requirement in women with hypothyroidism during androgen therapy for breast cancer. *Ann Intern Med.* 1994;121(4):247-251. PMID: 7518657

20 ANSWER: C) Cardiac tamponade

This patient has developed a large pericardial effusion (diminished heart sounds, low voltage on electrocardiography). Chest x-ray shows an enlarged cardiac silhouette (*see image*) (Answer C).

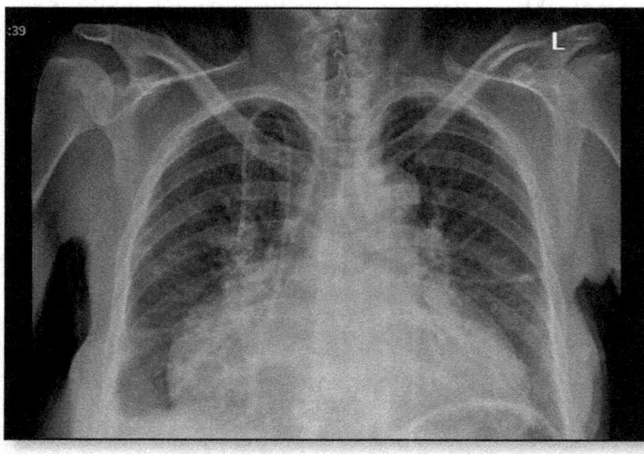

She is already being treated with corticosteroids to prevent adrenal insufficiency (Answer A).

Although she is at risk for developing cardiac ischemia (Answer B), as the thyroid hormone levels are increased, nothing in the scenario points to this diagnosis.

In the setting of hypothyroidism, there is decreased contractility and decreased pulse rate—both contributing to decreased cardiac output at a time when peripheral vascular resistance is increased. The patient is at risk for congestive heart failure (Answer D) from this mechanism, but again nothing in the scenario suggests this etiology for the decline in her cardiac function.

Although the TSH remains mildly elevated 48 hours after initiating intravenous levothyroxine treatment, the free T_4 is in the reference range. Thus, inadequate thyroid hormone replacement (Answer E) is unlikely.

In addition to being treated with levothyroxine, patient such as this may also require pericardiocentesis.

EDUCATIONAL OBJECTIVE

Identify signs of cardiac tamponade in a patient with myxedema coma.

REFERENCE(S)

Savage MW, Mah PM, Weetman AP, Newell-Price J. Endocrine emergencies. *Postgrad Med J.* 2004;80(947):506-515. PMID: 15356351

Karu AK, Khalife WI, Houser R, VanderWoude J. Impending cardiac tamponade as a primary presentation of hypothyroidism: case report and review of literature. *Endocr Pract.* 2005;11(4):265-271. PMID: 16006302

Wang J-L, Hsieh M-J, Lee CH, et al. Hypothyroid cardiac tamponade: clinical features, electrocardiography, pericardial fluid and management. *Am J Med Sci.* 2010;340(4):276-281. PMID: 20601858

21 ANSWER: B) Repeat thyroid function tests in 4 to 6 weeks

The primary differential in this patient is between Graves disease and gestational thyrotoxicosis. Gestational thyrotoxicosis is the most common cause of hyperthyroidism in the first trimester. It is typically seen in women with hyperemesis gravidarum and is caused by markedly elevated serum β-hCG levels. The concentration of β-hCG correlates with the severity of nausea, and gestational thyrotoxicosis is unusual in women without clinically significant nausea and vomiting. Gestational thyrotoxicosis resolves spontaneously as β-hCG levels fall after weeks 10 to 12 of gestation.

Graves disease is far more likely to be the cause of hyperthyroidism in this case because the thyrotoxicosis has not resolved after 12 weeks' gestation, T_3 is relatively elevated compared with T_4, the thyroid-stimulating immunoglobulin is positive, and she has no nausea or vomiting. However, her hyperthyroidism is subclinical: while the TSH level is low, the free T_4 and total T_3 levels are appropriate for her stage of gestation. Note that due to increasing levels of thyroxine-binding globulin, total thyroid hormone levels increase starting at week 7 of gestation until they plateau at week 16. A reasonable estimate for a gestational age–specific upper limit for total thyroid hormones can be derived by adding 5% to the upper limit of the nonpregnancy total thyroid hormone reference range each week starting at week 7. The upper limit will be 150% of the nonpregnancy reference range at week 16, and subsequently will remain stable for the rest of gestation.

Free T_4 assays generally do not perform well in pregnancy due to interference from high serum levels of binding globulins and esterified fatty acids. Although the effects of pregnancy are assay-specific, most assays provide artifactually low free T_4 values in the second and third trimesters. The free T_4 index, an older method in which both total T_4 and a test of serum thyroid hormone uptake such as the thyroid hormone–binding ratio are measured to calculate the free T_4 level may be more robust than commercial free T_4 immunoassays in pregnancy and is preferred by some for the estimation of free T_4 in pregnant women when available. Another option is to measure free T_4 using a tandem mass spectrometry assay, which may be more accurate than free T_4 immunoassays during pregnancy.

Large cohort studies suggest that there is no obstetric risk associated with subclinical hyperthyroidism in pregnancy. This patient should be monitored to watch for progression to overt hyperthyroidism (Answer B), but she does not need treatment now. Graves disease may sometimes temporarily remit during pregnancy, and this patient's TSH has improved slightly.

Both methimazole (Answer D) and propylthiouracil (Answer E) are teratogenic and should not be used in women without overt hyperthyroidism.

Thyroidectomy (Answer A) can be performed safely in the second trimester of pregnancy, but it is not warranted for subclinical hyperthyroidism.

While short-term use of β-adrenergic blocker in pregnancy is sometimes warranted for the reduction of hyperthyroid symptoms, atenolol (Answer C), which is a US FDA pregnancy category D drug, should not be used during pregnancy. Propranolol or labetalol are safer choices in pregnancy.

EDUCATIONAL OBJECTIVE

Diagnose and manage subclinical hyperthyroidism in pregnant women.

REFERENCE(S)

Alexander EK, Pearce EN, Brent GA, et al. 2017 guidelines of the American Thyroid Association for the diagnosis and management of thyroid disease during pregnancy and the postpartum. *Thyroid.* 2017;27(3):315-389. PMID: 28056690

Cooper DS, Laurberg P. Hyperthyroidism in pregnancy. *Lancet Diabetes Endocrinol.* 2013;1(3):238-249. PMID: 24622372

Lee RH, Spencer CA, Mestman JH, et al. Free T4 immunoassays are flawed during pregnancy. *Am J Obstet Gynecol.* 2009;200(3):260.e1-e6. PMID: 19114271

22 ANSWER: C) Omphalocele

Methimazole use in the first trimester of pregnancy is associated with embryopathy, including aplasia cutis, choanal atresia, esophageal atresia, tracheoesophageal fistula, omphalocele (Answer C), and dysmorphic facial features. Recently, a large population-based retrospective review of women exposed to either methimazole or propylthiouracil in early pregnancy (and prepregnancy) identified increased risks of embryopathy with *either* drug exposure, although the pattern of defects differed. Propylthiouracil is generally associated with less severe anomalies than methimazole. These include anomalies of the head and neck, urinary tract, and musculoskeletal systems.

These and other recent similar findings have prompted a call for a greater use of definitive therapy for Graves disease in women planning pregnancy to avoid exposure to either antithyroid drug during early gestation. Biliary atresia (Answer A), cleft palate (Answer B), placenta previa (Answer D), and spina bifida (Answer E) have not been associated with the use of antithyroid drugs in pregnancy.

EDUCATIONAL OBJECTIVE

Identify congenital birth defects associated with methimazole use in early pregnancy.

REFERENCE(S)

Andersen SL, Olsen J, Wu CS, Laurberg P. Birth defects after early pregnancy use of antithyroid drugs: a Danish nationwide study. *J Clin Endocrinol Metab.* 2013;98(11):4373-4381. PMID: 24151287

Rivkees SA. Propylthiouracil versus methimazole during pregnancy: an evolving tale of difficult choices. *J Clin Endocrinol Metab.* 2013;98(11):4332-4335. PMID: 24194618

Andersen SL, Knøsgaard L, Olsen J, Vestergaard P, Andersen S. Maternal thyroid function, use of antithyroid drugs in early pregnancy, and birth defects. *J Clin Endocrinol Metab.* 2019;104(12):6040-6048. PMID: 31408173

23 ANSWER: E) Suppressed serum TSH level

Drug-induced thyrotoxicosis, which occurs in up to 5% of patients treated with amiodarone, can present both diagnostic and therapeutic challenges. The diagnostic uncertainty is due to the dramatic effects that amiodarone has on thyroid function, even in euthyroid patients. A large iodine load is delivered with each dose (74 mg total iodine, 7.4 mg of free iodine per 200-mg tablet). Further, amiodarone inhibits both peripheral and central (intrapituitary) conversion of T_4 to T_3 through its action on type 1 deiodinase (DIO1) and type 2 5′-monodeiodinase (DIO2) enzymes, respectively. Amiodarone also has T_3 antagonistic effects at the nuclear level. The common pattern seen in euthyroid patients is a high free T_4, high total T_4, low-normal T_3, and high-normal TSH. Because of the potent inhibition of DIO2 and DIO1, either a suppressed TSH level or an elevated (rather than low) T_3 level is suggestive of amiodarone-induced thyrotoxicosis. An undetectable TSH value in this patient (Answer E) would be the most accurate indicator of thyrotoxicosis.

An elevated total T_4 level (Answer C) or free T_4 level (Answer B), as noted, can occur in euthyroid individuals. The degree of elevation of total and free T_4 in an individual who remains euthyroid on amiodarone is greater with the acute effects of amiodarone, which occur within the first 3 months (approximately 50% elevation). After 3 months, the chronic effect of amiodarone results in a 20% to 40% elevation in these hormones. Either of these degrees of elevation translates into these levels not being the most specific for detection of amiodarone-induced hyperthyroidism. The free T_4 level should be higher than expected (in the mid- to high-normal range), but this is not as helpful as the undetectable TSH value.

The radioactive iodine uptake (Answer D) is expected to be lower than normal even in a euthyroid patient on amiodarone because of the large iodine load.

Clinical signs and symptoms (Answer A) are insufficiently specific to make this diagnosis.

EDUCATIONAL OBJECTIVE

Identify the pattern of thyroid function test results in patients with amiodarone-induced thyrotoxicosis.

REFERENCE(S)

Trohman RG, Sharma PS, McAninch EA, Bianco AC. Amiodarone and thyroid physiology, pathophysiology, diagnosis and management. *Trends Cardiovasc Med.* 2019;29(5):285-295. PMID: 30309693

Basaria S, Cooper DS. Amiodarone and the thyroid. *Am J Med.* 2005;118(7):706-714. PMID: 15989900

24 ANSWER: C) Pyriform sinus fistula

Pyriform sinus fistulae (Answer C) have been identified in most patients with infectious thyroiditis, particularly in those with recurrent episodes from childhood or adolescence, as observed in this patient. The pyriform sinus is a recessed space in the normal pharynx at the level of the vocal cords. A pyriform sinus tract is a communicating channel between the pyriform sinus and a persistent brachial cleft cyst adjacent to the thyroid. Anatomic visualization of a pyriform sinus tract can be obtained with ultrasonography, barium swallow, CT, and MRI of the neck. Ultrasonography can show a hypoechoic area within the thyroid gland that can be misinterpreted as a thyroid nodule. The figure shows a schematic of a pyriform sinus passing through the thyroid gland where an abscess can form. The left side is more frequently affected than the right side. Surgical excision is required to prevent recurrence.

A thyroglossal duct cyst (Answer E) is typically located at the level of the hyoid bone in the midline.

Chronic sinusitis (Answer A) does not cause thyroiditis.

Intravenous drug use (Answer B), although rarely cited as a source of an isolated thyroid abscess, is much less common than a pyriform sinus fistula in cases of recurrent acute thyroiditis.

Finally, a dental abscess (Answer D) is not a likely source of contiguous spread of bacterial infection to the thyroid.

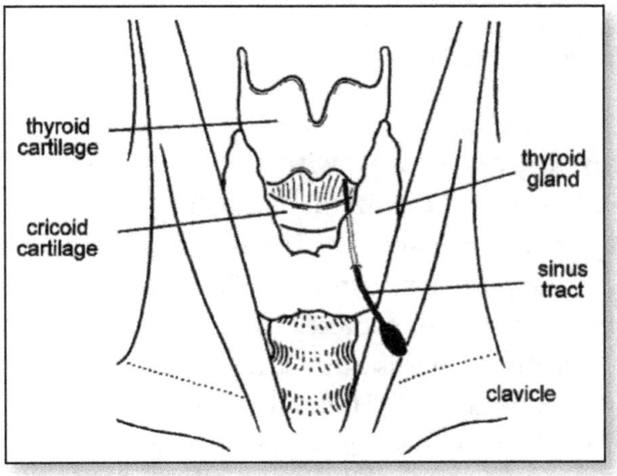

Reprinted from Park SW et al. *Am J Neuroradiol*, 2000; 21(5): 817-822. © American Society of Neuroradiology.

EDUCATIONAL OBJECTIVE

Identify pyriform sinus fistula as an etiology of acute thyroiditis.

REFERENCE(S)

Masuoka H, Miyauchi A, Tomoda C, et al. Imaging studies in sixty patients with acute suppurative thyroiditis. *Thyroid.* 2011;21(10):1075-1080. PMID: 21875365

Park SW, Han MH, Sung MH, et al. Neck infection associated with pyriform sinus fistula: imaging findings. *AJNR Am J Neuroradiol.* 2000;21(5):817-822. PMID: 10815654

Ahn D, Lee GJ, Sohn JH. Ultrasonographic characteristics of pyriform sinus fistulas involving the thyroid gland. *J Ultrasound Med.* 2018;37(11):2631-2636.PMID: 30099745

25 ANSWER: A) Stage II

Staging for thyroid cancer is uniquely related to patient age. In October 2016, the American Joint Committee on Cancer (AJCC) (cancerstaging.org) published the eighth edition of the AJCC/tumor, lymph node, metastasis (TNM) cancer staging system, replacing the seventh edition. There are several notable changes that were implemented, including the age cutoff used for staging being increased from 45 years to 55 years, minor extrathyroidal extension seen only on histology being no longer part of the definition of T3 disease, and N1 disease in an older patient (now older than 55 years) no longer upgrading a patient to stage III. The first change is relevant to this vignette.

Although in general, patients with thyroid cancer of all ages have an excellent prognosis, this is particularly the case for younger patients. Studies have shown conflicting data as to whether prognosis simply incrementally worsens with advancing age or whether there is a distinct cutoff that predicts a step up in risk. Based on the prevailing data, the American Joint Committee on Cancer retained an age cutoff in thyroid cancer staging but increased the age from 45 to 55 years. As a result, the most advanced stage category for patients younger than 55 in the American Joint Committee on Cancer system is stage II (Answer A) even with metastatic disease present. If this patient were 55 years or older, she would have IVB disease (Answer D).

Stage III classification (Answer B) would occur for a patient 55 years or older with a T4a tumor, which is a tumor with gross extrathyroidal extension invading subcutaneous soft tissues, larynx, trachea, esophagus, or recurrent laryngeal nerve from a tumor of any size.

In contrast, stage IVA classification (Answer C) would occur with gross extrathyroidal extension invading prevertebral fascia or encasing the carotid artery or mediastinal vessels from a tumor of any size.

With the eighth edition of TNM staging, stage IVC (Answer E) is reserved for anaplastic thyroid cancer.

This patient's age already approximates 55 years, but if she were a few months older, her stage would change from II to IVB. It remains to be seen whether this upstaging reflects a strength or a limitation of the AJCC staging system for differentiated thyroid cancer. It also remains to be verified over time whether this discontinuous staging, rather than a more continuous staging, reflects the nature of the disease.

EDUCATIONAL OBJECTIVE

Assign staging for differentiated thyroid cancer based on the eighth edition of the AJCC (American Joint Committee on Cancer) staging system.

REFERENCE(S)

Amin MB, Edge SB, Greene FL, et al, eds. AJCC Cancer Staging Manual. 8th ed. New York: Springer International Publishing; 2017.

Perrier ND, Brierley JD, Tuttle RM. Differentiated and anaplastic thyroid carcinoma: major changes in the American Joint Committee on Cancer eighth edition cancer staging manual. *CA Cancer J Clin.* 2018;68(1):55-63. PMID: 29092098

26 ANSWER: D) Start propranolol

The key to this question is recognizing that the case represents thyroid hormone resistance and that because of variable tissue sensitivity to thyroid hormone in this setting, the patient has symptomatic cardiac effects, which are amenable to treatment with a β-adrenergic blocker (Answer D). Thyroid hormone resistance occurs in approximately 1 in 40,000 live births. Thyroid hormone effects are seen at the cellular level through interaction with nuclear receptors, including THR-α and THR-β. Patients with thyroid hormone resistance most frequently are heterozygous for a defect in THR-β, which presents with elevated serum TSH, free T_4, and free T_3 levels. Symptoms are due to a combination of low thyroid hormone action in predominantly THR-β–expressing tissues (such as the liver) and TH overexposure in THR-α–expressing tissues (such as the heart, skeletal muscle, and brain). Goiter and tachycardia, as seen in this patient, are common presenting symptoms (*see table*).

Table. Clinical Features of Thyroid Hormone Resistance

Sign or Symptom	Frequency
Thyroid	
Goiter	66%-95%
Heart	
Tachycardia	33%-75%
Nervous system	
Emotional disturbance	60%
Attention deficit	40%-60%
Hearing loss	10%-22%
Growth and development	
Short stature	18%-25%

Data derived from Refetoff S & Dumitrescu AM. *Best Pract Res Clin Endocrinol Metab*, 2007; 21(2):277-305. © Elsevier Ltd.

This disorder presents with discordant TSH and free T_4 values, but there is a differential diagnosis to be considered, which includes a TSH-secreting pituitary adenoma; TSH or free T_4 assay interference; and medications such as amiodarone, which this patient is not taking. In this vignette, the α-subunit-to-TSH molar ratio less than 1.0 favors thyroid hormone resistance rather than a TSH-producing pituitary tumor (the MRI is also normal and most TSH-secreting tumors are macroadenomas). Heterophile antibodies may cause a falsely elevated TSH value in a patient with thyrotoxicosis, but this interference was eliminated by the test results provided.

The goals of treatment for patients with resistance to thyroid hormone are to improve the symptoms that are caused by excessive THR-α signaling, while minimizing symptoms caused by deficient THR-β signaling.

Of the options provided in this case, the best is to proceed with treatment with β-adrenergic blockade to reduce the palpitations. Other approaches such as radioiodine therapy (Answer E) and thyroidectomy (Answer B) would not be beneficial. They would cause hypothyroidism, which would be challenging to treat because the supraphysiologic levothyroxine dosing that would be required to achieve euthyroidism in THR-β–sensitive tissues would cause hyperthyroidism in the THR-α–sensitive tissues.

Methimazole (Answer C) would most likely improve palpitations, but it would worsen symptoms caused by deficient THR-β signaling.

Because he has symptomatic cardiac involvement, no treatment (Answer A) is also incorrect.

EDUCATIONAL OBJECTIVE

Diagnose thyroid hormone resistance and treat variable tissue sensitivity.

REFERENCE(S)

Dumitrescu AM, Refetoff S. The syndromes of reduced sensitivity to thyroid hormone. *Biochim Biophys Acta.* 2013;1830(7):3987-4003. PMID: 22986150

Refetoff S, Dumitrescu AM. Syndromes of reduced sensitivity to thyroid hormone: genetic defects in hormone receptors, cell transporters and deiodination. *Best Pract Res Clin Endocrinol Metab.* 2007;21(2):277-305. PMID: 17574009

27 ANSWER: C) Increased risk of dental caries

One of the common adverse effects of radioactive iodine therapy is salivary gland damage. This can lead to salivary gland pain and swelling, salivary gland infection and stones, and decreased saliva production. Decreased salivary production leads to xerostomia. Xerostomia can in turn result in excessive dental caries (Answer C). Patients can also experience difficulty eating certain foods and challenges with speaking for long intervals. Approximately 4% to 5% of patients have persistent xerostomia after radioiodine therapy. One study showed a 40% reduction in parotid gland function after doses of 270 mCi ^{131}I. An early study suggested that the use of sialogogues after radioiodine therapy (to increase clearance of isotope from the salivary glands) actually increased the rate of xerostomia. However, a subsequent well-performed study showed that lemon drops given several times daily do, in fact, reduce salivary gland exposure to radioiodine.

An alteration of taste, which occurs commonly after radioiodine therapy, is typically transient rather than permanent (Answer E). Patients may describe a metallic or chemical taste that sometimes persists for months after therapy.

Permanent hypoparathyroidism (Answer B) is a very rare consequence of radioiodine therapy, with only a handful cases described in the literature.

Transient depression of sperm counts occurs following radioiodine therapy, and there is a cumulative effect on the testes that is manifested as an elevation in serum FSH and a slight decrease in sperm count, but typically not azoospermia (Answer A). It is recommended that men desiring future fertility and receiving radioiodine doses greater than 400 mCi consider sperm cryopreservation.

Leukemia (Answer D) is a potential less common consequence of radioactive iodine therapy. In a recent study, radioactive iodine therapy was associated with increased risk of hematologic malignancies (relative risk, 1.51; 95% CI, 1.08-2.01), including leukemia (relative risk, 1.92; 95% CI, 1.04-3.56). An estimated 22 excess hematologic malignancies (95% CI, 4-41) were attributable to radioactive iodine therapy in a cohort of 27,050 thyroid cancer survivors younger than 45 years. Patients who receive the highest doses over the shortest intervals are most likely to develop this rare complication, with a latency period of less than 10 years. Ideally, patients requiring repeated treatments with radioiodine should receive this at intervals of at least 1 year, but patients with aggressive radioiodine-avid disease should not be denied therapy at shorter intervals when appropriate.

EDUCATIONAL OBJECTIVE

Identify adverse salivary gland effects associated with radioiodine therapy.

REFERENCE(S)

Van Nostrand D, Bandaru V, Chennupati S, et al. Radiopharmacokinetics of radioiodine in the parotid glands after the administration of lemon juice. *Thyroid.* 2010;20(10):1113-1119. PMID: 20883172

Jeong SY, Kim HW, Lee SW, Ahn BC, Lee J. Salivary gland function 5 years after radioactive iodine ablation in patients with differentiated thyroid cancer: direct comparison of pre- and postablation scintigraphies and their relation to xerostomia symptoms. *Thyroid.* 2013;23(5):609-616. PMID: 23153322

Singer MC, Marchal F, Angelos P, et al. Salivary and lacrimal dysfunction after radioactive iodine for differentiated thyroid cancer: American Head and Neck Society Endocrine Surgery Section and Salivary Gland Section joint multidisciplinary clinical consensus statement of otolaryngology, ophthalmology, nuclear medicine and endocrinology. *Head Neck.* 2020;42(11):3446-3459. PMID: 32812307

Pasqual E, Schonfeld S, Morton LM, et al. Association between radioactive iodine treatment for pediatric and young adulthood differentiated thyroid cancer and risk of second primary malignancies. *J Clin Oncol.* 2022;40(13):1439-1449. PMID: 35044839

28 ANSWER: B) Continued monitoring for compressive symptoms

This patient's ultrasound demonstrates a low-risk pattern (an isoechoic solid thyroid nodule with regular margins) and the nodule was benign on FNA biopsy on 2 occasions. The risk of false-negative FNA biopsy results is believed to be less than 3%, and the risk that a nodule will have false-negative results on more than one occasion is very close to zero. The risk of malignancy does not differ in thyroid nodules with low-risk ultrasonographic characteristics that grow compared with low-risk nodules that do not grow.

There is no clear rationale for continued ultrasonographic surveillance (Answer E) of nodules that are repeatedly benign on FNA biopsy and have low-risk ultrasonographic characteristics. There is certainly no rationale for repeated ultrasound in such a short timeframe.

Despite continued nodule growth, the risk of malignancy is very low in this patient, and repeated FNA biopsy (Answer A) is not warranted.

Core biopsy (Answer C) may be considered in patients with nodules that are repeatedly nondiagnostic on FNA biopsy, but there is no reason to pursue core biopsy in this patient who has had diagnostic results on FNA biopsy.

Thyroid lobectomy (Answer D) may ultimately be required if the patient develops compressive symptoms, but he is currently asymptomatic.

Continued monitoring for compressive symptoms (Answer B) is reasonable, since such symptoms would prompt consideration of surgery.

EDUCATIONAL OBJECTIVE

Guide the appropriate follow-up of benign thyroid nodules.

REFERENCE(S)

Haugen BR, Alexander EK, Bible KC, et al. 2015 American Thyroid Association management guidelines for adult patients with thyroid nodules and differentiated thyroid cancer: the American Thyroid Association guidelines task force on thyroid nodules and differentiated thyroid cancer. *Thyroid.* 2016;26(1):1-133. PMID: 26462967

Rosário PW, Purisch S. Ultrasonographic characteristics as a criterion for repeat cytology in benign thyroid nodules. *Arq Bras Endocrinol Metabol.* 2010;54(1):52-55. PMID: 20414548

Kim YY, Han K, Kim EK, et al. Validation of the 2015 American Thyroid Association management guidelines for thyroid nodules with benign cytologic findings in the era of the Bethesda system. *AJR Am J Roentgenol.* 2018;210(3):629-634. PMID: 29323546

Bahn RS, Castro MR. Approach to the patient with nontoxic multinodular goiter. *J Clin Endocrinol Metab.* 2011;96(5):1202-1212. PMID: 21543434

29 ANSWER: A) Continue current levothyroxine

This patient has had an incomplete biochemical response to therapy for her thyroid cancer, with persistently elevated serum thyroglobulin levels in the absence of localizable disease. Based on the lack of uptake on her most recent posttreatment scan, her disease does not appear to be radioactive iodine-avid and neither a repeat diagnostic iodine scan (Answer C) nor repeated radioiodine therapy (Answer D) is likely to be helpful. She has no evidence for measurable structural disease, her disease is not currently symptomatic or progressive, and kinase inhibitor therapy is associated with significant adverse effects; therefore, sorafenib therapy (Answer E) is not warranted now.

Overall, studies demonstrate a survival benefit for TSH-suppressive levothyroxine dosing in patients with high-risk tumors. However, TSH suppression is also associated with increased morbidity and mortality, particularly in patients who are older or who have cardiovascular disease, cardiovascular risk factors, or osteoporosis. A recent meta-analysis showed a significant risk of decreased lumbar spine bone mineral density in postmenopausal women undergoing TSH suppression therapy. Even though this patient has not sustained a fracture, she is likely at more risk for a fracture than she is from adverse consequences from her thyroid cancer. Of the available options, maintaining a moderate degree of TSH suppression (Answer A) is preferable to complete TSH suppression (Answer B) in this older patient with osteoporosis, whose thyroglobulin has been stable and who does not have known structural disease. It would also be appropriate to consider other bone-protective therapies in this patient, such as calcium, vitamin D, and bisphosphonate treatment.

EDUCATIONAL OBJECTIVE

Identify clinical characteristics informing the choice of TSH targets in the long-term follow-up of patients with differentiated thyroid cancer.

REFERENCE(S)

Biondi B, Cooper DS. Benefits of thyrotropin suppression versus the risks of adverse effects in differentiated thyroid cancer. *Thyroid.* 2010;20(2):135-146. PMID: 20151821

Parker WA, Edafe O, Balasubramanian SP. Long-term treatment-related morbidity in differentiated thyroid cancer: a systematic review of the literature. *Pragmat Obs Res.* 2017;8:57-67. PMID: 28553154

Haugen BR, Alexander EK, Bible KC, et al. 2015 American Thyroid Association management guidelines for adult patients with thyroid nodules and differentiated thyroid cancer: the American Thyroid Association guidelines task force on thyroid nodules and differentiated thyroid cancer. *Thyroid.* 2016;26(1):1-133. PMID: 26462967

Ku EJ, Yoo WS, Lee EK, et al. Effect of TSH suppression therapy on bone mineral density in differentiated thyroid cancer: a systematic review and meta-analysis. *J Clin Endocrinol Metab.* 2021;106(12):3655-3667. PMID: 34302730

30 ANSWER: E) No radioactive iodine

Current guidelines call for risk stratification postoperatively to inform decision-making about radioactive iodine and other additional therapies. This patient's tumor is considered low-risk because it is a classic papillary cancer smaller than 4 cm without aggressive histologic features (such as tall-cell or columnar variant), there was no tumor invasion of local structures, the tumor was fully resected, and there was no vascular invasion. The presence of fewer than 5 micrometastases (<0.2 cm) in cervical lymph nodes does not confer additional risk. In addition, these micrometastases do not merit additional surgery to further explore the central compartment (Answer D). Monitoring for recurrence can be achieved with thyroglobulin measurement and ultrasonography.

In patients determined to have low-risk tumors according to the American Thyroid Association criteria, radioactive iodine ablation has not been shown to reduce risk for disease recurrence or mortality and is not routinely recommended. Therefore, Answer E is correct and the other answers involving radioactive iodine administration (Answers A, B, and C) are incorrect because this patient's tumor does not meet criteria for intermediate or high risk. Radioactive iodine treatment has been associated with decreased risk for both tumor recurrence and for disease-specific mortality in patients with high-risk tumors (those with gross extrathyroidal extension, incomplete tumor resection, and known distant metastases or postoperative thyroglobulin levels suggesting distant metastasis). In patients with intermediate-risk tumors (microscopic extrathyroidal extension, vascular invasion, aggressive histologic features, or metastases in the neck), the evidence for benefit is less clear, but radioactive iodine should be considered and treatment should be individualized on the basis of patient and tumor characteristics.

EDUCATIONAL OBJECTIVE

Recommend the most appropriate postoperative therapy for thyroid cancer classified as low risk.

REFERENCE(S)

Haugen BR, Alexander EK, Bible KC, et al. 2015 American Thyroid Association management guidelines for adult patients with thyroid nodules and differentiated thyroid cancer: the American Thyroid Association guidelines task force on thyroid nodules and differentiated thyroid cancer. *Thyroid.* 2016;26(1):1-133. PMID: 26462967

Lamartina L, Durante C, Filetti S, Cooper DS. Low-risk differentiated thyroid cancer and radio-iodine remnant ablation: a systematic review of the literature. *J Clin Endocrinol Metab.* 2015;100(5):1748-1761.PMID: 25679996

Nixon IJ, Ganly I, Patel SG, et al. The results of selective use of radioactive iodine on survival and on recurrence in the management of papillary thyroid cancer, based on Memorial Sloan-Kettering Cancer Center risk group stratification. *Thyroid.* 2013;23(6):683-694. PMID: 23742290

31 ANSWER: B) Repeated FNA biopsy with flow cytometry

The image shows multiple uniform-appearing lymphocytes. Features of anaplastic carcinoma, another potential cause of very rapid thyroid growth, are not seen. Thyroid lymphoma is rare, comprising 2% or less of all thyroid malignancies. The mean age at presentation is 65 to 75 years, and this occurs more frequently in women. The risk for thyroid lymphoma is 40 to 80 times higher in individuals with Hashimoto thyroiditis than in the general population. The most common presentation of thyroid lymphoma is a rapidly enlarging, painless goiter, often with compressive symptoms. The enlargement may be nodular or diffuse. Cytopathology showing uniform-appearing lymphocytes may be consistent with either Hashimoto thyroiditis or thyroid lymphoma. FNA biopsy with flow cytometry (Answer B) is typically needed to confirm a diagnosis of lymphoma.

Treatment of thyroid lymphoma usually consists of chemotherapy with or without radiation. The role of thyroidectomy (Answer E) is controversial, but it has not been demonstrated to improve survival.

Radioactive iodine scan (Answer A) may demonstrate a cold nodule, but it would not be helpful in diagnosing thyroid lymphoma.

Gene classifier testing (Answer C) can be useful to predict the risk of differentiated thyroid cancer when an FNA biopsy result is indeterminate, but it is not useful in distinguishing between Hashimoto thyroiditis and thyroid lymphoma.

Similarly, testing for pathogenic variants associated with differentiated thyroid cancer (Answer D) may aid decision-making when the FNA biopsy result is indeterminate, but it would not be helpful here where the clinical scenario is suggestive of thyroid lymphoma.

EDUCATIONAL OBJECTIVE

Identify the association between Hashimoto hypothyroidism and thyroid lymphoma and recommend initial workup.

REFERENCE(S)

Walsh S, Lowery AJ, Evoy D, McDermott EW, Prichard RS. Thyroid lymphoma: recent advances in diagnosis and optimal management strategies. *Oncologist.* 2013;18(9):994-1003. PMID: 23881987

Mancuso S, Carlisi M, Napolitano M, Siragusa S. Lymphomas and thyroid: bridging the gap. *Hematol Oncol.* 2018 [online ahead of print] PMID: 29484690

Stein SA, Wartofsky L. Primary thyroid lymphoma: a clinical review. *J Clin Endocrinol Metab.* 2013;98(8):3131-3138. PMID: 23714679

32 ANSWER: B) Add prednisone to methimazole

This patient has amiodarone-induced thyrotoxicosis (AIT), which was initially diagnosed as iodine-induced thyrotoxicosis and was treated with methimazole, with minimal response. Two subtypes of AIT have been described: type 1, which is believed to be an iodine-induced thyrotoxicosis occurring in patients who often have preexisting thyroid autonomy, and type 2, which is a destructive thyroiditis. Distinguishing between the 2 subtypes can be difficult. The presence of hypervascularity on Doppler ultrasonography favors type 1, while low vascularity favors type 2. In this patient, ultrasound findings are indeterminate. Some patients who have mixed types of AIT respond best to combination therapy. Combination therapy is indicated in patients demonstrating an inadequate response to monotherapy, in patients in whom a subtype cannot be determined using available testing, and in patients with severe complications (generally cardiovascular compromise) in whom stepwise therapy would be inappropriate. Thus, adding prednisone to methimazole (Answer B) is the best option.

Replacing methimazole with prednisone or perchlorate (Answers D and E) is likely to be less effective than additive therapy in a refractory case in which types 1 and 2 cannot be differentiated. Furthermore, potassium perchlorate is no longer available in the United States.

Lithium (Answer A) has been used as a treatment for thyrotoxicosis and may provide some benefit, but prednisone is likely to be more beneficial if this patient has a mixed type of AIT.

Thyroidectomy (Answer C) in patients with uncontrolled thyrotoxicosis and underlying heart disease is a high-risk procedure and should be considered only when medical therapies have been exhausted. However, it may well be that this patient might ultimately need a thyroidectomy if he does not respond to medical management.

An algorithm for treating amiodarone-induced thyrotoxicosis is shown (*see image*).

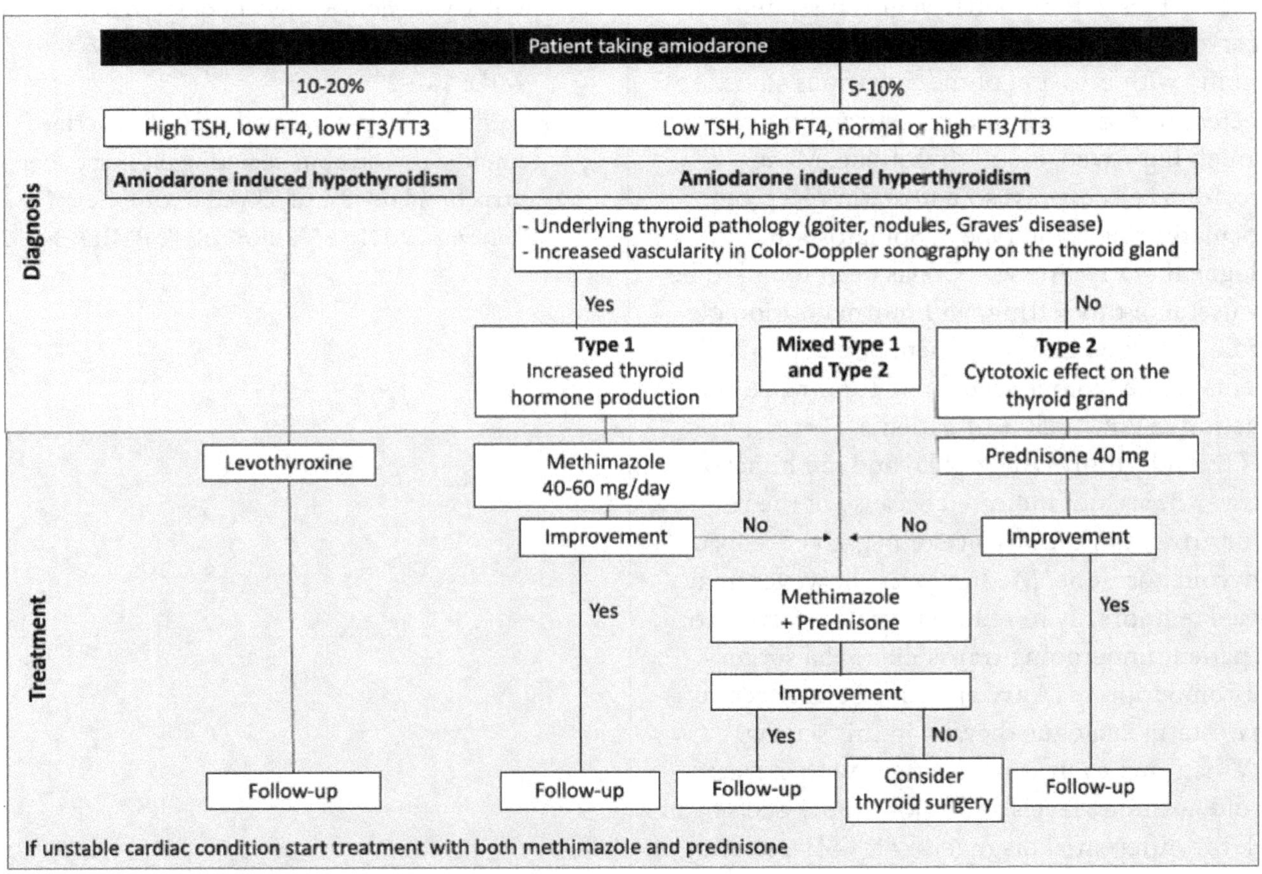

Reprinted from Ylli D et al. *J Clin Endocrinol Metab*, 2021; 106(1): 226-236. © The Endocrine Society.

EDUCATIONAL OBJECTIVE

Treat amiodarone-induced thyrotoxicosis.

REFERENCE(S)

Basaria S, Cooper DS. Amiodarone and the thyroid. *Am J Med.* 2005;118(7):706-714. PMID: 15989900

Schubert L, Bricaire L, Groussin L. Amiodarone-induced thyrotoxicosis. *Ann Endocrinol (Paris).* 2021;82(3-4):163-166. PMID: 32409004

Ross DS, Burch HB, Cooper DS, et al. 2016 American Thyroid Association guidelines for diagnosis and management of hyperthyroidism and other causes of thyrotoxicosis. *Thyroid.* 2016;26(10):1343-1421. PMID: 27521067

Ylli D, Wartofsky L, Burman KD. Evaluation and treatment of amiodarone-induced thyroid disorders. *J Clin Endocrinol Metab.* 2021;106(1):226-236. PMID: 33159436

33 ANSWER: C) Somatostatin analogue

This patient underwent transsphenoidal surgery for a large TSH-secreting pituitary adenoma with invasion of the cavernous sinus. As expected, resection was incomplete and the patient, although improved, is still thyrotoxic. Most thyrotroph cells express somatostatin receptors, particularly type 2 and type 5. Somatostatin analogue therapy (Answer C) has been found to be very useful in this setting, with normalization of thyroid hormone in most patients treated (>70% of patients treated in one study) and tumor size reduction in 20% to 50% of patients.

Thyroidectomy (Answer D) and methimazole (Answer B) are not indicated because of the risk of tumor growth in the absence of negative feedback of thyroid hormone. Methimazole, however, may be used temporarily to reduce thyrotoxicosis prior to a patient undergoing transsphenoidal surgery.

Bromocriptine (Answer A) is not as effective as somatostatin analogue therapy in this setting.

When first evaluating a patient with elevated thyroid hormone levels and a nonsuppressed serum TSH, the differential diagnosis of a TSH-secreting adenoma vs resistance to thyroid hormone is often considered. However, the diagnosis of a TSH-secreting pituitary adenoma is now confirmed in this patient.

Triiodothyroacetic acid (TRIAC) (Answer E) is a thyroid hormone analogue that has been used to treat some patients with thyroid hormone resistance, but it would not be an appropriate therapy for a TSH-secreting adenoma.

EDUCATIONAL OBJECTIVE

Recommend treatment for secondary hyperthyroidism.

REFERENCE(S)

Beck-Peccoz P, Persani L, Mannavola D, Campi I. Pituitary tumours: TSH-secreting adenomas. *Best Pract Res Clin Endocrinol Metab.* 2009;23(5):597-606. PMID: 19945025

Socin HV, Chanson P, Delemer B, et al. The changing spectrum of TSH-secreting pituitary adenomas: diagnosis and management in 43 patients. *Eur J Endocrinol.* 2003;148(4):433-442. PMID: 12656664

Amlashi FG, Tritos NA. Thyrotropin-secreting pituitary adenomas: epidemiology, diagnosis, and management. *Endocrine.* 2016;52(3):427-440. PMID: 26792794

De Herdt C, Philipse E, De Block C. Endocrine tumours: thyrotropin-secreting pituitary adenoma: a structured review of 535 adult cases. *Eur J Endocrinol.* 2021;185(2):R65-R74. PMID: 34132199

www.ingramcontent.com/pod-product-compliance
Lightning Source LLC
LaVergne TN
LVHW060057220926
848484LV00008BA/1993

* 9 7 8 1 9 3 6 7 0 4 1 7 0 *